HOMEOPATHY
A Comparative Materia Medica

(Part II)

HOMEOPATHY

A Comparative Materia Medica

(Part II)

S. Kumar

New Age Books

ISBN: 81-7822-040-7 (2 Pts.)

First Edition: Delhi, 2005

Published by
NEW AGE BOOKS
A-44 Naraina Phase I
New Delhi-110 028 (INDIA)
Email: nab@vsnl.in
Website: www.newagebooksindia.com

Printed in India
at Shri Jainendra Press
A-45 Naraina Phase-I, New Delhi-110 028

CONTENTS

Part II

Melilotus Alba	415
Mercurius Corrosivus	417
Mercurius Cyanatus	421
Mercurius Solubilis	423
Mezereum	431
Millefolium	435
Murex Purpurea	437
Muriatic Acid	439
Naja Tripudians	443
Natrum Arsenicum	445
Natrum Carbonicum	447
Natrum Muriaticum	449
Natrum Phosphoricum	459
Natrum Sulphuricum	461
Nitric Acidum	465
Nux Moschata	473
Nux Vomica	479
Opium	489
Petroleum	493
Petroselinum	497
Phosphoric-acid	499
Phosphorus	505
Phytolacca	513
Platinum	517
Plumbum	521
Psorinum	525
Pulsatilla	529
Rheum	537
Rhododendron	539
Rhus Toxicodendron	541
Rumex Crispus	549

Ruta Graveolens 551
Sabadilla 557
Sabina 559
Sambucus Nigra 561
Sanguinaria 563
Sanicula 567
Sarsaparilla 569
Secale Cornutum 573
Selenium 577
Sepia 579
Silicea 587
Spigelia 595
Spongia Tosta 597
Stannum 599
Staphisagria 603
Sticta Pulmonaria 611
Sulphur 613
Sulphuric Acid 625
Tabacum 629
Tarentula 631
Terebinthina 635
Theridion Curassavicum 639
Thuja Occidentalis 641
Trillium Pendulum 645
Tuberculinum Bacillinum 647
Valeriana 649
Veratrum Album 651
Veratrum Viride 657
Viburnum Opulus 659
Zincum 661

List of Remedies 665
Glossary of Medical Terms 673
Understanding Homeopathic Medicines 709
Index of Medicines 717
Index of Diseases and Symptoms 725

MELILOTUS ALBA

I. Introduction (Cow-486)

Synonym: Melilotus officinalis.
Natural Order: Leguminoseae.
Common Name: Sweet Clover, yellow (not white) Melilot.
Habitat: An indigenous plant of Europe and naturalised in the USA.
Preparation: Tincture from the fresh flowers.

II. General Analysis (Cow.)

Acts upon nervous system, producing a very severe headache with Bell. like symptoms. With epistaxis which rapidly relieves headache. Useful in sick headaches.

III. Suited to (Allen-186)

Congestion relieved by Haemorrhage. Engorgement of blood vessel, in any part of organ. Headache-Epistaxis gives relief (Bufo, Ferr. phos., Mag. s.).

IV. Clinical (Clarke-II-420)

Blushing, Congestion, Cough, Dysmenorrhoea, Epilepsy, Epistaxis, Fear, Haemoptysis, Headache, Insanity, Leucorrhoea, Melancholia, Ovarian neuralgia, Pneumonia, Shyness, Spasms.

V. Symptoms-Particular (Nash-453)

1. Fearful headaches and haemorrhage.
2. Congestion to Brain with intense red face.
   With throbbing carotid. > Epistaxis profuse.
   Meli., +++ congestion to brain is similar to that of Bell., Glon.
   Stram.—congestion to brain with loquacity.

3. Nose bleed—with intense red face. Blood hanging in clots from nose like icicles. (Merc. s.), if not clotted so markedly then Meli.
4. Strong head symptoms—Meli., Bell., Glon.

MERCURIUS CORROSIVUS

I. Introduction (Cow-502)

Synonyms: Mercurius sublimatus Corrosivus,
Bi-choride of Mercury, Mercuric Chloride.
Common Name: Corrosive sublimate.
Preparation: Corrosive sublimate is dissolved in alcohol one to 99 making 2x dilution, subsequent dilutions with alcohol.
It was proved by Hahnemann with other Mercurious preparations.

II. General Analysis (Cow.)

It acts pre-eminently upon mucous membranes with destructive energy, producing and intensely acute inflammation. Its action extends to serous membranes esp. peritoneum. Most marked feature of Merc. c. is phegedenic tendency of all inflammatory conditions.

III. Clinical (Clarke-II-459)

Antrum of Highmore-disease of, Aphthae, Appendicitis, Bone affections, Bright's disease, Cancrum oris, Chancre, Diarrhoea, Dysentery, Eczema, Enteric fever, Eye affections, Gums-affections of, Intestines ulcerated, Intussusception, Iritis, Jaundice, Kidneys-inflammation of, Labour-puerperal fever, Measles, Miscarriage, Mouth affections, Mumps, Neuralgia-supraorbital, Oesophagus-constriction of, Paralysis, Paraphimosis, Pemphigus, Perimetritis, Peritonitis, Prosopoplagia, Rigg's disease, Syphilis, Tabes mesenterica, Taste disordered, Tenesmus, Throat inflamed, Tongue-affections of, Uvula elongated.

IV. Symptoms-General (Nash-43)

1. Most persistent and terrible tenesmus before, during and after stool; stool scanty, mucous turgid with blood.
2. Tenesmus of bladder and rectum at the same time; urine passed in drops with much pain.
3. Throat intensely inflamed, swollen burning with swollen gums, which bleed easily.

V. Symptoms-Particular (Nash-43)

1. Skin troubles—works better.
2. Incessant tenesmus of rectum.
   Stool does not relieve (Nux. v.—better after stool)
   Tenesmus may begin in rectum, extend to Bladder and vice versa.
   (Canth., Caps., Nux. v.—tenesmus of bladder)
3. Throat inflamed, swollen, burning; swollen, bleeding Gums.
4. IInd stage gonorrhoea—very efficient remedy. Burning and tenesmus continues with greenish discharge.

VI. Black Letter Symptoms (Tyler)

- Slow in answering questions. Memory weak.
- Face earthy-coloured, puffy.
- Teeth black, loose.
- Carious teeth. Decay of teeth, they become loose in succession-blackened, laid bare, loose and carious.
- Teeth become denuded of the gum and turn black, with nightly pain in teeth, jaws and head.
- Violent toothache, with swelling of gum and salivary glands.
- Gums red and bleeding at slightest contact, spontaneously.
- Gums have a bright red margin; small ulcers at intervals.
- Gums spongy and bleeding sore.
- Tongue black with red edges. Tongue red, swollen.
- Coated tongue, showing impress of teeth upon the margin.

- Tongue swollen and its movements difficult.
- Bad odour from the mouth; foetid odour; sweetish.
- Violent stomatitis and salivation.
- Speech difficult on account of the trembling of the mouth and tongue. Speech stammering.
- Tremor of hands. Trembling.

MERCURIUS CYANATUS

I. Introduction (Clarke-II-465)

Synonym: Bycyanide of Mercury.
Preparation: Trituration.

II. Clinical (Clarke-II-465)

Diphtheria, Dysentery, Enteric fever, Haemorrhage, Kerato-iritis syphilitica, Phlebitis, Throat sore, Varicosis.

III. Symptoms-Particular (Nash-44)

1. Remarkable prostration.
2. Sore throat of Public speakers—raw, sore, and broken-Merc. proto.
3. Tongue coated thickly; diphtheria.

IV. Symptoms-Particular (Tyler)

1. Almost specific for diphtheria.

MERCURIUS SOLUBILIS

I. Introduction (Cow.-491)

Synonym: Mercurious Vivus.
Common Name: Quick silver, Mercury, Mercurious Solubilis Hahnemanne.
Preparation: (1) Triturations of precipitated black oxide of mercury with Nitric Acid and Ammonia gives Mercurius Solubilis Hanemanni. (2) Trituration [Decoction: water in which Quick Silver has been boiled for half an hour] gives Mercurius Vivus-Hahnamann preferred the use of Merc. Vivus over Merc. Sol. Similarity between the two is so great that usually no distinction is made in practice (Clarke-II-438-439).
Hahnemann proved its Homeopathic use. (Pierce).

II. General Analysis (Cow.)

Acts profoundly upon entire organism. Pre-eminently upon vegetative system altering its functional power causing increased secretion and absorption, secretions are thinner, acrid and excoriating. Upon organic system it acts more, especially upon mucous/serous membranes, glandular system paranchymatous organs, fibrous and osseous tissues and the skin. The most characteristic feature of action is like that of syphilitic poisoning, though Merc. attacks long bones, while syphilis flat bones. Chief characteristic is aggravation of all symptoms at night and from the warmth of the bed.

III. Suited to (Allen-190)

Light-haired person/ skin muscle lax. Bone disease/pains worse < night. Great weakness from least exertion. Catarrah- < night, damp, with much sneezing. Toothache < warm, evening, shoot to face, ear, tearing, pulsating. Root intact crown decay (Crowns intact roots decay-Mez.) > rubbing the cheek. Tongue-takes the imprint of teeth, large, flabby. Profuse perspiration, in almost all complaints, does not relieve (Relieves—Nat. m., Psor., Verat.) Diseases of men, Syphilitic, ulcers, with corroding acrid pus, Bright's disease. Tenesmus of rectum not > by stool (< by stool Nux. v.), incessant, persistence, stool-hot, scanty, bloody, slimy, offensive. Tenesmus of bladder, burning in urethra.

IV. Clinical (Clarke-II-438)

(*The letters 's' and 'v' indicate the preparation—Solubilis or Vivus mentioned in connection with the name of the malady which they follow. They do not indicate a preference of one over the other).* Abscess(s), Anaemia, Aphthae, Appendicitis, Balanitis*(s)*, Bone disease *(s)*, Brain-inflammation of, Breath offensive*(s)*, Bronchitis *(s)*, Bubo*(s)*, Cancrum oris, Catarrh*(s)*, Chancre, Chicken-pox*(s)*, Cold*(s)*, Condylomata, Cough*(s)*, Dentition abnormal*(s)*, Diarrhoea*(s)*, Dysentery, Dyspepsia*(s)*, Ecthyma*(s)*, Eczema, Emaciation, Excoriation*(s)*, Eyes-affections of*(s)*; gouty inflammation of, Fainting, Fever, Fissures, Glandular swelling(s), Gout(s), Gum-boil*(s)*, Gums unhealthy*(s)*, Heart affections*(s)*, Herpes*(s)*, Hydrophobia, Jaundice *(s)*, Joints-affections of*(s)*, Leucorrhoea-in little girls, Liver-affections of*(s)*, Lumbago*(s)*, Mania, Measles *(s)*, Melancholia *(s)*, Meningitis, Mollities ossium, Mucous patches, Mumps, Noises in the head*(s)*, Odour of body-offensive*(s)*, Ovaries-affections of, Pancreatitis*(s)*, Parametritis*(s)*, Parotitis, Peritonitis, Perspiration abnormal*(s)*, Phimosis*(s)*, Pregnancy-affections of*(s)*, Prostate-disease of*(s)*, Purpura *(s)(v)*, Pyaemia*(s)*, Ranula*(s)*, Rheumatism *(s)(v)*, Rickets, Rigg's Disease, Salivation*(s)*, Scurvy*(s)*, Small-pox*(s)*, Stomatitis, Suppuration*(s)*, Surgical fever, Syphilis *(s)*, Taste disordered*(s)*, Teeth-affections of*(v)*, Throat-deafness*(s)*, Throat sore,*(v)*, Tongue-affections of *(s)(v)*; mapped*(v)*, Toothache*(s)*, Tremors*(s)*, Typhus fever*(v)*, Ulcers*(s)*, Vaccination*(s)*, Vomiting*(s)*.

V. Symptoms-General (Nash-39)

1. Swollen, flabby tongue taking imprint of the teeth, gums also swollen, spongy bleeding, breath very offensive.
2. Sweats day and night without relief in many complaints.
3. Creeping chilliness in the beginning of a cold or threatened suppuration.
4. Slimines of mucous membranes.
5. Moist tongue with intense thirst.
6. Glandular swelling, cold, inclined to suppurate, ulcers with lardaceus base.
7. Modalities; < at night in warmth of bed, while sweating, < lying on right side.
8. Bone disease, pains worse at night.
9. Dysentery; stools slimy, bloody, colic, fainting: great tenesmus during and after followed by chilliness and a "cannot finish sensation".
10. The more blood and pain the better indicated.
11. Affects lower lobe of right lung; stitches through to back (Chel., Kali c.).
12. Intense thirst, although the tongue looks moist and the saliva is profuse.
13. In low potencies, hastens suppuration, in high, aborts suppuration, as in quinsy.

VI. Symptoms-Particular (Nash-39-43)

1. Tongue, swollen, takes print of teeth, gums swollen, spongy, often bleeding.
   Ars.,
   Chel.,
   Podo.,
   Rhus t.,
   Stram.
2. Very offensive mouth odour, moist mouth with intense thirst-with saliva Soapy or stringy. Key-No other remedy has this condition of the mouth to this degree.

3. Perspiration without relief profuse and persistent.
    Merc. s.,
    Verat.,
    Ars.
    Nat. m. } Perspiration relieves.
    Psor.
4. Fever chill—Creeping chill in the beginning of taking cold-indication of cold been taken, if left alone then sore throat, coryza may follow. But a dose will abort all these troubles. Chilliness is felt mostly in the evening and increases into night. It alternates with the flushes of heat (Ars.). Often felt in single parts, in abscesses.
5. < Night esp. warmth of bed.
    Led.,
    Merc. s..
6. Sweats—Profuse, don't relieve like inflammatory sweats do, but they increase complaints (Tilia.). This condition is found in any disease.
7. Discharges, from nose to diarrhoeic.
    Merc. c.—thin, excoriating in the beginning, then thicker (Puls.)
    < Night leucorrhoea.

VII. Black Letter Symptoms (Tyler-541-544)

- Hurried and rapid talking.
- Memory weak: forgets things.
- Itching on the hairy scalp.
- The whole HEAD is painful to touch.
- Tearing, drawing pains, in periosteum, head and face: rheumatic headaches.
- Congestion to head: feels it will burst: fullness of brain.
- As if contracted by a band: as if in a vice.
- External head painful to touch.
- Black insects seem to be always flying before the sight.
- Mist before one or both EYES, Dimness of sight.

- The light of the fire dazzles the eyes greatly.
- The eyes cannot bear the light of the fire or delight.
- A fog before one or both eyes.
- If she attempts to look at anything she can't distinctly recognize it, and then the eyes are involuntarily drawn together; the more she tries to restrain the contraction, the less able is she to prevent it: she is obliged to lie down and close the eye.
- Lachrymation profuse, burning, excoriating.
- Muco-purulent discharges, thin and acrid.
- Blepharites: lids red, thick, swollen, worse open air: worse cold applications.
- Aching in the eyes: itching in the eyeballs.
- Roaring in the EARS.
- Ear inflamed internally and externally, with cramp like, sticking pain, and a feeling as if stopped by swelling.
- Bloody and offensive matter flows from right ear, with tearing pain.
- Epistaxis, Nose bleed during sleep.
- Offensive odour from the NOSE as in violent coryza.
- Acrid matter flows from nose, Green foetid pus.
- Nasal bone is painful when taken hold of.
- Corners of MOUTH ulcerated and painfully sore.
- Looseness of teeth which are very painful when touched by tongue. A feeling as if all the teeth were loose.
- Tongue white, as if covered with fur: great swelling of tongue.
- A kind of Aphthae in mouth.
- Violent toothaçhe at night followed by great chilliness over whole body.
- Jerking toothache at night-jerking from teeth of lower jaw into ear, and from upper jaw into head, with painfullness of gums.
- Gums swollen; separate from the teeth.
- Bleeding of gum from slightest touch. Gum painful when touched and on chewing.
- Tongue coated white, with whitish swollen gums that bleed when touched.

- Tongue swollen and so soft on the margin that it showed the imprint of the teeth in scallops, which looked ulcerated.
- Corners of mouth ulcerated and sore.
- Pain and swelling of salivary glands.
- Constant epistaxis.
- Sweetish taste in the mouth.
- THROAT constantly dry: hurts as if to tight posteriorly: a pressure in it if he swallowed, yet constantly obliged to swallow because the mouth was always full of water.
- Something hot rises to her throat.
- When swallowing, shooting pain in tonsils.
- Suppuration of the tonsils, with sharp, sticking pain in fauces when swallowing.
- (*Sensation of apple-core sticking in throat.*)
- Very salt TASTE on the lips, salt taste on tongue.
- Salt expectoration.
- Taste of rotten eggs when he moves the tongue and then involuntary swallowing.
- Slimy taste in the mouth.
- At night (1 AM) much water flows into the mouth, at the same time nausea, so that he wakes up from at and must vomit; something very bitter comes up.
- Frequent HICCOUGH.
- Extremely violent THIRST. Extraordinarily intense thirst.
- Burning pain in scorbiculus cordis.
- Swelling of inguinal GLANDS, with circumscribed redness.
- Ignuinal gland becomes red and inflamed; is painful when touched and walking.
- Ineffectual urging to STOOL every moment, with tenesmus in the rectum.
- Along with soft stools, burning pain in anus.
- Bloody stools with painful acrid sensation at anus.
- Green slimy acrid stools that excoriate the anus.
- Green diarrhoea: diarrhoea of green mucous with burning and protrusion of anus.
- Greenish, painless gonorrhoea, especially at night.

- Burning in URETHRA.
- Constant desire to urinate; indeed every ten minutes; but only a little passed.
- Urine immediately after being passed very turbid and depositing a sediment.
- He passes much more urine than the liquid he has drunk.
- Too frequent and too profuse urination.
- Nocturnal seminal emission mixed with blood.
- Catamenia too profuse.
- Greenish biting leucorrhoea with much scratching, especially evening and night, with violent burning after scratching.
- Frequent sneezing without coryza.
- Stitches in chest with sneezing or coughing.
- A stitch in anterior upper chest, extending through to back.
- During the cough, inclination to vomit.
- Sticking in small of back on breathing.
- Weakness and wearing of all limbs.
- Trembling of the hands .
- Ankle joint as if sprained.
- As if bruised in the limbs.
- Profuse perspiration when walking.
- Perspiration on every movement.
- Complaints increase during sweat.
- Constant cold hands and feet.
- Perspires day and night, through more at night.
- Profuse perspiration at night. Very profuse.
- Fatty and oily perspiration at night.
- Profuse, offensive perspiration, soaking the bedclothes.
- Large ULCERS bleed and when touched there is a pain affecting the whole body. Their margins everted like raw meat and their bases covered with a caseous coat.
- Bleeding of an ulcer that had previously existed.
- Dropsical patients (so-called) very rapidly lost the swelling and got instead foetid, rapidly decomposing ulcers on the legs.

- Frequent waking from sleep.
- Great weariness.
- Very much exhausted after a stool.
- As soon as he went to bed in the evening, the pains recommenced and banished sleep.

MEZEREUM

I. Introduction (Cow 510)

Synonym: Daphne Mezereum.
Natural Order: Thymelaceae.
Common Name: Spurge Olive.
Habitat: A small shrub, native of Northern and Central Europe.
Preparation: Tincture from the fresh bark.
It was proved by Hahnemann, whose companion was Dr. C Hering, then a medical student. (Pierce-601).

II. General Analysis (Cow.)

Acts especially upon the skin, mucous membranes of the genitourinary organs and alimentary tract producing a high degree of inflammation in all these. It resembles the action of Mercury upon the long bones and periosteum of the jaw and syphilitic poisoning.

III. Suited to (Allen-194)

Hypochondriacal, despondent, indifferent to everything. Angry at trifle then sorry. Eczema and itching after vaccination. Winter skin complaints (eruption) every January or February. Head covered with thick leather like crust. Toothache < night > open mouth drawing air in. Light haired, irresolute persons with phlegmatic temperaments.

IV. Clinical (Clarke-II-481)

Bone affections, Coccygodynia, Constipation, Crusta lactea, Ear affections ; sensitive to air, Erythema, Exostosis, Eye affections, Glands enlarged, Gleet, Gonorrhoea , Haematuria, Hernia, Herpes zoster, Impetigo, Irritation, Leucorrhoea, Mercury-effects of, Neuralgia, Osteoma, Pediculosis, Pityriasis, Prolapsus ani, Pruritus senilis, Rheumatism, Scrofula,

Syphilis, Teeth-affections of, Tendons contracted, Tinea capitis, Tinea versicolor, Tongue-affections of; swelling of, Ulcer, Vaccination.

V. **Symptoms-General** (Nash-467)

1. Pains in the long bones, especially tibia.
1. Facial neuralgia or toothache when the pains are greatly < by eating or motions of the jaws > by radiate heat.
2. Nose; vesicular eruption, with excoriation, formation of thick scabs, < at night; Zona.

VI. **Black Letter Symptoms** (Tyler-551-552)

- Hypochondriac and despondent. Takes no pleasure in anything.
- Everything seems to him dead, and nothing makes a vivid impression upon his mind.
- Very violent HEADACHE: Head painful to slightest touch (after a slight vexation).
- Bone pain in bones of skull, especially aggravated by contact.
- Cranial bones pain, are swollen and sensitive to cold and contact: worse from motion and in the evening. Caries.
- Itching and burning of SCALP.
- Head covered with a thick leather-like crust, under which thick white pus collects here and there and hair is glued together.
- On the head, great elevated white scabs, under which ichor collects in quantity, and which begins to be offensive and to bread vermin.
- EYES: sensation of dryness.
- Obstinate jerking of the muscles of left upper lid.
- EAR: Sensation of air distending the right external meatus (Then the left)
- TEETH: feel blunt and elongated: painful on biting or from fresh air.

- VIOLENT BURNING in mouth.
- Heat and scraping in fauces.
- Burning in THROAT and pharynx: dryness in fauces, hacking cough; anxious oppression of breath, loosening of scanty mucous on coughing.
- Vomits Beer, which has a bitter taste (Not water).
- Pain in periosteum of long BONES, especially tibia: worse at night in bed; least touch is intolerable. Worse in damp weather.
- Bones inflamed, swollen, especially shafts of cylindrical bones; after abuse of Mercury and venereal disease.
- Eczema, itching intolerably, copious serous exudation.
- Neuralgia and burning after zona.
- The SKIN of face is of a deep inflammatory redness and the eruption is "fat" and moist.
- The child scratches the face continually; it becomes covered with blood.
- In the night the child scratches its face so that the bed is covered with blood in the morning; and face is covered with a scab which the child keeps constantly tearing off a new, and on the spots thus left raw, large (fat) pustules from.
- Ulcers covered with thick whitish-yellow scabs, under which thick, yellow pus collects.
- Vesicles appear around the ulcers, itching, violently and burning like fire. After eight days these vesicles dry up, leaving scabs, the tearing off of which causes great pain and retards healing.

MILLEFOLIUM

I. Introduction (Cow.-516)

Synonym: Achillea Millefolium.
Natural Order: Compositae.
Common Name: Yellow Milfoil.
Habitat: A perennial herb growing in old fields in N. America and Europe.
Preparation: Tincture from fresh leaves.
It was first proved by Nenning, one of the provers of Hahnemann (Pierce-605)

II. General Analysis (Cow.)

Acts upon venous capillaries causing haemorrhage from pelvis region organs and from nose and lungs. More active haemorrhage than in Ham. It affects mucous membranes causing irritation, slight congestion, gastric and abdominal pain, diarrhoea and enuresis.

III. Suited to (Allen-195)

Ailments of over-lifting, over exertion, or a fall. Vertigo—when moving slowly. Haemorrhage—painless, without fever. Wounds bleed profusely especially after a fall (Arn., Ham.).

IV. Clinical (Clarke-II-490)

Asthma, Cancer, Chlorosis, Consumption, Dentition, Diarrhoea, Dysmenorrhoea, Enuresis, Epilepsy, Fistula lachrymalis, Haematemesis, Haematuria, Haemoptysis, Haemorrhage, Hypochondriasis, Hysteria, Leucorrhoea of children, Lochia-too profuse; suppressed, Milk-absence of, Nipple sore, Nose-bleed, Puerperal convulsions, Puerperal fever, Rodent ulcer, Sterility, Sycosis Hahnemanni, Tetanus, Varices.

V. **Symptoms-Particular** (Nash-220)

1. Causes-nose bleed haematuria.
2. Blood-bright red-without anxiety (Acon.-with anxiety).
3. Bleeding after a fall/injury when Arn. fails-Mill.

MUREX PURPUREA

I. Introduction (Clarke-II-505)

Synonym: Murex Purpura.
Common Name: Purple Fish.
Natural Order: Gasteropoda. Muricidae (Allen)a

Preparation: Trituration or tincture of fresh juice.
It was first proved by Dr Petroz of Spain in 1841 (Pierce-608).

II. Suited to (Allen-196)

Persons of melancholic temperament. Suffering during climacteric (Lach., Sep., Sul.). Great depression of spirit. Persons with violent sexual excitement. Excessive desire for embrace. (Reverse-Sep.).

III. Clinical (Clarke-II-505)

Abortion, Breasts painful, Cervix uteri-affections of, Climacteric sufferings, Diabetes, Dysmenorrhoea, Leucorrhoea, Menorrhagia, Metrorrhagia, Nymphomania, Pregnancy-affections of, Uterus-prolapse of.

IV. Symptoms-Particular (Nash-207)

1. Comparable with Sep. with following difference.
   Sep.—aversion to sex, esp. with prolapsus.
   Mur. p.—uncontrollable sexual desire.
2. Common points are—bearing down sensation; sinking all gone sensation. Sensation as if internal organs would be pushed out; must sit and cross limbs to ameliorate the pressure.
3. Sore pain in uterus (Helon. d.), womb is so tender and sore that she feels it when she moves.
4. Nymphomania:
   Lil. t.,
   Plat.,
   Mur. p.

MURIATIC ACID

I. Introduction (Cow.-518)

Synonym: Hydrochloric Acid, Hydrogen chloride.
Common Name: Muriatic Acid.
Preparation: A solution in distilled water is called 1x dilution, from 3x onward with dilute alcohol.

It was first proved by Hahnemann (Pierce-609).

II. General Analysis (Cow.)

Acts upon ganglionic nervous system, and through it upon blood, skin, and alimentary canal, especially mouth and anus. Essential feature is low adymanic condition similar to that of low putrid fever, in atonic conditions with extreme weakness with low reaction (Pierce-609).

III. Suited to (Allen-197)

Persons with black hair, dark eyes, dark complexion. Irritable, peevish, disposed to anger (Nux. v.), restless. Great debility—as soon as closes his eyes, lower jaw hangs down. Diseases with moaning, unconsciousness, fretfulness. Haemorrhoids sensitive and painful to touch.

IV. Clinical (Clarke-II-508)

Anus-prolapse of, Cerebral deafness, Chilblains, Chorea, Diphtheria, Enteric fever, Ephelis, Feet-soles painful, Gastric disorders, Haemorrhoids, Hemiopia, Impotence, Measles, Mercurial ulceration, Mouth-aphthae; psoriasis of tongue; ulcerated, Scarlatina, Scurvy, Tendo Achilles-affections of, Tongue-affections of; psoriasis of, Typhus, Varices, Whooping-cough.

V. Symptoms-General (Nash-245)

1. Moaning or sliding down in bed from excessive weakness. (Typhoid).
2. Tongue dry, leathery and shrunken; one-third its natural size. (Typhoid).
3. Haemorrhoids: swollen and blue, and so sensitive to touch that they can't bear the contact of the sheet.
4. Great debility; as soon as he sits down his eyes close; lower jaw hangs down; slides down in bed.
5. Malignant affections of mouth: ulcers, deep, dark, base bluish, offensive, foul breath.
6. Diarrhoea: stool involuntary while urinating. Can't urinate without having bowels move at the same time.

VI. Symptoms-Particular (Nash-245-6)

1. Typhoid—excessive weakness, lower jaw fallen, eyes closed, tongue dry, leathery, shrunken; stools involuntary when urinating. One of best remedies for Typhoid. Nearer to Carb. v.; (higher grade Typhoid-Phos. ac.).
2. Haemorrhoids—swollen and blue.
   Sensitive to touch. Rectum prolapse easily (Mur. ac., Ign., Rut.). Can't urinate without it coming down.
3. Urine passes slowly; must press until rectum protrudes.
4. Cannot bear the least touch, not even sheets on genitals.

VII. Black Letter Symptoms (Tyler-564-565)

- Diarrhoea with protrusion of blue or dark purple haemorrhoids, especially when occurring in feeble children suffering from gastric atony, muscular debility and threatened marasmus.
- Haemorrhoids swollen, blue; painful to touch; appear suddenly in children; protruding, reddish blue, burning, too sore to bear the least touch, even sheet is uncomfortable.

- Slow emission of urine; bladder weak, must wait a long time; has to press so that anus protrudes.
- Leucorrhoea with backache; sore anus from piles or Fissure.
- Great debility; as soon as he sits down his eyes close; lower jaw hangs; slides down in bed.
- Typhus. Constant restlessness of stupid sleep; unconscious; loud moaning or confused talking; wishes to uncover; lower jaw dropped; aphthous ulcers in mouth, foetid, sour smelling; tongue coated at edges, shrunken, dry like leather, paralysed. Thin, offensive smelling evacuations; involuntary stools while passing urine; rapid, weak, rattling respiration; sliding down in bed; urine dark, but clear; bleeding from anus; haemorrhage of dark, liquid blood; mouth full of dark blue ulcers; pulse omits every third beat; legs flexed, feet drawn up, skin hot and dry. Typhoid fever also.
- Scarlatina; redness intense and rapidly spreading; Eruption, scanty interspersed with petechiae; skin purplish.
- One of the greatest remedies of very bad cases of typhoid, diphtheria, scarlet fever, etc.

NAJA TRIPUDIANS

I. Introduction (Cow-523)

Synonym: Naja.
Class: Reptile.
Order: Squamata.
Family: Elapidae.
Common Name: Cobra virus.
Preparation: The poison obtained is triturated.

It was first proved by Dr. Stokes of England, 1853 (Pierce-610).

II. General Analysis (Cow.)

Like Lach. and other serpent poisons, it affects profoundly the cerebrospinal system, the pneumogastric and glossopharyngeal nerves causing difficult respiration, cardiac oppression and usual decomposition and fluidity of the blood resulting in ecchymosis and haemorrhage and other general effects resulting from all serpent poisons.

III. Suited to (Allen-199)

Suicidal insanity, broods constantly over imaginary troubles. Simple hypertrophy of heart.

IV. Clinical (Clarke-II-523)

Angina pectoris, Asthma, Dysmenia, Hay-fever, Headache, Heart affections, Oesophagus-spasmodic stricture of, Ovaries-affections of, Plague, Spinal irritation (of nucha), Throat sore.

V. Symptoms-Particulars (Nash-124-125)

1. Affections of heart—very decisive use, esp. weak heart (Nux. v.-Tired feeling).

2. Diphtheria with impending heart failure or paralysis.
3. Dyspnoea and prostration with weak heart.
4. Sympathetic cough in organic diseases with weak heart action (sympathetic dry cough in heart affections-Spon.)
5. Palpitation and bad feeling in heart < walking.

NATRUM ARSENICUM

I. Introduction (Cow-526)

Synonym: Sodium Arsenate.
Common Name: Arsenate of soda.
Preparation: Triturations.

II. General Analysis (Cow.)

Affects upon mucous membrane causing irritation, congestion, sub-acute catarrhal inflammation. It resembles more of Nat. m. than Ars.

III. Clinical (Clarke-II-534)

Coryza, Diphtheria, Eyes-inflammation of; granular lids, Haemoptysis, Interscapular pain, Miner's asthma, Nose-affections of; pain in root of, Oesophagus-constriction of, Pityriasis rubra, Post-nasal catarrh, Testicles-neuralgia of, Tuberculosis.

NATRUM CARBONICUM

I. Introduction (Cow-529)

Common Name: Carbonate of soda.
Preparation: Triturations.

It was proved by Hahnemann as Herring one of his provers (Pierce-611).

II. General Analysis (Cow.)

Through ganglionic nervous system, acts upon mucous membranes of nasal cavity, eyes and digestive tract including liver, producing inflammation. Chief indication-catarrhal conditions, weak memory, especially from over study, bad effects of a sunstroke.

III. Suited to (Allen-199)

Constitutions averse to open air and dislike to exercise, mental or physical, great debility caused by heat of summer chronic affects of sun stroke. Emaciation with pale face with blue rings around eyes. Headache from slightest mental exertion, from sun, working under gas light. Intolerable melancholy and apprehension.

IV. Clinical (Clarke-II-537)

Albuminuria, Anidrosis, Ankles weak, Burns, Cornea-ulceration of, Corns, Coryza, Deafness, Dysmenia, Dyspepsia, Goitre, Hands chapped, Headache, Heel blistered, Herpes, Iris-circinatus, Hypochondriasis, Hysteria, Ichthyosis, Lisping, Moles, Nose-swollen; eruptions on; red, Ozaena, Post-nasal catarrh, Presbyopia, Priapism, Rheumatism, School-headache, Scrofula, Stammering, Sterility, Sunstroke-chronic effects of, Throat-mucus in, Toothache, Warts.

V. Symptoms-Particular (Nash-336)

1. Worse by mental exertion. Any mental labour brings headache.
   Arg. n.,
   Nat. c.,
   Saba.
2. Headache from over heating from sun or gas light
   Nat. c.—greatly depressed in spirits, wholly occupied with sad thought.
   Glon.,
   Lach.,
   Lyss.
3. Chronic nasal catarrh extending to posterior nares and throat (Nat. c.).
4. Violent hawking and spitting of thick mucous which collects again and again.
   Nat. c.,
   Coral. r.
5. Weakness of ankles from childhood (Nat. c.).
6. Bearing down pains with sadness, over sensitiveness to noise, music.

NATRUM MURIATICUM

I. Introduction (Cow.-534)

Synonym: Chloride of sodium.
Common Name: Common salt.
Preparation: Trituration.

It was proved by Hahnemann first (Pierce-613).

II. General Analysis (Cow.)

Acts upon the blood, the lymphatic system, mucous lining of the digestive tract, liver and spleen. It causes through deterioration of the blood, ulcers, eruption on the skin, destructive inflammation of mucous and glandular tissues. Dyscrasia of a scorbutic character. Chief expression-condition of system which results from long lasting cases of agues, intermittent fever.

III. Suited to (Allen-201)

Anaemic and cachetic persons, whether from loss of vital fluids, profuse menses etc. or mental affections. Great emaciation, losing fresh white living well (Abrot., Iod.). Great liability to take cold (Calc. c., Kali c.). Irritable child—cross when spoken to. Marked disposition to weep (Puls.).

IV. Clinical (Clarke-II-541)

Addison's disease, Anaemia, Aphthae, Atrophy, Brain-fag, Catarrh, Chorea, Constipation, Cough, Cracks in skin, Debility, Depression, Diabetes, Dyspareunia, Dropsy, Dyspepsia, Epilepsy, Erysipelas, Eye affections, Eye-strain, Face-complexion unhealthy, Gleet, Glossopharyngeal paralysis, Goitre, Gonorrhoea, Gout, Headache, Heart affections, Hemiopia, Hernia, Herpes, Herpes circinatis, Hiccough, Hodgkin's disease, Hydroa, Hypochondriasis, Intermittent fever, Leukocythemia, Leucorrhoea, Lips-eruption on, Lungs-oedema of, Menstruation disordered, Mouth-inflammation of, Nettlerash, Pediculosis, Ranula, Seborrhoea, Self-abuse, Somnambulism, Speech embarrassed, Spermatorrhoea, Spinal irritation, Spleen enlarged, Sterility, Stomatitis, Sunstroke, Taste-lost; disordered, Tongue-blistered; white coated; heavy; Trifacial-nerve paralysis, Ulcer, Varices, Vaginismus, Vertigo, Warts, Whooping-cough, Worms, Yawning.

V. **Symptoms-General** (Nash-325)

1. Melancholy, depressed, sad and weeping; consolation aggravates.
2. Great emaciation, even while living well; shows most in the neck.
3. Anaemia with bursting headaches, especially at the menses; also school girls headache.
4. Great dryness of mucous membranes from lips to anus; lips dry cracked, especially in the middle; anus dry, cracked, fissured; constipation.
5. Heart palpitates, flutters, intermits, pulsates violently, shaking the whole body; < lying on left side.
6. Itching Eruption, dry or moist; < at the margins of the hair.
7. Modalities: < 10 to 11 AM (many complaints), especially malarial affections; lying down, especially on left side; heat of sun or heat in general; abuse of Quinine, > relieved by sweat.
8. Tongue: mapped with red insular patches.
9. For bad effects of anger, nitrate of silver; too much salt; craves salty things
10. Hang nails; skin around the nails dry and cracked; herpes about the anus, in border of hair.
11. Warts on palms of hands (sore to touch-Nat. c.).

VI. **Symptoms-Particular** (Nash-326-334)

1. Anaemia—one of the best remedies, irrespective of cause.

   Nat. m.—general paleness, emaciation, throbbing headache, shortness of breath when going upstairs.

China. } due to loss
Kali c. } of fluid.
Puls.—due to menses, irregularities.
Phos. ac. } due to loss
China. } of semen

2. Depression (weeping) of spirit is characteristic of this medicine.
   Puls. -> by soothing
   Nat. m.-< by soothing.
3. Flutter, palpitation, intermittent action of heart, hypochondriac.
   Nat. m.—loss of weight while eating well.
   Spig.—violent pulsating of heart, shaking body.
4. Chronic Headache (one of the best remedies).
   (a) with sore eyes esp. when turning them.
      Nat. m.—throbbing, pale face.
      Bell., Nux. v., Meli.—face red, eyes red or burning, beating or throbbing nature.
   (b) Headache of school girls, often brought on by eye strain.
      Calc. phos. } anaemic
      Nat. m. }
      Rut. } asthenopia with
      Arg. n. } headache.
   (c) After menses.
      Nat. m., } after the menstrual period
      China. } with throbbing headache.
5. Dryness of lips to anus.

Nat. m.	—dryness, lips and corners of mouth ulcerated or cracked (condurango).
Nat. ars.	—anus dry, ulcerated, cracked, fis sured, often bleeding.
Graph.	—Both mouth and anus affected exematous.
Ant. c.	—milder than Graph.
Nat. m.	—Sense of dryness without actual dryness.
Merc. s.	—thirst with moist mouth.
Puls.	—dry mouth with no thirst.

6. Dryness in Mouth.
   Nat. m. —sense of dryness without actual.
   Merc. c. —wet mouth with thirst.
   Puls. —Dry mouth with no thirst.
7. Loss of taste.
   Nat. m. } common
   Puls. } butter taste
8. On Tongue sensation of HAIR.
   Sil.,
   Nat. m.,
   Kali. bich.
9. Pearl like blisters around mouth.
   Nat. m.,
   Bell.,
   Calc. c.
10. Scorbutic (tiny bleeding spots) gums.
   Nat. m.,
   Mur. ac.,
   Merc. c.,
   Carb. v.
11. Numbness tingling of lips, tongue, nose (with liver).
   Nat. m..
12. Tongue-Mapped.
   Nat. m.,
   Lach.,
   Ars.,
   Nit. ac.,
   Tarax.
13. Paralysis of muscles of deglutition (part diphtheria).
   Lach.,
   Caust.,
   Nat. m.
14. Hungry, yet loss of flesh while eating well.
   Nat. m.—after food sleep and weary
   Acet. ac., Abrot.,
   Iod.—after food feels better.
   Sanic., Tuberc.
15. After eating, better.
   Anac.—eating but eats again, as the stomach ache returns.

Chel.—liver symptoms with
Petr.
Iod.
Nat. m. } fills up quickly followed by fullness,
China. } distress, and flatulence follow.
Lyc. } Better after digestion process is over.

16. Abnormal Craving for salt.
    Nat. m.—with intense thirst.
    Caust.

17. Diabetes with thirst/salt craving.
    Nat. m.

18. Stool and Rectum.
    (a) Constipation/stool dry crumble.
        Nat. m.,
        Amm. mur. stools, dry crumbling.
        Mag. m.
    (b) Inactively of Rectum (constipation from).
        Nat. m.,
        Alumina,
        Verat.,
        Sil.
    (c) Anus contracted, torn, bleeding, smarting, and pain after stool.
        Nat. m.,
        Nit. ac.
    (d) For want of moisture.
        Bry.,
        Op.
    (e) Much soreness.
        Ign.,
        Nit. ac.,
        Alumen,
        Nat. m.

19. Cholera infantum. Loose stool with hunger, emaciation, thirst.
    Nat. m.—in neck, emaciation.
    Amm. mur.,
    Arg. n.,
    Abrot.—in leg, emaciation.

20. Increased and involuntary urine. Cutting and burning after act, urine clear and watery.
    Caust.,
    Puls.,
    Zinc.,
    Nat. m.,
    Nit. ac.
    When Nit. ac. fails-Lac can.,
    Sarsa.
21. Uteric Symptoms with back pain > lying down (like Rhus t.) bearing down. Must sit down to prevent prolapsus. (Sep.-cross legs) < moving.
22. Periodicity of aggravation.
    Nat. m.- 10-11 AM.
    Eup. perf.- 7 AM.
    Apis.- 4 PM.
    Lyc.- 4-8 PM.
    Ars.- 1-2 AM / PM
23. Sweating, fever, headache, and all other symptoms of Nat. m. and Ars.
24. 'Hang Nails'—skin near nails cracked.
25. Numbness and tingling in finger and toes, tongue, lips.
26. Weak ankle—child walks late.
27. Painful Tension in bends of limbs, sensation of as if cords were too short.
    Caust.,
    Guaic.,
    Cimex. (actual),
    Nat. m.
28. Spine-general weakness better by hard pressure, sensitive to touch (best medicine).
29. Skin eczema worse on hair line (Raw, inflamed).
30. Tetters at the bands of joints.
31. Urticaria
    Apis.,
    Hep. s.,
    Calc. c.,
    Nat. m.

Nat. m., Lach., Caust. are most efficient in high potency.

32. Strong action upon heart and circulation—
    —fluttering of heart with weak faint feeling < lying down
    —Irregular intermission of heart beats and pulse > lying left side > by sweating.
    —violent pulsation of heart which shakes the body (Spig.).

VII. Black Letter Symptoms
(Tyler-572-573)

- Very much inclined to weep and be excited.
- Depression. Hurriedness with anxiety and fluttering at heart.
- Sad and weeping mood without cause. Involuntary weeping.
- Sad and weeping: consolation aggravates.
- Melancholy; mood, preferred to be alone.
- the more he was consoled, the more he was affected.
- Hypochondriacal, tired of life.
- Trifles provoke anger.
- Indifferent.
- Distraction: disinclined for mental work.
- Head dull, heavy.
- Pressing pain, as if head would burst.
- When coughing, as if forehead would burst.
- Redness of whites of eyes with lachrymation.
- Eyes give out in reading; writing.
- Pressure in eyes when looking intently.
- Unsteadiness of vision. Letters and stitches run together.
- Ophthalmia, after abuse of nitrate of silver.
- Spasmodic closure of lids.
- Upper lip swollen.
- Great swelling lower lip followed by large vesicle.
- Crack in middle of lower lip.
- Blisters on tongue.
- Bitter taste in mouth.
- Loss of taste: food has no taste.
- Tongue coated, with insular patches.

- Tongue heavy difficult speech. Children, slow in learning to talk (talk the next day after a dose of Nat. m.).
- Very violent thirst. Unquenchable thirst.
- Great longing for bitter things, beer; for farinaceous food; for sour things; for salt, oysters, fish, milk.
- Aversion to meat, bread, coffee.
- Acid eructation and malaise after eating.
- Chronic diarrhoea, watery; with fever, dry mouth: worse as soon as he moves about, and after farinaceous food. With much flatus. Sensation of contraction in rectum during stool; hard faeces evacuated with greatest exertion, so that anus is torn, bleeds, and is sore.
- Constipation. Obstinate retention of stool. Seat worms.
- An unusually hard, dry, crumbly stool.
- Increased desire to urinate, with very light watery urine.
- Involuntary escape of urine while walking, coughing, sneezing.
- Intermittent heart beat.
- Heart's pulsations shake the body.
- Emaciation: great emaciation.
- Easily fatigued.
- Great weakness and relaxation of all physical and mental power from exertion or after long talking.
- Paralysis from intermittents, nervous exhaustion, sexual excesses, from diphtheria, from anger or emotions; from pain: of flexors.
- Dreams: anxious: vivid: frightful, of robbers in house, will not believe the contrary till search is made.
- Eruption especially margin of hair at nape of neck.
- Herpes about mouth, arms and thighs.
- White scales on scalp: dandruff.
- Nettle-rash; large red blotches with violent itching.
- Tetters, bends of joints, oozing of an acrid fluid; crusts with deep cracks. Scaly Eruption on flexor surfaces.
- Fever with headache: much heat in face; great thirst, drinks much and often; with nausea and vomiting: stitches in head: unconsciousness: blindness, blurred sight; faintishness; aversion to uncover; without chill, 10 to 11 AM.

- Or chill predominates, with thirst, yawning, severe headache bursting headache: nausea and vomiting; tearing pains in bones; chattering of teeth; internal as from want of animal warmth.

NATRUM PHOSPHORICUM

I. Introduction (Clarke-II-565)

Synonym: Phosphate of Soda.
Preparation: Trituration. Solution.

II. Clinical (Clarke-II-565)

Acidity (infants), Conjunctivitis, Diabetes, Dyspepsia, Enteralgia, Erysipelas, Gastralgia, Glands-scrofulous swelling of, Goitre, Gout, Intertrigo, Leukocytosis, Leucorrhoea, Morphinomania, Phthisis, Post-nasal catarrh, Rheumatism, Scrofula, Sighing, Sterility, Threadworms, Urticaria, Worms.

III. Symptoms-General (Nash-473)

1. Excess of acidity.
2. Yelleo creamy coating at the back part of the root of the mouth.
3. Sour eructation and vomiting.

IV. Black Letter Symptoms (Tyler-576)

- Thin, moist coating on Tongue.
- Soft palate has yellowish, creamy look.
- Sour eructation, sour vomiting, greenish diarrhoea; pains spasms and fever with acid symptoms.
- Gastric derangements with symptoms of acidity.
- Yellow, creamy coating of back part of roof of mouth.

NATRUM SULPHURICUM

I. Introduction (Cow-542)

Synonym: Sodium Sulphate.
Common Name: Glauber's salt. Sulphate of soda.
Preparation: Triturations.

It was first proved by Schreter of Austria and Nenning of Austria in 1832-33. (Pierce-622).

II. General Analysis (Cow.)

Hydrogenoid constitutions of Dr. Grauvogl, acts directly upon the blood through which it causes inflammations, catarrhal and rheumatic, worse from damp influences.

III. Suited to (Allen-204)

Patients who feel every change from dry to wet. Can't tolerate sea air, or eat plants near sea. Recovery slow from every sickness. Ailments which are by or which depend upon dampness of weather, damp houses (Aran.). Every spring skin affection reappear (Psor.). Ailments which are worse by or which depend upon dampness of weather or house.

IV. Clinical (Clarke-II-571)

Asthma, Biliousness, Brain-injuries of, Condylomata, Debility of drunkards, Diabetes, Dyspepsia-of drunkards, Enuresis, Epilepsy-traumatic, Epistaxis (menstrual), Fistulous abscesses, Gonorrhoea, Headache, Hydraemia, Influenza, Leukemia, Liver enlarged, Malaria, Migraine, Nephritic scarlatina, Ophthalmia, Panaritium, Phlegmasia alba dolens, Photophobia, Phthisis, Sciatica, Scrofulous ophthalmia, Spleen-affections of, Sycosis, Warts.

V. Symptoms-General (Nash-323)

1. Diarrhoea, acute or chronic < in the morning on beginning to move (Bry.) with much flatulence (Aloe. and Calc. phos.) and rumbling in abdomen, especially right ilco-caecal region.
2. Loose cough, with great pain in the chest; < in lower left chest.
   (right-Chel.)
3. Modalities: < in cold, wet weather; damp cellars; hydrogenoid (diarrhoea, rheumatism, asthma).
4. Mental effects from injuries to the head.
5. Chronic effects from blows, falls.
6. Toothache > by cold water, cool air.
   Coff.,
   Puls.
7. Gonorrhoea , greenish, yellow, painless, thick discharge (Puls.).

VI. Symptoms-Particular (Nash-323-325)

1. Acute/chronic diarrhoea.
2. Morning diarrhoea < on beginning to move.
   Nat. s.,
   Rum. c.,
   Bry.-< on move
   Nuph.
   Sul.—(drives patient out of bed).
   Nat. s.—Rumbling of flatus in the bowels.
   Aloe.—especially on right side of abdomen in Nat. s.
3. Stool accompanied with a profuse emission of flatus.
   Nat. s.,
   China,
   Arg. n.,
   Cal.,
   Agar.,
   Aloe.
   Nat. s.—< Damp weather (Rho.).
   Nat. s.—warm to cold weather, whether damp or dry.

4. Loose cough with soreness and pain through left chest.

   (Right—Kali c.)

   Nat. s.—loose cough

   Bry.—dry cough
5. Right lower chest pain.

   Kali c.
6. Chronic asthma < damp
7. Toothache > (better) cold water or air.

VII. Black Letter Symtoms (Tyler)

Mention only taluzid symptoms, which need further proving, hence not included here.

NITRIC ACIDUM

I. Introduction (Cow-546)

Synonym: Hydrogen Nitrate. Aqua Fortis.
Common Name: Nitric Acid.
Preparation: On decimal scale in distilled water makes 1x dilution and subsequent dilutions in Alcohol.
It was proved under Hahnemann's directions (Pierce-624).

II. General Analysis (Cow.)

Acts upon the blood, mucous membranes, glands, bones, skin, its special action upon muco-cutaneous outlets of the body—mouth, rectum, anus and vagina, Intense irritation to inflammation, ulceration and then destruction of part, whole scene is that of violent dyscrasia or poison resembling syphilitic, sycotic or mercurial miasmas.

III. Suited to (Allen-206)

Persons of thin rigid fibres, dark complexioned, black hair and eyes, nervous temperament. Persons suffering with chronic diseases, take cold easily, disposed to diarrhoea, rarely to those who suffer from constipation. Excessive physical irritability in old people with weakness and diarrhoea. Pains sticking, pricking as from splinter. Strong smelling urine. The mucous outlets of the body where skin and mucous membranes join; mouth, nose, rectum, anus, urethra, vagina (Mur. ac.).

IV. Clinical (Clarke-II-587)

Actinomycosis, Anus-fissure of, Axilla-offensive perspiration of, Bladder-chronic catarrh of, Breath offensive, Bright's disease, Bronchitis, Bubo, Chancre, Cheloid, Chilblains, Choking easy, Climacteric, Cold easily taken, Condylomata, Constipation, Corns, Cough, Dysentery, Dyspepsia,

Ear affections, Epilepsy, Eye affections, Feet perspiring, Fistula lachrymalis, Freckles, Frost-bite, Glandular swellings, Gleet, Gums sore, Haematuria, Haemorrhage, Herpes, Herpes preputialis, Toenail-ingrowing, Iritis-syphilitic, Irritation, Jaw-cracking in, Menstruation profuse, Metrorrhagia, Mouth sore, Mucous patches, Muscoe volitantes, Myopia, Nails-affections of, Ozaena, Paralysis (left side), Perspiration abnormal, Phimosis, Polypi, Proctitis, Prostate-suppuration of, Ranula, Rectum-affections of, Rickets, Salivation, Spine-injury to, Syphilis, Taste disordered, Tongue ulcerated, Ulcer, Warts, Wens, Whooping-cough.

V. **Symptoms-General** (Nash-247)

1. Has a particular affinity for mucous outlets, where skin and membranes join; cracks; rhagades, Fissure.
2. Pricking pains as of a splinter in the parts.
3. Urine strong smelling; like horse urine.
4. Haemorrhage from all outlets of the body; blood bright red.
5. Pricking ulcers; excrescences; condylomata; fig-warts (sycosis).
6. Nervous, irritable, dark complexioned persons.
7. Modalities; > riding in carriage.

VI. **Symptoms-Particular** (Nash-247)

1. Most effective antidote of Mercury dosing.
   Hep. s.,
   Nit. ac.,
   Calc. c.
2. Affinity for the outlets of the mucous surfaces, where skin and membrane join. Corners of mouth, nose, anus. In mouth-corners cracked, ulcerated and scabby, also aphthel stomatitis, swelling of gums, etc.

a. Swollen and spongy gums.
b. Anus—great pain even after soft stool, agony lasts for an hour or so after (Ratan.).

Nit. Ratan.	} as if splinter inside the anus, anus fissured and cracked.

Nux. v.—Pain ceases after stool (Difference with Nit. ac.).

Merc. s.—Pain before, during, after stool (Difference with Nit. ac.) Pricking pain as if splinter in the part.

3. Haemorrhage—from all outlets-blood bright red.
4. Chronic Diarrhoea-Trio-

   Thuj.,
   Staph.,
   Nit. ac.
5. Offensive Urine.

   Benz. ac.—dark
   Nit. ac.—horse like
   Sep.—sourish

VII. Black Letter Symptoms
(Tyler-589-93)

- Depressed and very anxious in the evening.
- Anxiety, as if engaged in a lawsuit or quarrel exciting uneasiness. Anxiety about his disease, with fear of death. Morbid fear of cholera.
- Anxious about his illness: constantly thinks about past troubles.
- Mind weak and wandering.
- Hopeless despair.
- Nervous, excitable, especially after abuse of Mercury.
- Vexed at least trifle.
- No disposition to work, to perform any serious business.
- Great weakness of memory.
- After continued loss of sleep, long-lasting anxiety-over-exertion of mind or body from nursing the sick (Compare Cocc.)—great anguish of mind from loss of dearest friend.
- VERTIGO on rising in the morning: had to sit down.
- Heaviness, obtrusion, fullness in HEAD. Head as if surrounded with a tight bandage.
- Sensation, "Head in a vice from ear to ear over vertex".

- Painful tension inside head extending to eyes: with nausea.
- Head very sensitive to pressure of hat: < evening, and part lain on. As if contused all over, or in spots. Right side skull painful.
- Profuse falling out of hair: especially vertex: from congestion of blood to scalp: from syphilis: nervous headaches, debility, emaciation.
- Double vision.
- Stitches in EYES; smarting.
- In morning difficult to open eyes and to raise upper eyelids. (Compare Sep., Caust.)
- Ophthalmia: neonatorum: scrofulous: gonorrhoeal: syphilitic: from abuse of Potash and Mercury.
- (*Curious symptom, eyelashes of right side all point stiffly towards nose.*)
- Roaring in EARS. Cracking when chewing.
- (*Deafness: riding in carriage or train (compare Graph.): with induration tonsils: after abuse of Mercury: syphilitic.*)
- Violent itching in NOSE. Nose-bleed. When eating, small pieces of food get into posterior nares; are not got down till swallowed with saliva. (Compare Gels.).
- Nasal catarrh; acrid, watery at night, yellow, offensive; corroding: with swelling upper lip. with scarlet fever, diphtheria; or syphilitic.
- (*Ozaena: green casts every AM with ulcers; syphilitic, involving upper lip, which is swollen and honeycombed with ulcers.*).
- Ulceration of nostrils, scurfy; of inner nose with frequent bleedings.
- Corners of MOUTH ulcerated and scabby: with sticking pain.
- Cracking in articulation of jaw when chewing and eating.
- Foul, cadaverous smell from mouth.
- Ulcers, mouth, with sticking pain as from a splinter: within cheeks: edges of tongue: deep eating: at first lardaceous, later discoloured, dark, dirty, putrid, destructive: syphilitic.

- Mucous membrane gets between teeth, easily bitten swollen ulcerated: with pricking pains: especially after abuse of Mercury; aphthous, covered with white or thin yellow-grey membrane.
- Saliva; profuse; foetid, acrid, makes lips sore; bloody.
- Swelling of parotid and sub-maxillary glands with loose teeth and bleeding gums, after abuse of Mercury.
- Looseness of teeth when chewing. (Compare Merc.c.).
- Putrid smell from mouth.
- Small painful pimples on sides of tongue.
- THROAT. A morsel sticks in pharynx. When eating, as if pharynx constricted.
- Swallowing very difficult: distorts face and draws head down: can't swallow even a teaspoonful of fluid: causes violent pain extending to ear.
- Tonsils red, swollen, uneven, with small ulcers; yellow streak; white patches.
- Stinging pains in swollen throat.
- Sticking, painful, sore throat.
- Longing for fat: herring: chalk: lime: earth. (Calc. c.) Bread disagrees.
- Jaundice: pain, region of LIVER: urine scanty and strong smelling.
- Awakened at midnight with crampy pains in small intestines chilly: pain worse if he moved.
- Stitches, region of Liver.
- Abundant, flatulence: rumbling in abdomen.
- Nausea after a MEAL. Sweat all over after a meal.
- Eructation before and after a meal.
- Constant desire for STOOL: unsuccessful.
- Colic, sometimes drawing, before stool.
- Profuse discharge of blood during stool.
- Burning of the varices of ANUS.
- Itching of the rectum.
- Burning: itching: of the anus, moisture.
- Sticking in rectum and spasmodic contraction in anus, during stool, lasts many hours.
- With stool pain, as if something in rectum would be torn asunder.
- Diarrhoea: great straining, but little passes; as if stayed in rectum and could not be expelled: with soreness and rawness of anus.

- Constipation: painful, hard, difficult irregular stool: stool in hard masses: with every stool, protrusion of haemorrhoids with profuse bleeding: great pain during and after stool, as though there were fissure of anus. Piles bearing down on standing.
- Haemorrhoids: constant pressing out: painful or painless: prolapsing with every stool.
- Needle-like stitches in orifice of URETHRA.
- Ulcers in urethra: bloody mucous or purulent discharge.
- SEXUAL ORGANS much affected: with small itching vesicles: ulcers exuding an offensive moisture: bleeding when touched: sharp stitches.
- Condylomata: foetid bleeding when touched: moist: resembling cauliflower: on thin pedicles: oozing: after abuse of Mercury.
- Gonorrhoea: discharge yellowish or bloody: bloody mucous: horrible pain. Condylomata about genitals and anus (Thuj.).
- Itching, swelling and burning.
- Haemoptysis, COUGH: dry, barking; tickling in larynx and pit of stomach with complete ptosis of both eyes from coughing.
- Chronic dry, laryngeal, with stinging smarting, as if small ulcers were in larynx, generally felt on one side.
- Sputum seems to stick like glue: greenish-white casts as if from air cells: expectoration by day of dark blood mixed with coagula: or yellow, acrid pus of offensive odour. Pain low down in lungs as if something were tearing away.
- HEART, fourth beat intermits: alternate hard, rapid and small beats.
- Want of breath, palpitation of heart and anguish when going upstairs. Sudden want of breath and palpitation when walking slowly. Panting breathing.
- Stitches in and between scapulae.
- Neuralgic pains up back, especially left side.
- Herpes between fingers.
- Paronychia (applied in its incipiency).

- Drawing all limbs, stretching being very agreeable.
- Stitches in all parts of the body: drawing pains in all parts of body, suddenly appearing and disappearing.
- Tearing in bones of lower extremities, especially at night.
- Syphilitic nodes upon shin bones, with severe nightly pains.
- Weak: almost constantly obliged to lie down. Loss of breath and speech.
- Weakness: trembling: shocks on going to sleep depressed.
- Great debility, heaviness and trembling of limbs: < in AM.
- PERSPIRATION, in the morning.
- Night sweats every other night; or every night.
- Profuse perspiration on the soles, causes soreness of toes and balls of feet, with sticking pain as if walking on pains.
- Drowsiness by day.
- Wakes at 2 O'clock every night and is unable to fall sleep again.

NUX MOSCHATA

I. Introduction (Cow.-554)

Synonym: Myristica Moschata.
Common Name: Nutmeg.
Natural Order (Clarke): Myristicaceae.
Habitat: Cultivated in tropical and semi tropical countries. A native of Molucca island.
Preparation: Tincture from the dried, coarsely powered nutmeg.

It was proved firstly by Dr. Helbig of Germany (Pierce-629).

II. General Analysis (Cow.)

Affects particularly, through nervous system digestive tract, ovaries, uterus and produces only nervous symptoms, no organic changes. Chief expression-sleepy drowsy condition with all complaints.

III. Suited to (Allen-209)

Especially women and children of a nervous and hysterical temperament (Ign.): to people with a dry skin, who rarely perspire, complaints, of pregnancy, weakness of old age, dyspepsia of old people. Complaints which cause sleepiness. Great dryness of mouth (Apis., Lach.).

IV. Clinical (Clarke-II-604)

Abortion, Apoplexy, Asthma-hysteric, Brain softening; infantile affections of, Catalepsy, Chilblains, Cholerine, Clairaudience, Clairvoyance, Convulsions, Cough, Debility, Deltoid rheumatism, Dysmenia, Dyspepsia, Eructations, Eyesight weak, Fainting, Flatulence, Freckles, Frost-bite, Gastralgia, Haemorrhage, Headache, Head-convulsive movement of, Hiccough, Hoarseness, Hysteria, Intermittent fever, Locomotor ataxy, Lumbago, Marasmus, Menopause, Menorrhagia, Menses suppressed, Metrorrhagia, Mind-affections of Pelvis-congestion of, Perspiration-bloody; hysterical, Pregnancy-affections of, Ptosis, Puerperal convulsions; Renal colic, Rheumatism, Sleep overpowering, Speech disordered, Stammering, Strangury, Toothache, Turpentine-effects of, Typhoid-haemorrhage in, Uterus-prolapse of, Worms.

V. **Symptoms-General** (Nash-348)

1. Stupor, insensibility, unconquerable sleep; sleepy with most all complaints.
2. Excessive dryness of the tongue, mouth, lips and throat; no thirst.
3. And, < cold damp weather, getting wet, or washing; after eating (bloating); > in room, dry weather.
4. Changeable humour; one moment laughing, the next crying.

VI. **Symptoms-Particular** (Nash-349-351)

1. Stupor and insensibility unconquerable sleep interrupted by piercing screams.
2. (a) Vanishing of thought while speaking etc.

    Nux. m.,
    Camph.,
    Cann. ind.,
    Lach.

    (b) Changeable Mood and fitful disposition.

    Nux. m.,
    Acon.,
    Ign.,
    Croc.,
    Plat.

    (c) Loss of memory.

    Acon.,
    Lyc.,
    Bry.,
    Sul.,
    Nat. m.

(d) Absence of mind.

Anac.,
Kreas.,
Lach.,
Nat. m.,
Merc. s.,
Nux. m.
} (Hysteric medicines)

(e) Sleepiness, Dullness or Stupor.

Op.-fullness of blood vessels, due to,
Nux. m.-benumbing of very nervous due to

3. Excessive dryness of lips, tongue with no thirst.

Apis.,
Puls.,
Lach.,
Nux. m.-Strongest

4. Abdomen distended-immediately after eating.

(a) immediately after food.

Nux. m.,
Kali bich..

(b) after an hour or two.

Nux. v.,
Anac.

(c) everything turns into gas and fill the stomach so full as to cause pressure on heart and abdomen.

Iod.,
Kali c..

(d) Diarrhoea. Efficacious in Cholera infantum, without thirst yet mouth dry, yellow watery stool with bloating of abdomen.

VII. Black Letter Symptoms (Tyler-596-597)

- Mentally: Stupor and insensibility: unconquerable sleep.
- Vanishing of thoughts while talking, reading, or writing.
- Weakness and loss of memory.
- Uses wrong words (during headache).
- Surroundings seem changed; fanciful, dreamy images; does not recognize the known street. (Opium).

- Inclination to laugh at everything, more in open air.
- Sensation as if all vessels were pulsating, especially in HEAD: a throbbing, pressing pain, confined to smell spots, principally to left supra-orbital ridge.
- Severe tearing in occiput, towards nape of neck.
- Dryness of EYES: too dry to close lids.
- TONGUE PARALYSED: difficult to move tongue: dry, feels as if gone to sleep or leather covered. At night dry, as if would fall into powder; sticks to roof of mouth; great complaint of its dryness; in reality not very dry.
- Mouth so dry that tongue sticks to roof, yet no thirst (evening).
- Greatly troubled with dryness of mouth and throat while sleeping; always wakes with a very dry tongue, but without thirst.
- STOMACH: No thirst with dry mouth.
- Eating a little too much causes headache.
- Vomiting: spasmodic; during pregnancy; from irritation of pessaries; from acid stomach; flatulence.
- Fullness in stomach impeding breathing: during pregnancy.
- STOOL: soft but difficult; rectum inactive; slow; undigested; with great sleepiness.
- MENSES irregular in time and quantity: too early and profuse; too late, preceded by pain in back. Flow generally dark, thick. Pain in small of back, as if a piece of wood were lying crosswise and being pressed out, unconquerable drowsiness: mouth dry: hysteric laughter.
- Threatened abortion; hysterical females disposed to fainting; feel chilly and catch cold easily; fears she will abort; continued and obstinate flooding.
- Hoarseness from walking against wind.
- Difficult inhalation: hysteric asthma.
- Dyspnoea with feeling of weight in CHEST.
- Stitches in chest: tightness; spitting of blood.
- Pains now in BACK: now in sacrum; knees very tired: worse during rest. Lumbago.
- Pain in sacrum when riding in a carriage.

- HANDS cold as if frozen: tingling under nails, on entering a warm room.
- NERVES: Drowsiness: torpor: lethargy.
- Spasms: hysterical in inner parts: chronic hysteric fits: convulsive motions.
- Hysteria: exhausted from least effort.
- Complaints cause sleepiness: irresistibly drowsy; sleepy, muddled, as if intoxicated; coma, lies silent, immovable: eyes closed: strange feeling on waking.
- Want of sweat: skin cool and dry.

NUX VOMICA

I. Introduction (Cow.-558)

Synonym: Strychnos Nux Vomica.
Natural Order: Loganiaceae.
Common Name: Poison Nut.
Habitat: A tree indigenous to India, Burma and North Australia.
Preparation: Tincture or Triturations from the finely pulverised seeds.

First proved by Hahnemann who called it a poly chrest (medicine of many uses) (Pierce-630).

II. General Analysis (Cow.)

Acts pre-eminently upon spinal cord including motor and sensory centres at the base of the brain and affects reflex action on causing violent tetanic contractions. But through these horrible convulsions the mind remains unaffected. Affects profoundly the organs and functions of nutrition presenting picture of gastric, hepatic and intestinal affections. This same irritation produces constipation in the alimentary canal, dry catarrhal condition in respiratory sphere; obstruction in nasal passage and dry cough. In genito-urinary sphere-first increased activity, followed by relaxation and depression. Chief expression-disorders of digestion from especially long continued errors of diet, highly seasoned foods stimulating drinks, hot mediums, especially in persons with sedentary habits.

III. Suited to (Allen-211)

Thin, irritable, careful zealous person, dark hair bilious or sanguine temperament. Disposed of to be quarrelsome, spiteful Nervous melancholic. Prone to haemorrhoids, constipation. Impatient temperament, sanguine, sedentary life-style, oversensitive to external impressions; to noise, odours, light or music (Nux. m). Trifling ailments unbearable (Cham.), every harmless word offends (Ign.).

IV. Clinical (Clarke-II-613)

Acne rosacea, Alcoholism, Amaurosis, Amblyopia, Anger-effects of, Apoplexy, Asthma, Bilious attack, Biliousness, Bladder affections, Bone-nodes on, Brain-affections of, Breath sour, Carriage-sickness, Catarrh, Clavus, Colds, Colic, Constipation, Convulsions, Cough, Cramps, Delirium, Diarrhoea, Dysentery, Dyspepsia, Emissions, Epilepsy, Erotomania, Eyes-affections of; gouty inflammation of, Gall-stones, Gastrodynia, Gout, Haemorrhoids, Headache, Heart affections, Hernia, Hydrocele, Hypochondriasis, Impotence, Intermittent fever, Lisping, Liver disorder, Locomotor ataxy, Lumbago, Masturbation, Muscoe volitantes, Myelitis, Night-blindness, Nightmare, Nose affections, Nymphomania, Paralysis-spastic, Paraphimosis, Pregnancy-affections of; spurious, Pylorus-disease of, Renal calculi, Sea-sickness, Sexual perversion, Sleep abnormal, Speech disordered, Spermatorrhoea, Strabismus, Taste disordered, Tea-effects of, Tenesmus, Tobacco-habit, Tongue-affections of, Trachea-affections of, Urethra-spasm of, Urine-frequent passing of, Uterus-prolapse of, Vagina-prolapse of, Vertigo, Water-brash, Worms, Yawning.

V. Symptoms-General (Nash-13-14)

1. For very particular, careful, zealous persons, inclined to get excited or angry, spiteful, malicious disposition, mental workers or those having sedentary occupations.
2. Over-sensitiveness, easily offended; very little noise frightens, can't bear the least even suitable medicine; faints easily from odours, etc.
3. Twitching, spasms, convulsion, < slightest touch, Chilliness, even during high fever, least uncovering brings on chilliness. Very red face.
4. Persons addicted to stimulants, narcotics, patent medicines, nostrums, debauchees, etc.

5. Frequent and ineffectual desire for stool or passed little at a time > after stool.
6. Modalities: < uncovering, mental work, after eating, cold air, dry weather, stimulants, 9 AM > wet weather, warm room, on covering; after stool.
7. Spasm (from simple twitching to the clonic from); sensitiveness, nervous and chilliness are three general characteristics of this remedy.
8. Anxiety with irritability and inclination to commit suicide, but afraid to die.
9. Sleepy in the evening, hours before bedtime; lies awake for an hour or two, at 3 AM or 4 AM, then wants to sleep late in morning.
10. Awakens tired and weak and generally worse, with many complaints.
11. Stomach: pressure in hour or two after eating as from a stone. (Immediately after-Kali bich., Nux. m).
12. Convulsions with consciousness (Strych.): < anger, emotion, touch, moving, alternate constipation and diarrhoea (Ant. c.).
13. Menses: Too early, profuse and lasting too long, with aggravation of all other complaints during their continuance.
14. Nux Vomica acts best when given at night, during repose of mind (Sul. in the morning).

VI. Symptoms-Particular (Nash-14-22)

1. Nervous temperament (over sensitiveness, harmless word offends, little noise frightens).

   Nux. v.,
   Cham.,
   Ign.,
   Staph.
2. Sedentary habit with costiveness.
3. Hypochondria but little irritation breaks, arises out of hypochondirac gloom.

   If does not then-Aur. m., Nat. m.
4. Frequent and ineffectual desire to defecate or passing little quantities of faeces.

Nux. v.-irregular peristaltic action.

Bry.-No desire at all stool dry and hard as if burnt.

5. Dysentery also has the symptom of ineffectual desire.

   Nux. v.-greatly relieved after stool for a while.

   Merc. c.-pain and Tenesmus continue after the stool.

6. Menses-too long, copious, before time, with complaints to continue even after (with characteristic rectal trouble) the onset, which remain till it is over.

   Calc. c.,
   Puls.,
   Sep.

7. Inefficient labour pain, pressing downward, extends to rectum or urination Nux 200, Makes them efficient.

8. Menorrhagia with costive gastric < morning-sure remedy-Nux. v.

   (a) Worse in the morning.

   Nux. v.,
   Lach., } soon after
   Nat. m. } awakening.

   (b) After mental exertion.

   Nux. v.,
   Nat. c. (vertigo)
   Calc. c., } Occipital
   Sil. }

   (c) < After eating (Anac.-reverse).

   (d) < In cold Air (Puls.-reverse).

9. Fever-whole body burning hot, face red hot, yet can't uncover or move without chill.

10. Gastric troubles.

    Kali bich., }
    Nux. m., } < after eating.
    Nux. v. }

    (a) Sour Taste, heaviness after one hour or two afterword with Hypochon-driacal mood, tightness about waist. Must loose clothing.

    Lach.,
    Calc. c.,
    Lyc.

(b) Can't use mind 2-3 hours after a meal, epigastrium bloated as if stone.

(c) Immediately after food.

Nux. m.,
Kali bich.

(d) Pressure as from stone.

Bry.,
Puls.,
Nux. v.

(e) Broken Rest from long Night watching, too high living.

Nux. v.,
Cocc.,
Cupr.,
Nit. ac.

11. Headache, Backache from:

(a) Mental exertion, chagrin or anger, in open air (Puls.-reverse).
(b) On awaking in morning.
(c) After eating.
(d) Abuse of coffee, spirits.
(e) Sour stomach.
(f) On opening eyes (moving-Bry.).
(g) From coughing, high living or highly seasoned food.
(h) Stormy weather, after drugging.
(i) Constipation, masturbation.

(*These headaches may or may not localise.*).

12. Backache-peculiar:

(a) Must sit up to turn over in bed.

Nux. v.-turning or twisting worsens.
Sul.-< standing.

(b) < Sitting.

Puls.,
Nux. v.,
Rhus t.,
Cobalt,

Zinc.

(c) < Lying.
Nux. v.,
Staph.

(d) Pains in lumber region with haemorrhoids.
Nux. v.
Aesc. hip. < when walking (with haemorrhoids).

13. Backache by masturbation-Cobalt < sitting; Staph. < lying at night.

VII. Black Letter Symptoms
(Tyler-1002-1007)

- Worse dry wind.
- Exaggerated sensitiveness and irritability.
- Excessive uneasiness.
- Moral exaltation and excitability with extreme sensitiveness to least pain, to least smell, nose or movement.
- Insane desire to kill.
- Takes everything amiss; readily breaks out into scolding and abuse.
- He is hasty. Looks malignantly at anyone who asks him anything without answering.
- It seems as if he would like to strike anyone in the face who speaks a word to him, so irritable and uncontrollable is his disposition.
- Every harmless word offends. Peevish. Malevolent. Fiery, excited temperament. Ill-humour, vexation and anger, breaking out in acts of violence.
- Extravagant and frantic actions.
- Quarrelsome, even to violence.
- Extraordinary anxiety. Sadness.
- She can't get over the smallest evil.
- Much disposed to scolding crossness.
- Much given to reproach others for their faults.
- He feels everything too strongly.
- Oversensitive to impressions of the senses.
- Can't bear strong odours and bright light.
- Can't bear any nose or speaking.

- Music and singing affect him strongly.
- Irresolution.
- Can't endure the slightest ailment.
- Very hypochondriac, and affected by the slightest thing, after eating.
- Dread of literary work at which one must think and employ the ideas.
- Intoxication.
- Drunken confusion in the head.
- Dullness of head after dinner, which recurred 24 hours afterwards.
- In the morning, drunken, giddy heaviness of the head.
- Aching pain in occiput in the morning immediately after rising from bed.
- Squeezing headache.
- Dullness, headache, felt even before opening the eyes.
- Worse moving the eyes.
- Morning headache, as if head had been beaten with an axe.
- Headache, worse after eating, with nausea and very sour vomiting.
- Attacks of vertigo, as if it turned round in the brain, with momentary loss of consciousness.
- Drunken confusion of the head.
- Profuse discharge of mucus from one nostril, that seems obstructed by dry catarrh.
- Frequent coryza in the morning.
- Coryza fluent during the day, and stopped at night.
- Frequent discharge from both nostrils obstructed by dry catarrh.
- Real coryza, with scraping in the throat, crawling and creeping in the nose, and sneezing.
- Catarrh with headache-heat in face, chilliness and much mucous in throat.
- Sneezing in bed: after rising, sudden fluent coryza.
- Throat rough from catarrh. Painful, raw and sore, at the palate.
- Rawness in throat that provokes cough.

- Sore throat. Scraped throat.
- Rawness and scraped feeling in larynx. Provokes cough.
- Violent cough before rising in the morning, with expectoration of clotted blood, and soreness in chest.
- Very early morning cough.
- Dry cough, from midnight till daybreak.
- Scraping in chest, causing hawking.
- Cough which bring on headache as if the skull would burst.
- Cough which cause bruised pain in epigastrium.
- Asthmatic constrictive tightness transversely through the chest, when walking and going up hill.

  Among the feverish symptoms of Nux. v. are:
- After drinking, immediately shivering and chilliness.

Digestive tract symptoms

- Putrid taste in the morning, but food and drink taste right.
- Bitter taste. Putrid taste on coughing.
- Repugnance of food. And to the accustomed tobacco and coffee.
- Eructation of bitter and sour liquid.
- Nausea-in the morning: after eating.
- Smoking makes him nauseated and qualmish.
- After a meal he is qualmish, anxious, nauseated and sick as after a violent purge.
- Inclination to vomit. Vomiting of sour mucous.
- Retching, as if to vomit, while hawking mucous from fauces.
- Tension above stomach.
- Pressure, as from a stone in epigastrium: worse walking.
- Pressure in stomach, after eating a little, in the morning.
- A metallic, herby taste returns.
- Pressure as from overloading the stomach, immediately after eating.
- Violent gastric symptoms.
- Scraped sensation in stomach.

- Flatulent distension of abdomen, after eating.
- Colic, as if diarrhoea from taking cold would come on.
- Cutting colic, with qualmishness. Colic that causes nausea.
- Colic speedily disappearing during rest, sitting or lying.
- Pain in abdominal ring, as if a hernia would become incarcerated.
- Sensation of weakness in abdominal ring, as if a hernia would occur.

Intestine

- Pinching, tearing abdominal pain as if diarrhoea from a chill would occur.
- Needle pricks, cutting pains, pinching pains.
- After bellyache evacuations of dark-coloured mucous, which caused smarting burning at anus.
- Sensation of weakness in the abdominal ring, as if a hernia would occur.
- Forcing down towards the genitals in the lower abdomen.
- Development of a tendency to inguinal hernia.

The rectum and anus are extremely affected by Nux

- Blind haemorrhoids.
- Sharp pressive pain in the rectum, after a stool and after a meal, especially on exerting the mind, and studying.
- Tearing sticking and constricting pain, as from aggravated blind piles, in the rectum and anus, after a meal and after exerting the mind and reflecting.
- After a stool it seemed as if some remained behind and could not be evacuated, with a sense of constriction in the rectum, not in the anus.
- Discharge of bright blood with faeces, with a sensation of constriction and construction in the rectum during stool.
- With the stool it always seemed as if it were not

enough, and as if the evacuation were incomplete.

- Anxious desire for stool.
- Frequent ineffectual desire for stool as if the evacuation were incomplete.
- Diarrhoea of a dark colour, especially in the morning and immediately after dinner.
- Obliged to go to stool three or four times a day: it was often ineffectual, and the stool when passed was soft.
- Constipation, as from constriction and contraction of the intestines.
- Urging to urinate. Frequent desire to urinate: constantly called out he would be better if he could pass water.
- Painful, ineffectual desire to urinate.
- Violent straining: the effects to urinate were constant and most painful, without being able to pass a single drop.
- Urine passed with difficulty.
- Whilst urinating, a burning and tearing pain in the neck of the bladder.
- Whilst urinating an itching in the urethra.
- Menses three days early with Cramp in abdomen.
- During the menses-nausea in morning, with chilliness and attacks of fainting.
- In the convulsion of Nux, one observes the strychnine element.
- The slightest touch of the hand immediately brought on spasms.

OPIUM

I. Introduction (Cow-575)

Synonym: Papaver somniferum.
Natural Order: Papaveraceae.
Common Name: White poppy. Opium.
Habitat: Native plant of Asia.
Preparation: Tincture from inspissated Juice.

Hahnemann first proved it in MMP. He mentions its power as pain destroyer ("No medicine has done more harm, with preliminary apparent relief, than this opium") (MMP) (Pierce-630).

II. General Analysis (Cow.)

Acts upon the cerebro-spinal and sympathetic nervous system producing brief excitation, rapidly followed by depression, and paralysis of all functional activity. Stupor ensues; mucous membranes become dry and congested, breathing slow and irregular, hearts, action retarted, death or passing off, leaves deranged digestion, headache, sleeplessness and constipation (no desire). Its universal use as palliative is not homeopathic and condemned. Extremely valuable in Apoplexy, Delirium tremens, Intestinal obstruction, Faecal vomiting, Aphonia from fright, Retention of urine.

III. Suited to (Allen-214)

Especially to children and old people; (Baryt. c., Mill.) Persons with light hair, lax muscles, and want of bodily irritability. All complaints: with great sopor; painless, complaints of nothing; wants nothing. Ailments that originate from fear (Acon., Hyo.) Charcoal vapours. Lack of vital reaction, the well chosen remedies make no impact (Carb. v., Laur., Valer.).

IV. Clinical (Clarke-II-664)

After-pains, Apoplexy, Bladder-paralysis of, Brain-affections of, Cancer, Catalepsy, Chilblains, Colic, Constipation, Diabetes mellitus, Dreams, Dysmenia, Epilepsy, Fear-effects of, Foetus-excessive movements of, Hernia incarcerated, Hystero-epilepsy, Ileus, Intestines-obstruction of, Labour pains abnormal, Lead colic, Marasmus, Measles, Melancholia, Meningitis, Paralysis, Puerperal convulsions, Sighing, Sleep abnormal, Snoring, Starting, Sunstroke, Tympanites, Uraemia, Urine-suppression of; retention of, Uterus-inertia of, Veins-fullness of, Whooping-cough.

V. Symptoms-General (Nash-344)

1. Abnormal painlessness.
2. Want of susceptibility, trembling, lack of vital reaction.
3. Blunted morals, worst liars in the world.
4. Reversed peristalsis and faecal vomiting.
5. Fright; the fear of fright remaining.
6. Sleepy but can't sleep, Hears sounds not ordinarily noticed.
7. Very hot skin with sweating; perspiration.
8. Profound stupor with dark-red face and stertorous breathing.
9. Bed feels so hot she can't lie on it; moves often in search of a cool place; must be uncovered.

VI. Symptoms-Particular (Nash 344-348)

1. Stupid/comatose sleep with strenuous (loud) breathing, with red face, eyes, half closed, lower jaw dropped, skin hot sweat. (No response to light etc.).
   Lach., } in typhoid with
   Hyo. } above symptoms.
2. Sleeplessness with acuteness of hearing:
   Op., (Tick of watch etc. keep awake)
   Cimicif. r.,
   Coff.—due to excitement in bed.
3. Searches cool places.
   Op.,
   Sul.

4. Banishing of pain (Laur.)
5. Paralysing effects in intestines-faeces lie there hard, black balls, must be removed mechanically. NO DESIRE AT ALL.
6. Urinary-Paralysis of fundus of bladder, can't pass water, involuntary urination or stool.
7. Delirious-wide open eyes, glistening face, red puffed, vivid imagination exaltation of mind.
8. Nervous irritability, easily frightened.

VII. Black Letter Symptoms (Tyler-616)

- Fear of impending death. Expression of fright and terror.
- Complete insensibility. Impossible to excite any sign of uneasiness by pulling the hair, or pinching the skin, or sudden effusion of cold water.
- Insensibility with complete apoplectic respiration.
- Unconscious: eyes glassy, half closed, face pale, deep coma.
- Mania a potu: senses dull; sopor with snoring. Sees animals coming towards him. People want to hurt him; Creeps under covers: wants to jump out of bed. Believe themselves murderers or criminals, to be executed. Want to run away.
- Staring look: facial muscles twitch. Lockjaw. Tremor.
- Ailments from excessive joy, fright, anger, shame.
- Ailments after fright, the fear of the fright remaining.
- Trembling limbs after a fright. Spasm from emoting, fright, etc.
- Face pale. Face flushed.
- PUPILS dilated, insensible to light; or contracted and sluggish.
- Paralysis of tongue with difficult articulation.
- Great thirst; unquenchable thirst.
- Colic: transient: very violent: griping, with constipation, as if intestines cut to pieces. Painters colic.
- Stools: involuntary after fright; fluid, frothy; burning in anus; tenesmus. Hard, round, dry, black balls: like sheep dung: feels as if rectum were closed; come down and recede. (Sil.).

- Almost unconquerable chronic constipation.
- Cholera Infantum; Stupor, snoring, Convulsion, contracted pupils.
- Well selected remedy refuses to act. Want of susceptibility to drugs, want of vital reaction.
- Painlessness in all ailments. Complains of nothing; wants nothing.
- Paralysis: insensibility: after apoplexy-in drunkards-old people.
- Weakens expulsive power of bladder; which is unable to expel its contents; retention of urine.
- Frequent involuntary deep breathing. Respirations long, sighing or stertorious respirations.
- Pulse show, with slow stertorious respirations: exceedingly red face: extremely profuse perspiration. Convulsion.
- Whining in sleep. Drowsy, difficult to keep awake; at night, restless with much perspiration.
- Sleepless with acute hearing; clocks Striking and cocks crowing at a distance, keep her awake.

PETROLEUM

I. Introduction (Cow-589)

Synonym: Oleum Petrae. Naphtha Montana.
Common Names: Rock oil. Coal oil.
Preparation: Tincture on centiminal scale. (1 part crude oil to 99 parts alcohol=2x dilution).

First proved by Hahnemann-776 symptoms (Pierce-649).

II. General Analysis (Cow.)

Acts upon skin and mucous membrane producing irritation, eczema and herpes especially behind ears, occiput and hands, with raw, moist surface with thick scabs. Occipital headache, nausea and vomiting, intermittent fever with climacteric headache and bladder atony with dribble. Chief action on skin especially eczema and herpes of behind ears, on occiput, on hands. Bladder intermittent.

III. Suited to (Allen-217)

Persons with light hair and skin, quarrelsome disposition (Nux. v.), easily offended at trifles (Ign., Medo.); vexed at every thing. Ailments-from riding in a carriage, worse before and during a thunder storm (Nat. c., Phos., Psor.).

IV. Clinical (Clarke-III-742)

Addison's disease, Albuminuria, Anaemia, Angina pectoris, Anus-fissure of, Bed-sores, Breath offensive, Burns, Chilblains, Chlorosis, Constipation, Cracks in skin, Deafness, Diarrhoea, Dysmenia, Dyspepsia, Ear affections, Eczema, Face rough, Facial paralysis, Feet-soles painful, Fester-tendency to, Fistula, Frost-bite, Gastric ulcer, Gonorrhoea, Haemorrhoids, Hands chapped, Headache-occipital, Herpes, Herpes preputialis, Irritation, Jaw-easily dislocated, Myopia, Nose sore, Otorrhoea, Perspiration offensive, Pregnancy-sickness of, Presbyopia, Prostatitis, Psoriasis, Rheumatism, Sea-sickness, Skin-affections of, Sprain, Syphilis, Tabes mesenterica, Toothache, Urethra-stricture of; chronic inflammation of, Varices, Vomiting, Warts.

V. **Symptoms-General** (Nash-396)

1. Eczema on scalp, behind ears, scrotum anus, hands, feet, legs, hands chap and bleed; all < in winter; get better in summer Diarrhoea preceded by colic, only in the daytime.
2. Headache or heaviness like lead in the occiput; sometimes with nausea on vomiting; < by motion, as in riding in boat or carriage.

VI. **Symptoms-Particular** (Nash-396)

Anti Psoric medicine-one of the best with Sul., Graph., Caust., Lyc.

1. Skin-Eruption on scrotum, anus, etc. < Winter, > summer.
   Petr., Aloe., Alumen, Psor.
2. Chronic Diarrhoea preceding colic only in daytime.
3. Chilblains.
   Petr.,-(burning, itching, swelling in cold weather).
   Agar.,
   Hep. s.-slight scratch suppurates. < Cold weather.
4. Headache-heaviness on top (occipital).
   < motion, riding in carriage, boat, etc.
5. Pain in stomach < eating relieves. (Petr., Chel., Anac.).
6. Sea-sickness (Cocc.).
7. Cracking of Joints (Caust.).
8. Chronic Rheumatism (Caust.).

VII. **Black Letter Symptoms** (Tyler-633)

- Delirium: thinks another person lies alongside of him, or that one limb is a double.
- Out of humour and angry; becomes vehement easily.
- Forgetful, and not disposed to think.
- Heaviness like lead in occiput: pinching in occiput.

- Great pressure in eyes.
- Conjunctivitis pustulosa, with acute inflammation of lids. Lids red, inflamed, covered with scabs or scrufs. Surrounding skin rough: blennorrhoea of lachrymal sac: pain in occiput.
- Inflammation of lachrymal sac, when suppuration has commenced and a fistula has formed.
- Eustachian tubes affected, causing whizzing, roaring and cracking noise, with hardness of hearing.
- Redness, soreness and humour behind the ears.
- Pustule in nose. Bleeding nose.
- Nausea and qualmishness all day: every AM, after walking, could not eat breakfast.
- In the morning accumulation of water in mouth sudden on walking: from riding in carriage: after so violent that it takes away the breath, without vomiting; violent, with cold sweat, incessant: with vertigo and vomiting.
- Seasickness.
- After a slight meal, feels giddy and head swims.
- Heartburn towards evening.
- Nausea and qualmish the whole day.
- Obstinate, itching herpes on perineum; itching, redness and moisture, scrotum. Skin cracked, rough and bleeding.
- Hoarseness: cough from dryness in throat.
- Sharp pains, shooting up dorsal spine into occiput.
- Painful chilblains on hands.
- Tips of fingers rough, cracked and fissured.

PETROSELINUM

I. Introduction (Cow-594)

Synonym: Apium Petroselinum.
Natural Order: Umbellifarae.
Common Name: Parsley.
Habitat: A native plant of S. Europe.
Preparation: Tincture from fresh plant.

II. General Analysis (Cow.)

Acts upon urethral mucous membrane, producing irritation and inflammation. In sub-acute Gonorrhoea and Gleet.

III. Suited to (Allen-218)

Sudden urging to urinate (Canth.). Child suddenly seized with desire to urinate, jumps up and down, trys to hold on. Burning, tingling from perineum throughout whole urethra. Thirsty and hungry, yet as soon as they begin to eat desire disappear; (Reverse of Calc. c.). Intermittent fever-traumatic or chronic urethrities or stricture.

IV. Clinical (Clarke-III-751)

Catheter fever, Cystitis, Dysuria, Gleet, Gonorrhoea, Gravel, Intermittent fever, Night-blindness, Priapism.

V. Symptoms-Particular (Nash-443)

1. Great sudden desire to urinate (like desire for stool in Aloe.).
2. Itching in urethra, must put a stick to scratch there.
3. Burning, tingling-from perineum throughout whole urethra.

PHOSPHORIC-ACID

I. Introduction (Cow-595)

Common Name: Glacial Phosphoric acid.
Preparation: dilution on centicimal scale in distilled water and alcohol.

It was first proved by Hahnemann (Pierce-652).

II. General Analysis (Cow.)

Acts mainly upon nervous system producing debility without erethism (with erethism-Cinchona rub.) giving rise to conditions like continued grief (Ign.), exhaustion of mind and body. Its main effects are upon kidney and sexual organs, bones and skin.

III. Suited to (Allen-219)

Persons of originally strong constitutions, debilitated by loss of vital fluids, sexual excesses. (China), violent acute diseases, disappointed love, grief etc. Ailments from care, chagrin grief, home sickness (Ign.), sleepy, disposed to weep, mild yielding (Puls.). Pale sickly complexion, eyes sunken and surrounded by blue margins. Listless, apathetic. Children and young people who grow too rapidly (Calc. c., Calc. phos.).

IV. Clinical (Clarke-III-762)

Amblyopia, Asthma, Boils, Brain-fag, Bronchitis-capillary, Chancre, Chilblains, Cholera, Climacteric flushes and vertigo, Coccygodynia, Condylomata, Corns, Cough, Coxalgia, Debility, Diabetes, Diarrhoea, Dyspepsia, Emissions, Enteric fever, Enuresis, Feet sore, Flatulence, Ganglion, Gout, Gravel, Hair falling off, Headache of school children, Hectic, Herpes, Hip-joint disease, Homesickness, Impotence, Joints scrofulous, Lactation defective, Levitation,

Lienteria, Locomotor ataxy, Love-disappointed, Masturbation, Mind-weakness of, Mercurial syphilis, Navel-pains in, Neurasthenia, Nymphomania, Osteo-myletis, Perspiration profuse, Phosphaturia, Physometra, Pimples, Pregnancy-diarrhoea of; nausea of, Prepuce-warts on, Psoas abscess, Puerperal eclampsia, Purpura, Rheumatism, Sciatica, Scurvy, Self-abuse, Spermatorrhoea, Spinal caries, Sycosis Hahnemanni, Syphilis, Tetters, Typhus fever, Ulcer, Urine phosphatic, Uterus-prolapse of, Varices, Vertigo, Warts, Wens, Worms.

V. **Symptoms-General** (Nash-240)

1. Drowsy, apathetic; unconscious of all surroundings, but can be aroused to full consciousness.
2. Chronic effects of grief; hair turns grey, hopeless, haggard look.
3. Grows too fast and too tall; young persons with growing pains in bones.
4. Great physical and mental weakness from ovarian or sexual excesses.
5. Diarrhoea-white, watery, painless, with rumbling; meteorism; but not so much weakness as would be expected.
6. Very profuse, watery, or milky urine.
7. Modalities: < bad news, depressing emotions; masturbation or sexual excess; draft; wind; snowy air; > after short sleep.
8. Headache of schoolgirls from eyestrain, or overuse of eyes, occipital. Chest-weak from talking or coughing; cough, purulent, offensive expectoration, and pains in chest. Salty expectoration in proving.

VI. **Symptoms-Particular** (Nash-241-244)

1. Lies in stupor-unconscious of surrounding-when aroused is fully conscious.
   Ign.-Sighs, nervous twitch,
   Phos.-Stupefied, No sighing or twitch.
2. Grows too fast, overtaxed mentally and physically.
   Phos.-too fast and tall.
   Calc. c.-too fat.

3. Student's headache, esp. of those growing too fast.
   Phos. ac.-(relived by urine-Gels.)
   Nat. m.,
   Calc. phos.
4. Depression (Typhoid)-unique medicine in this sphere.
   Phos. ac.-+++, no ecchymosis, terribly offensive stool and urine.
   Arn.-indifferent but profound depression, ecchymosis.
   Bap.-goes to sleep while answering.
   Op.-surpasses all medicine in stupying.
   Rhus t. } stupid but different in
   Hyo. } other symptoms.
5. White profuse stool-diarrhoea yellow, painless, without exhaustion, rumbling in abdomen.
   Phos. ac.-without debility.
   China-debility with diarrhoea.
6. Weak feeling in chest from talking.
   Phos. ac.,
   Stan.,
   Sul.
7. Cough.
   Phos. ac., -Copious, purulent, offensive.
   Stan. -thick, heavy sweetish.
8. URINE.
   Phos. ac.-Profuse, clear or milky, excess of phosphate.
   > Headache with flow.
   Ign. -hysterical.
   Phos. ac.-Not hysterical.

VII. Black Letter Symptoms
(Tyler-637-639)

- Quiet, indifferent.
- Loss of ideas, and weakness of mind.
- He can't collect his thoughts in proper manner.
- He speaks unwillingly: talking is irksome.
- Speaks little and answers questions unwillingly.
- Listless, apathetic: remarkable indifference to everything in life, especially if there be emaciation and debility.

- Ailments from care, grief, chagrin, homesickness, or disappointed love: particularly with drowsiness, night sweats towards morning emaciation.
- He looks very ill humoured and sullen.
- Sad humour, on account of concern for the future.
- He becomes very cheerful and well disposed: (secondary, curative reaction).
- Schoolgirl's headache from overuse of eyes.
- Occipital headaches and pain nape of neck from exhausted nerve power or excessive grief. Confusion of whole head. Headache like stupidity; buzzing in head.
- Constant headache.
- On the slightest shock or noise pains in head become extremely violent.
- Hard pressure on left side forehead.
- Squeezing pressure right temple, more violent on moving.
- Squeezing pain in both parietal bones: worse on moving.
- Pain as if temples were pressed towards one another, as if violently pinched by forceps.
- Drawing pressure in right parietal and occipital bones, more violent when moving.
- Tearing and squeezing pain in brain, here and there.
- Tearing pressure in occiput, worse noise and slightest movement.
- Violent shooting pain, right temporal, extending into right eye.
- Burning, sore pain on the side of nape.
- Vertigo towards evening, when standing and walking.
- Vertigo in the morning, making him fall when standing.
- Transient burning left eye, as if something pungent had been smelt.
- Pain as if eyeballs were forcibly pressed together and into head.
- Itching in the point of nose: must scratch.
- Violent burning pain in right lower lip, persisting when moved.

- Bleeding gums.
- Dry feeling-palate. Nausea-palate.
- When swallowing food, shooting in throat:
- An almost insatiable thirst for cold milk.
- After eating, pressing down weight in stomach and aching.
- In navel, a periodical aching, squeezing.
- Loud rumbling in abdomen, especially upper part.
- Extremely violent pinching contraction of bowels from both sides of the umbilical region.
- Pressure on several parts of hypogastrium. Distress in the abdomen.
- Thin, Whitish-grey stools.
- White or yellow watery diarrhoea, chronic or acute, without pain or marked debility or exhaustion.
- Stools involuntary.
- Urging to urinate, with scanty discharge of urine.
- Quite pale urine which immediately forms a thick whitish cloud.
- Very profuse emissions.
- Onanism with distress, at its culpability.
- Great hoarseness.
- Difficult inspiration, from pressure and oppression behind the sternum. Pain in chest from weakness.
- Pressive pain in middle of the chest, most severe when expiring.
- Felt as if sternum would be pressed out: pain more violent on pressing hand on sternum, stooping, coughing, etc.
- Dry cough from tickling low down just above pit of stomach.
- Feels bruised in hips, thighs, arms and nape: like growing pains: with single tearing stitches in all these parts at once.
- Exhaustion in legs when walking. Formication right leg.
- Squeezing pressure in soles (one or other).
- Here and there, a creeping, like ants running about.
- Itching creeping in body and hands, evening, lying down.

- Drowsy in the morning: can hardly be roused from sleep.
- Deterioration of health from nursing.
- Weak and prostrated: weak and apathetic in the morning.
- Neurasthenia: cerebrospinal exhaustion from overwork: least attempt causes heaviness in head and limbs.
- Interstitial inflammation of bones: scrofulous, syphilitic or mercurial.
- Periosteal inflammation, with burning, gnawing, tearing pains.
- Scrofulous affections of children:. hip disease, curvature of spine, rickets, FEELING AS IF BONES WERE SCRAPED WITH A KNIFE.
- Children and young people who have gown too rapidly: all slender, slim: pains in back and limbs as if beaten: growing pains.

PHOSPHORUS

I. Introduction (Cow-600)

Common Name: Phosphorus.
Preparation: A saturated solution prepared in Alcohol.

It was Homeopathically proved by Hahnemann and is a tissue remedy of the first rank (Pierce-655).

II. General Analysis (Cow.)

Acts powerfully upon vegetative system and the blood, in each tending disorganisation and destruction. First is violent erethism leading to congestion and inflammation then to torpor and paralysis. The characteristic action is upon blood, maxillary bones, lungs and teeth–haemorrhage and ecchymosis caries and necrosis; and in lungs sanguinous infiltration while fatty degeneration especially in kidney, heart and liver. In all mucous membranes it causes inflammation all along the alimentary and respiratory tracts.

III. Suited to (Allen-221)

Tall slender persons of sanguine temperament, fair skin, delicate eye lashes, fine blond or red hair, quick perceptions, and very sensitive nature, young people who grow too rapidly. Inclined to stoop (Sul.), anaemic, old people with morning diarrhoea. Restless fidgety, moves continually, cannot sit or stand still a moment (fidgety feet-Zinc.). Over sensitive to external impressions light, sound, odours, touch etc.

IV. Clinical (Clarke-III-772)

Alopecia areata, Amaurosis, Amblyopia, Anaemia-acute; pernicious, Anus-fissure of, Antrum-disease of, Arteries-disease of, Asthma, Bone disease, Brain-affections of;

softening of, Brain-fag, Breast-abscess of; fistulae of, Bronchitis-membranous, Cancer-of bone, Cataract, Catarrh-intestinal; nasal, Chilblains, Chlorosis, Chorea, Ciliary neuralgia Coccygodynia, Colds, Constipation, Consumption, Corpulency, Cough, Croup, Dandruff, Diarrhoea, Dropsy, Ecchymosis, Enteric fever, Ephelis, Epilepsy, Erotomania, Exophthalmos, Exostosis, Eye affections, Fainting, Fatty degeneration, Fistula, Flatulence, Fungus haematoides, Gastritis, Glaucoma, Gleet, Gums-ulceration of, Haemoglobinuria, Haemorrhagic diathesis, Headache, Heart-degeneration of; murmurs of, Hydrocele, Hydrocephalus, Hysteria, Impotence, Intussusception, Jaundice-malignant; of pregnancy; of anaemia, Jaw-disease of, Joint affections, Keratitis, Lactation disordered, Laryngitis, Levitation, Lightning-effects of, Lienteria, Liver-diseases of; acute yellow atrophy of, Locomotor ataxy, Lumps-haemorrhage from; oedema of; paralysis of, Marasmus, Menorrhagia, Menstruation-symptoms before, Mollities ossium, Morphoea, Muscoe volitantes, Naevus, Nails-ulceration of, Neuralgia, Nightmare, Nipple sore, Nose-bleed, Numbness, Nymphomania, Odour of body-changed, Oesophagus-pain in, Ozaena, Pancreas-disorders of, Paralysis-pseudo-hypertrophic; general of insane, Periostitis, Perspiration abnormal, Petit mal, Plague, Pneumonia, Polypi, Pregnancy-vomiting of, Proctalgia, Proctitis, Progressive muscular atrophy, Pruritus ani, Psoriasis, Puerperal convulsions, Purpura, Pylorus-thickening of, Retinitis, Rheumatism-paralytic, Rickets, Screaming, Scurvy, Shivering, Sleep disordered, Somnambulism, Spine-curvature of, Spleen enlarged, Sprain, Stammering, Sterility, Syphilis, Syringo-myelia, Throat-mucus in, Tobacco-habit, Trachea-tickling in, Tuberculosis, Tumours-erectile; polypoid; cancerous, Typhus fever, Ulcer, Urethra-stricture of, Vaccinia, Variola, Voice lost, Whitlow, Wounds, Yellow fever.

V. Symptoms-General (Nash-190-191)

1. Tall, slender, narrow-chested, phthisical, delicate eyelashes, soft hair, or nervous, weak persons who like to be magnetised, waxy, half anaemic, jaundiced persons.

2. Anxious, universal restlessness can't stand or sit still. < dark or left alone before a thunder storm.
3. Burning prominent in every place as in mouth, stomach, small intestines, anus, between scapulae, intense, running up spine, palms of hands, heat begins in hands, spreads to face.
4. Craving for cold things, ice cream, which agrees, or cold water, which is thrown up as it gets warm in the stomach. Must eat often or he faints. Must get up at night to eat (Psor.).
5. Sinking, faint, empty feeling in head, chest, stomach and abdominal cavity.
6. Cough, < twilight till midnight, < lying on left side, > on right side. Right lower lobe most affected.
7. Diarrhoea, profuse, pouring out as from a hydrant; watery with sago like particles of dysenteric, with side open anus.
8. Apathetic, unwilling to talk, answers slowly, moves sluggishly.
9. Constipation: faeces slender, long, dry, touch and hard like a dog's; voided with difficulty.
10. Haemorrhagic diathesis; slight wound bleeds profusely, haemoptysis; metorrhagia worse, vicarious, from nose, stomach, anus, urethra in amenorrhoea.
11. Can't talk, the larynx is so painful; cough, going from warm to cold air, laughing, talking, eating, lying on left side (Dros., Stan.).

VI. Symptoms-Particular (Nash-190-199)

1. BURNER-Trio

   Phos.-burning often occurs in diseases of spine and nervous system, but not necessarily so.

   Ars., Sul.

2. Patient moves continuously to get relief from burning.

   Anxiety, esp. at twilight, fidgety all over.

3. Anaemia.

   Phos.-all around bloating of the face

   Kali c.
Apis. } pale or bloodless appearance, oedema on face.

Kali c.-Upper lids bloat.

Apis -more bloating of lower lid.

4. Oedema.

Kali c.-Upper Eye lid bloats.

Apis. -More lower lid.

Phos. -especially whole face bloat, all around eyes.

5. Slight wound bleeds much as well in fungoids, Cancer etc.

(Purpura haemorrhagica).

6. Mental:

(a) Great anxiety and restlessness.

Phos.,-anxiety and restlessness precedes another state.

Acon.,

Ars.

(b) Apathy, sluggishness talks slowly, or is indifferent.

(c) Fears to be left alone. Fears darkness.

(d) Stupor or slow muttering delirium,

> Sleep-Phos.,

< Sleep-Lac can.

(e) Loss of ambition-Mental.

Mental and physical labour is shunned.

(f) Amative (Shameless exposure).

Hyo.,

Phos.-maniacal sexual desire; strong desire but can't perform.

7. Vertigo of the aged (Best).
8. Attacks by preference lower half of right lung. Oppression of breathing.
9. Heaviness as from a weight on chest.
10. Heat running up the back (characteristic symptom).
11. Heat between scapula (Lyc.).
12. Deafness to Human voice.
13. Nasal catarrh with blood when blowing the nose.
14. Food tube-stricture of-Food swallowed comes up in.
15. Hungry esp. in night/after meal. Craving for salt (Nat. m.).

Phos.,

Iod.,

Chel.,
Petr.,
Acon.

16. Thirst-peculiar, cold things (Puls.), but as soon as they get warmed, vomited.
17. Great oppression of breathing in both acute and chronic affection of lungs.
18. Pneumonia—one of the best remedies., attacks by preference the LOWER HALF OF RIGHT LUNG.
19. Circumscribed Redness on cheek.
    Phos.-one side of lung inflamed (Sang.).
20. 'Empty', gone feeling in whole abdomen.
    Phos.-whole abdomen, most strong feeling.
    Ign.,
    Hydras.,
    Sep.
21. Stool (constipation).
    Phos.-Dog like, slender, dry.
    Sel.-Large.
22. Dysentery with stool profuse, watery, pouring away as from hydrant + mucous threads + Blood streaks, open anus, great Tenesmus, involuntary stool and oozing from Anus.
23. Female sexual organs.
    Haemorrhagic tendencies, vicarious bleeding in place of menses, from nose or lungs.
    "Phos. is bound to bleed".
24. Respiratory organs (one of the best remedies).
    Voice and larynx-Phos. causes great hoarseness and cures.
    < Fore part of night.

    Croup:
    Phos.
    Acon., } when they fail,
    Spon. } Phos. comes in.

    Cough from evening to midnight-Speaking, singing, reading (Arg. m.).
    < lying on left, whole body trembles. Cough hurts.
    Lung lower Right (Best) heaviness.
25. Burning of hands. (characteristic)-as strong as burning of feet of Sul.

26. Menses-vicarious bleeding from nose or lung instead. Cancer of womb and breasts. They bleed easily.

VII. Black Letter Symptoms

(Tyler-645-647)

- Respiration very difficult.
- Great apathy: unwilling to talk.
- Answers slowly and sluggishly.
- Fatigue, disinclination to work, without cause.
- Disinclination to study, or work, or converse, or think.
- Slow ideas.
- Vertigo; as soon as he made any efforts to rise, the vertigo returned (Bry.).
- Could see better when pupils were dilated by shading the eyes (Phos. has great photophobia).
- Nose-bleed. Nose swollen and dry.
- During the prostration of Phos. poisoning, tuberculosis frequently develops; at times also lobar pneumonia, terminating in gangrene of lung and pyaemia. (Great use of Phos. in severe pneumonias.).
- Vomiting of food. Pressure, as from a hard substance, in stomach.
- Emptiness and sensation of weakness in abdomen.
- Diarrhoea. Evacuations as if involuntary the moment anything entered the rectum. Stool grey-whitish grey.
- Menses earlier and scantier.
- Rawness larynx and trachea. With frequent hacking cough and hawking.
- With suffocative pressure in upper part of chest.
- Voice rough, husky-can hardly speak above a whisper.
- Cough with oppression of chest.
- Violent dry cough when reading aloud.
- Frequent dry cough, with slight dullness in right lower portion posteriorly, with diminished respiratory murmurs and fine vesicular rales (Both lungs, especially right side.).
- Tenacious, purulent mucous.

- Violent oppression of chest.
- Cough from constant tickling in throat. Cough with difficult respiration.
- Bloody expectoration, with mucous.
- Bloody expectoration from the lungs.
- Mucous rales both lungs, more noticeable in lower lobes.
- Respiration anxious, panting, oppressed. Very laboured.
- Difficult respiration is impeded by rapid walking.
- Great dyspnoea.
- Tubercles of the lungs develop, with hectic fever.
- Great oppression of chest, so that the patient, during attack of cough, must sit up in bed, when she experiences great pain, with a constrictive sensation under sternum.
- Heaviness of the chest, as if a weight were lying on it.
- Distressing anxiety and pressure in chest amounting to real suffocation, so that deep inspiration was difficult, but not impossible.
- (*It is one of our greatest remedies for pneumonia and phthisis.*).
- Anxiety about heart and a peculiar sensation of hunger, somewhat relieved by eating, distressing her even in bed.
- Violent palpitation.
- Burning pain between scapulae.
- The spinous processes of the dorsal vertebrae between the scapula became extremely sensitive to pressure.
- Weakness of all limbs.
- "Fingers all thumbs".
- Extensive gangrenous periostitis of tibia, with severe febrile disturbance, periosteum peeled off from a large area upwards, as far as knee-joint; the bone was rough.
- Exaciation.
- Lay constantly on the right side. He lay only one the right side at night.
- Mucous membranes pale.

- The blood from the Haemorrhage was very fluid and difficult to coagulate.
- Sense of suffocation.
- Small wound bleed very much.
- Lax muscular system.
- Great weariness. Weakness. Weak and oppressed. Weak and prostrate. Excessive exhaustion.
- Heaviness of whole body.
- Lying on left side causes anxiety.
- Ulcers bleed.
- Constant sleepiness. Great sleepiness. Even by day.
- Can't fall asleep before midnight.
- Flushed checks (in fever) especially the left one.
- Evening chilliness.
- Cold knees constantly, at night, in Bed.
- Heat at night without thirst.
- Febrile heat and sweat at night with ravenous hunger.
- Profuse perspiration over whole body.
- Profuse sweats on slight exertion.
- Exhausting profuse sweats every morning.
- Perspiration in the morning in bed-with feeling of anxiety.
- "Of one hundred seventy workers in match factories (mostly boys) one hundred and twenty were attached with typhus, often complicated with pneumonia and bronchitis, that often developed into consumption" (Russian Medo. Zeit. 1850).

PHYTOLACCA

I. Introduction (Cow-616)

Synonym: Phytolaca Decandra.
Natural Order: Phytolaccaceae.
Common Names: Poke weed. Poke root. Garget.
Habitat: An indigenous perennial plant.
Preparation: Tincture from the fresh roots.

Dr. Hale introduced this remedy to Homeopathy (Pierce-662).

II. General Analysis (Cow.)

Acts especially upon the glandular system, particularly of the throat and mammae, and serous, fibrous and mucous tissues. Upon kidney-general lithaemia. Upon periosteum and skin, like Mercury, Iodide of Potash or syphilitic poison. The general condition of Phyt. is one of inflammation in fibrous tissue of rheumatic nature, and in mucous and glandular ulceration and suppuration. In stomach and bowels it produces emesis and purging.

III. Suited to (Allen-227)

Rheumatic diathesis of both fibrous and periosteal (around bone). Irresistible desire to bite gums on teeth together (Podo.), during dentition. Sore throat. Vertigo when rising from bed (Bry.).

IV. Clinical (Clarke-III-802)

Abortion threatened, Albuminuria, Angina pectoris, Anus-fissure of, Asthma, Barber's itch, Boils, Bone disease; tumours of, Breasts-affection of, Cancer, Cholera, Cicatrix, Ciliary neuralgia, Constipation, Corpulence, Cough, Dentition difficult, Diarrhoea, Diphtheria, Diplopia, Dysentery, Dysmenia, Ear affections , Erythema nodosum, Eustachian tubes-affections of, Glands enlarged, Gleet, Glossitis, Gonorrhoea , Gout, Granular conjunctivitis, Haemorrhoids, Headache, Hearing altered, Heart-affections of; hypertrophy of; fatty, Impotence, Influenza, Intestinal catarrh, Itch, Lactation abnormal, Laryngismus, Leucorrhoea, Lichen, Liver-affections of, Lumbago, Lupus, Mercury-effects of, Mouth ulcerated, Mumps, Neuralgia, Nipples-sore; painful, Nursing painful, Orchitis, Ozaena, Panophthalmitis, Paralysis-diphtheritic, Parotitis, Prostate-affections of, Rectum-cancer of, Respiration abnormal, Rheumatism-syphilitic; gonorrhoeal, Ringworm, Rodent ulcer, Salivation, Sciatica, Sewer-gas poisoning, Spinal irritation, Spleen-pain in, Stiff-neck, Syphilis, Syphilitic eruptions, Tetanus, Throat-sore; diphtheritic; herpetic; granular, Toothache, Tumours, Ulcer, Uterine affections, Warts, Wens.

V. **Symptoms-General** (Nash-446)

1. Tonsils red, swollen, with white spots which sometimes coalesce and form patches; pains run up into ears, and aching, bruised, sore feeling in head, back and limbs; < on motion, but must move; he aches and is so sore.
2. Irresistible inclination to bite the teeth or gums together (Dentition).
3. Breasts very hard, swollen, not and painful; pain radiates all over the back when the child nurses.

VI. **Symptoms-Particular** (Nash-446-449)

1. Acts prominently on:
   Throat.
   Tonsils.
   Gums.
   Breasts.
2. Sore throat-tonsils red with white spots. Sharp pains extending to the ears.
   (Phyt.-is the best indicated).
3. Intense backache and headache with bruised feeling all over.
   Rhus t.-must move for relief.

Bry.-move makes dizzy.

Arn.-Heat on head face, limbs cool, in fever.

4. Irresistible inclination to bite teeth or gum together.
5. Mastitis (breast pain) when child nurses. Pain radiates all over body.

   Phyt., with fever, great pain in head and back.
   Bry.,
   Crot. t—pain runs through back (Sil., Puls.).
   Sil.,
   Phallan.—pain runs through milk ducts when nursing.
   Lac can.—least jar hurts breasts, Patient holds them in hand. Sore.
6. Suspicious Lumps or tumours in the breast.

   Phyt.— > CM dose once a mouth, during the wave of the moon (448).
7. Sciatica.

   Phyt.,
   Kali hydro.,
   Arn.
8. Periosteal rheumatism.
9. Every chemical remedy has a close relation to the vegetable kingdom. Phyt. occupies midway place between Bry. and Rhus t.

Chemical	Vegetable	Chemical	Vegetable
Kali hydro.,	Phyt.,	Bell.,	Calc. c.,
Aloe.,	Sul.,	Ipec.,	Cupr.,
All. c.,	Phos.,	Bry.,	Alumen,
Cham.,	Mag. phos.,	Mez.,	Merc. c.,
China,	Ferr.,		

VII. Black Letter Symptoms

(Tyler-653-654)

- When rising from bed feels faint (Opium.).
- Painful pressure on forehead and upper part of both eyes.
- Disposition to bite teeth together.

- Throat sore; the isthmus congested and of a dark red colour; dryness of throat, with some swelling of tonsils.
- Diphtheria; sick and dizzy when trying to sit up; frontal headache; pains shooting from throat into ears, especially on trying to swallow; face flushed; tongue much coated, protruded; thickly coated at back, fiery red at tip, breath foetid, putrid; vomiting difficulty of swallowing; tonsils swollen, covered with membrane, first upon left, three or four patches, tonsils, uvula, and back part of throat covered with ash-coloured exudation; tonsils covered with dirty white pseudo membrane; small white or yellow spot on tonsils coalesce and form patches of membrane; membrane has appearance of dirty wash leather; exudation pearly or greyish white; great thirst; < from hot drinks; dyspnoea; ropy, offensive mucous lining mouth and throat; glands of neck very tender; pain in neck and back. Body sore as if bruised, groans with pain, exp. when trying to move or turn in bed; aching limbs; great prostration; violent chill, soon followed by high fever; fever without chill; pulse 120, 140, weak, rash on skin; remarkably nervous phenomena; consecutive paralysis; leaves vision impaired, hearing dull; in cold weather generally epidemic; usually of catarrhal or rheumatic origin, brought on by exposure to damp and cold atmosphere or sleeping in damp, ill-ventilated rooms.
- ABSCESSES or Fistulous ulcers of mammae.
- MAMMARY GLAND full of hard, painful nodosities.
- Breast shows an early tendency to cake; especially useful when suppuration is inevitable; when child nurses pain goes from nipple all over body.
- Caked breasts; nipples cracked and excoriated.
- Barber's itch (local application of tincture).
- Ringworm; herpes circinatus.
- Squamous eruption, pityriasis; psoriasis.

PLATINUM

I. Introduction (Cow-625)

Synonym: Platinum Metallicum.
Preparation: Triturations of precipitated Platinum.

Staff and Gross proved this remedy for Hahnemann. (Pierce-666).

II. General Analysis (Cow.)

Acts chiefly upon nerve centres depressing sensorism, mostly in women in deranged sexual health, hysterical conditions and melancholic (Haughtiness and pride or melancholia, nervous deafness, pain in umbilical region, spasm from sexual erethism).

III. Suited to (Allen-229)

Women of rigid fibre thin, sanguine temperament, who suffer early and too profuse menses, sexual organs exceedingly sensitive, goes into spasm during examination, can't endure coition, cries easily (Croc., Ign., Puls.) Arrogant, looks down upon people usually respected. Sensation-growing large in every direction (Head-profound vexation from trifles (Ign., Staph.). Constipation-while travelling (at sea-Bry.). Stools adhere to anus like soft clay (Alumina).

IV. Clinical (Clarke-III-842)

Amenorrhoea, Chlorosis, Constipation, Convulsions, Delusions, Dentition, Depression of spirits, Dysmenia, Erotomania, Fear, Gout, Haemorrhage, Haemorrhoids, Hysteria, Lead poisoning, Masturbation, Melancholia, Menorrhagia, Menses suppressed, Mind-affections of, Neuralgia, Neurasthenia, Numbness, Nymphomania, Ovaries-affections of, Pruritus vulvae, Rheumatism, Sexual perversion, Spasms, Tape-worm, Uterus-induration of, Vaginismus, Yawning-spasmodic.

V. Symptoms-General (Nash-187)

1. Pride and over estimation of one's self, looking down on others; things look small to her.
2. Genitals exceedingly sensitive, but excessive sexual desire, nymphomania, with ovarian troubles; prolapsus or profuse menses.
3. Pains increase gradually and as gradually decrease (Stan.); sometimes attended with numbness (Cham.).

VI. Symptoms-Particular (Nash-187-189)

1. It has three relations.
   (a) Mental-everything seems small.
   (b) Nervous.
   (c) Sexual.

(a) Changing moods-Gay and sad mood alternate. All persons, mentally and physically inferior.

Plat.,
Ign.,
Nux. m.,
Acon.

Physical symptoms disappear and mental symptoms appear.

(b) Nervous Symptoms.

Pains (i) increase and decrease gradually (Stam.).
(ii) numbness of parts (Cham.).

Stan., Plat., Cham. } But patient is not as weak as in Stam. Bell. is exactly opposite. But in Plat. patient is not so ugly as in Cham.

Constipation-Soft stool adheres to anus.

Plat., Alumina } similar

(c) Sexual: Nymphomania aggravated lying in; titillation up into abdomen. Excessively sexual, or excessive development of sexual instinct. Genitals excessively sensitive-can't bear to be touched, goes into spasm during examination, faints during intercourse.

VII. Black Letter Symptoms
(Tyler-660-661)

- Illusions of fancy as if everything about her were very small and all persons physically and mentally inferior, but she herself physically large and superior.
- Arrogant, proud feeling.
- Contemptuous, pitiful looking down on people usually venerated with a kind of casting them off. (She thought she had no place in the world, life was wearisome but she had a great dread of death, which she believed near at hand.).
- Pride and over estimation of one's self: looking down with haughtiness on others.
- The room seemed gloomy,unpleasant, with apprehensive and fretful mood.
- A numb sensation in forehead, as if constricted.
- Cramp-like drawing constriction in the head from time to time.
- Tense, numb sensation in the zygomata and mastoid processes, as if the head were screwed together.
- *Head-shocks* followed by a numb sensation, as if too tightly bound.
- Crawling, like formication, on right temple, afterwards extending down along the lower jaw, with a feeling of coldness in it.
- Headache-gradually increasing till very severe, then decreasing as gradually.
- Painful cramp-like sensation of numbness in the left malar bone.
- Fermentation in the epigastric region.
- Constipation; after lead poisoning; while travelling; frequent urging with expulsion of small portions after great straining, after failure of Nux. v.
- Painful pressing downwards towards genitals, as during menstruation.
- *Urging with scanty stool* with a painful sensation of weakness.
- Voluptuous crawling in genitals and abdomen.
- Painful sensitiveness & constant pressure in the mons veneris and genitals.

- Emission of much clotted blood during first day of menstrual period.
- Menses about fourteen days too early and very profuse.
- Menses six days too early.
- While sitting a sensation of numbness in coccyx.
- Tightness of thighs as if too tightly wrapped.
- Tremulous crawling and uneasiness in legs while sitting; a sensation of numbness and rigidity.
- Great numbness, painful numb sensation, as from a blow, here and there.
- The parts affected by cramp-like pain are painful to pressure as if bruised.
- Sensation of coldness, crawling and numbness in the whole right side of face (in fever).

PLUMBUM

I. Introduction (Cow.-629)

Synonym: Plumblum Metallicum.
Common Name: Lead.
Preparation: Triturations from precipitated lead.

It was first proved by Hart Laub for Hahnemann (Pierce-670).

II. General Analysis (Cow.)

Acts with great power upon spinal nerve centres, increased sensibility, neuralgic spasms and convulsions and other affections of nervous system. Acts directly upon kidneys producing albuminuria and other renal affections. May cause degeneration of heart, liver and other organs. Chief feature-lead colic with spasmodic pain in abdomen (retracted to spine) with obstinate constipation.

III. Suited to (Allen-231)

Diseases from spinal origin (Phos., Pic. ac., Zinc.) Assumes strange attitudes and position in the bed. Delirium alternating with colic. Excessive and rapid emaciation. Violent colic, as if abdominal wall was drawn to the spine. Distinct blue line on the margin of gum. Stools-hard, lumpy, black, like sheep dung. (Chel., Op.).

IV. Clinical (Clarke-III-855)

Amaurosis, Anaemia, Anaesthesia, Aneurism, Anidrosis, Appendicitis, Asthma, Atrophy, Bone-exostoses on, Brain softening; tumour of, Bright's disease, Colic, Constipation, Cystitis, Depression of spirits, Diplopia, Dropsy, Dysmenorrhoea, Dysuria, Emaciation, Epilepsy, Epulis, Eyes inflamed, Ganglion, Gout, Haemoptysis, Haemorrhoids, Headache, Hernia strangulated, Hyperaesthesia, Hypopion,

Ichthyosis, Intermittent fever, Intestines-obstruction of, Intussusception, Jaundice, Jaw-tumour of, Kidneys-affections of; granular, Liver-affections of, Lockjaw, Locomotor ataxy, Melancholia, Metrorrhagia, Myelitis, Nephritis, Numbness, Oesophagus-constriction of, Paralysis-diphtheritic; agitans, Perichondritis, Proctalgia, Progressive muscular atrophy, Prolapsus ani, Sciatica, Spine-diseases of; sclerosis of; tumour of, Spleen-affections of, Stricture, Tabes mesenterica, Tobacco-habit, Tongue-paralysis of, Typhlitis, Umbilicus-abscess of; hernia of, Uric-acidaemia, Vagina-spasm of, Vaginismus, Veins-varicose.

V. **Symptoms-General** (Nash-305)

1. Abdomen retracted toward the spine, as if drawn in by a string, both objective and subjective.
2. Distinct blue line along margin of the gums.
3. "Wrist-drop" paralysis of the extensor muscles.

VI. **Symptoms-Particular** (Nash-305-306)

1. Blue line on margins of gums.
2. Abdomen drawn to spine-sensation or actual.
3. Stool sheep dung-Plumb., Ratan.
4. Excessive sensitive skin (China, Hep. s.) (Hyperaesthesia of skin).
5. Excessive pain in abdomen radiating to all parts of the body (Diosc.) in colic, uterine troubles, constipation.
6. Jaundice, whites of eye, skin, stool all yellow.
7. Paralysis with Plumb. symptoms, 'Wrist drop'.
8. Key-excessive emaciation, general or partial paralysis; blue gum-line.

VII. **Black Letter Symptoms** (Tyler-668-669)

- Slow of perception.
- Loss of memory, so that while talking he was often unable to find the proper word.
- Headache.
- Complexion sallow. Sallow pale face.

- Distinct blue line along the margins of gums. Dark blue line on the gums.
- Gums pale, swollen; show a lead-coloured line; blue, purple or brown; painful, with hard tubercles.
- Breath foetid.
- Constrictions of the throat.
- Loss of appetite.
- Nausea.
- Vomiting. Frequent vomiting. Constant Vomiting.
- Vomiting of food.
- Extremely violent pains in the umbilical region, that shoot to other parts of the abdomen, somewhat relieved by pressure.
- The navel seems to adhere to the spine.
- Violent colic.
- Excessive pain in abdomen, radiating thence to all parts of the body.
- Constipation: stools hard, lumpy, like sheep's dung, with urging and terrible pain from constriction or spasm of anus.
- Difficult micturition.
- Urine albuminous.
- Urine dark coloured and scanty, evacuated drop by drop.
- Morbus Brightii; contracted kidney.
- Vaginismus.
- Violent pains in the extremities; especially in the evening and night: especially in the muscular part of the thighs.
- Neuralgic pains in the limbs.
- The pains in the limbs are worse by paroxysms, which are so severe that he cries out.
- Jerking, trembling, numbness of limbs.
- Pains in the extremities.
- Pains in the limbs aggravated at night.
- Wrist-drop.
- Very sharp neuralgic pains.
- Extremely acute and paroxysmal pains.
- Lightning-like pains in the lower limbs.
- Emaciation.

- Anaemia.
- Convulsion.
- Paralysis.
- General prostration.
- Lassitude.
- Faintness.
- Uneasiness.
- Excessive hyperaesthesia.
- Anaesthesia.
- Arthralgia.
- Pain in trunk and limbs.
- Emaciation extreme, with anaemia and great weakness, of paralysed parts followed by swelling.
- Muscular atrophy; from sclerosis of spinal system.
- Dry skin.
- Yellow skin.
- Sleeplessness (entire sleeplessness).

PSORINUM

I. **Introduction** (Clarke-III-891)

Synonym: Psoricum. The Nosode of Psora.
Preparation: Triturations.

II. **Suited to** (Allen-233)

Especially adapted to Psoric conditions when well selected remedies fail to relieve or cure in chronic cases (in Acute diseases-Sul.) Child plays all day, restless, troublesome screaming at night. Body has filthy smell even after bathing. Great sensitiveness to cold air, change of weather. Restless for days before or during thunderstorm (Phos.) Dry scaly eruptions disappear in summer return in winter. Ailments from suppressed itch or other skin diseases, (when Sul. fails), severe from slight emotion, nervous, restless, easily startled. Religious melancholy, very depressed, sad suicidal thoughts, despondent headache preceded by flickering before eyes, by dimness of vision or blindness (Lac. def., Kali bich.). hair dry, tangles easily, glues together (Lyc.). Scalp dry scaly or moist foetid. Suppurating eruption oozing a sticky offensive fluid (Graph., Mez.) Hungry in the middle of the night. All excretions have a carrion like smell.

III. **Clinical** (Clarke-III-891)

Acne, Adenoids, Anus-itching in. Asthma, Backache, Boils, Cancer, Cholera infantum, Cough, Constipation, Cornea-ulcers of, Crusta lactea, Crusta serpiginosa, Debility, Diarrhoea, Diphtheria-after effects of, Dyspepsia, Eczema rubrum, Enuresis, Eruptions-moist; itching, Gleet, Gonorrhoea, Gout, Haemorrhages, Haemorrhoids, Hair-dry; tangling, Hay-fever, Headache, Head-congestion of, Hernia, Hydrocele, Impotence, Influenza, Injuries, Itch, Itching,

Leucorrhoea, Lienteria, Liver-affections of; chronic inflammation of, Melancholia-religious, Nose-redness of, Odour of body-foetid, Ophthalmia-scrofulous, Otorrhoea-foetid, Ozaena, Pediculosis, Peritonitis tubercular, Plica polonica, Polypus, Quinsy, Sciatica, Scurvy, Skin-affections of, Spina bifida, Spleen-affections of; induration of, Sprains, Syphilis, Throat-mucus in, Tinea capitis et faciei, Tonsils-concretions in, Ulcers.

IV. **Symptoms-General** (Nash-287)

1. Very sad, hopeless, despondent, "bluest of blue."
2. Great debility, sweats on slightest movement, wants to give up and lie down.
3. Eruption on the skin, dry or moist, or skin scaly or dry as parchment, dirty or the great unwashed, unwashable.
4. Intense itching of skin < in warmth of bed.
5. Discharges and exhalations exceedingly offensive.
6. Very sensitive to cold air, wears a fur cap in summer.
7. Modalities: < in cold air, < in warmth of bed (itching), sitting up or motion, > bringing arms down close to the body, > lying down (even the dyspnoea), wrapping up warm, psoric manifestations.
8. Great weakness and debility, from loss of fluids, remaining after acute diseases, without any organic lesion or apparent cause.
9. Cough and dry scaly Eruption return every winter.
10. Quinsy, to eradicate the tendency.

V. **Symptoms-Particular** (Nash 288-291)

1. Chief action is upon the skin, where it resembles Sul.

a. Itching when the body becomes warm.
b. Itching intolerable in warmth of bed (Merc. s).
c. Itching scratches until it bleeds.
d. Itching between fingers and in back of joints (Sep.).
e. Dry scaly Eruption which disappear summers and return winters.
f. Repeated outbreaks of Eruption.

g. Skin has a dirty dingy look and body has a filthy smell even after a bath.
2. Consequences of suppressed Eruption-When other anti psorics fail.
3. Resemblance with Graph.
a. Very depressed mind.
b. Great despondency especially after acute diseases like Typhoid (Psor. is better).
c. Stools dark brown, watery, intolerably offensive odour. (Cholera Infantum, chronic Diarrhoea).
d. Psor. Eruption are not as glutinous or sticky as with Graph.
4. Weakness or debility during convalescence from severe acute diseases. Sweats profusely when taking least exercise. Skin is dry inactive and sweats rarely. In stools choice remains between Psor. and China. Psor. has itching Eruption or tendency there to, before or during the sickness, while China has loss of fluids, suppuration etc.
5. Very sensitive to cold air or change of weather (Hep. s.) Wants to wear a fur cap, overcoat or shawl even in the hottest weather.
6. Chronic complaints following or dating back for years to some imperfectly cured or suppressed acute diseases (Carb. v.).

VI. Black Letter Symptoms (Tyler-675-676)

- Anxious: full of fear: melancholic.
- Very depressed, sad , suicidal thoughts.
- Driven to despair by excessive itching.
- Moist, suppurating, foetid, also dry Eruption on scalp.
- Tinea capitis et faciei.
- Discharge of foetid pus from ear.
- Otorrhoea, with headache, thin ichorous and horribly offensive, like rotten meat. Very offensive, purulent, with watery stinking Diarrhoea. Brown offensive, from left ear, for almost four years.

- Chronic cases following scarlet fever.
- Humid soreness behind ears, scrufs on ears, and humid scrufs behind ear.
- Swelled upper lip.
- Tongue very dry.
- Sensation or plug or lump in throat, impending hawking.
- Great hunger.
- Eructation tasting of rotten eggs.
- Stool, dark brown, very fluid and foul smelling.
- Cough, with expectoration of green mucus, nearly like matter.
- He perspires freely while walking, profuse sweat with consequent debility.
- Skin has a dry dingy look, as if patient never washed; in some places looks coarse as if bathed in oil. Sebaceous glands secrete in excess.
- Eczema behind ears, on scalp, in bends of elbows and armpits, accompanied by abscesses affecting bones.
- Itch, dry on arms and chest, most severe on finger joints, followed by boils; inveterate cases of tuberculosis, repeated outbreak of single pustules after main Eruption gone. Suppressed Eruption.

PULSATILLA

I. Introduction (Cow.-639)

Synonym: Pulsatilla Nigricans.
Natural Order: Ranunculaceae.
Common Name: Wind flower. Meadow Anemone. Pasque flower.
Habitat: A plant of snunny, elevated places, pasture grounds in sanday soils and in clear pine forests in Central Northern Europe.
Preparation: Tincture from the fresh plant.

It was proved by Hahnemann (Pierce-681).

II. General Analysis

Acts prominently upon all mucous membrances of the body, upon synovial membranes the vains, eyes, ears, and generative organs of both sexes esp. female. In mucous membrances catarrhal process is established, disturbing the functions of organs to whom secretions are supplied, thus symptoms of deranged digestion, respiratory troubles, genito uninary disturbances, catarrhal affections of ears and eye. Vericose venis. On synovial membrenes if produces Rheumatic inflammations, and in veins varicose conditions.

III. Suited to (Allen-237)

Indecisive, slow, phlegmatic temperament, sandy hair, blue eyes, paleface, affectionate mild, gentle timid, yielding. More to women easily moved to to ears to laughter affections, wild, gentle, yielding woman weeps easily. Furst health impairment to public age never better since.
Rapidly shifting Pains - One part to another-Kali Bi, Lack, Mang. Appear suddenly, go gradually.

Symptoms ever changing - no two stools, chills, moods etc. alike.

IV. **Clinical** (Clarke-III-907)

Acne. Amaurosis. Amenorrhoea. Anaemia. (Appetite, depraved. Bladder, catarrh of, Blepharospasm, Breasts, pain behind, Bronchitis, Cataract, Catarrh, Chaps, chest, pains in. Chilblains, Clavus, Cold. Cough. Biarrhoea; of phthisls, Distension, Dysmenia. Dyspepsia, Earache, Epilepsy, Epistaxis, Eyes, lachrymal sac, inflammation of; granular ophthalmia. Fear, Feet, sores, painful, Fbetus, mal-position of. Erechles, Gonorrhoea, Gout. Haemorrhoids, Hands, pains in Heart, palpitation of Heartburn. Hydrocele; congenital, Hysteria, Intermittent fever. Joints, synovitis of Labour, spurious pains of Lactation, disorders of. Leucorrhoea, Measles, Menstruation, abnormal; vicarious, Moles, Mumps. Neuralgia, Nymphomania. Ovaries, pain in; inflammation of. Phlegmasis alba dolens. Pregnancy; bladder trouble of; sickness of; heartburn of; diarrhoea of. Priapism, Prostate, inflammation of. Prostatorrhoea. Puerperal convulsions. Puerperal fever. Puerperal mania. Retained placenta. Rheumatism; gonorrhoeal. Side, pain in Smell, illusions of. Spine, curvature of. Stye, Synovitis. Tapeworm. Taste; depraved; lost. Tongue, coated, Toothache; Urine, incontinence of. Uterus; inflammation of; prolapse of. Veins. inflammation of; varicose. Whitlow. (Synovia- a lubricating fluid secreted in the joints of bones.)

V. **Symptoms-General** (Nash-23)

1. Mild, gentle, yielding disposition; sad and despondent, weeps easily, sandy hair, blue eyes, pale face, mucles soft and flabby.
2. Changeable remedy, pains travel from one joint to another, haemorrhages flow and stop and flow again, no two stools alike, no two chills alike, no head nor tail to the case-mixed.
3. Bad taste in the mouth, < mornings, with great dryness, but no thirst.
4. Stomach easily disturbed, especially by cakes pastry or rich fat foods.
5. Thick bland discharges from all mucous membrances.
6. Catamenia to late scanty or suppressed, particularly by wetting the feet.

7. Modalities: < in warm room, warm applications, or Iron, chillness with the pains, > by cool open air, walking slowly around, cold food or drink, tying up tightly > headache.
8. Pains accompanied with constant chilliness, and the more severe the pain the harder the chill (with profuse sweating, cham; with fainting, Heparsulph; with frequent micturition, Thuja; with delirsum-Verat. alb.

VI. Symptoms–Particulars (Nash-23)

Opposite of Nux (Male).
Pul-Female.
SIL is chronic of Pul.

1 (a) *Changeableness* of symptoms. Marellous with Pul temperament.
Pul.
Ig–hysterial contradictory symptoms (another women's remedy).
Nux. M–

(b) Rheumatism.
Mag acet
Lac C
Lali Bi
Kalm L
Pul

(c) *Changeableness* of mood.

(d) *Flows stop* and then flow.

(e) *Stool changes* in colour (Sani). No two stools alike, often found in cholera infenttum or entero colities of children in hot weather (24).

2. *Indigestion*-Bad taste in mouth esp. early morning.
Pul–No Thirst.
Bry- with thirst and coated tongue.

(b) < Cake, pastry, rich food, Fats.
Pul < hot food > cold things.
Nux > hot food < cold things.

3. *Thirst.*
Pul - No thirst with dry mouth.
Merc - Thirst with wet mouth.
Nux M - moist mouth with no thirst.

4. *Discharges* (almost all)

Pul - Bland, thick, yellowish green, from every mucous out-let of the body.

Car. V.
Lyc.
Paris
Phos
Sul.
} Also have greenish discharges, esp. expectoration.

5. *Female genital* organs-27

Menstruation:-

(a) Catminia too late & scanty, suppressed esp. getting feet wet (it is of prime importance).

Pul
Kali C.
Tuber C.

(b) Painful Messes with great restlessness.

Flow stops and flows, stops and flows again

Mag P- Excellent when symptoms telly (< cold air water, touch, heat, warmth, pressure bending double. Cramping pain).

Pul-also Menorrheagia

Delayed Menses of young girls.

Caulo
Cimi

6. *Expectoration*- Taste.

Pul - Green, thick, bland, taste bitter
Stan - Sweat
Kalihy
Sep
} Salty

Kali Sul (Biochemic) greatly resembles.

Pul in-Discharges
Wandering pains
evening aggrevations
better in cool open air
Kali Hydro is also worse in warm room.

7. Modahlis:- Better in cold air and cold applications in any ailment general or local.

(a) > walking slowly in open air

Pul
Ferr-moving slowly about

Rhus T- > general motion in warm air, dry while pul in cold open air only.

(b) Worse: Warm air, of warm application.
Pul
Mer C.-Even warmth of Bed.
Pul-retains cold drinks, vomits hot.

8. *Headache > pressure.*
Pul > by pressure or tying up head tightly.
Arg N.
Apis M.
9. *Increased inclination to urination < when lying.*
10. *Chilly yet wants* room cool.
11. Inflammed parts bluish.
Lach
Taran
Cub
Bell Red
12. *One sided sweats.*
13. Chronic affections after Measles.
Poulsatilla.
14. Metastasis- of Gonorrhoea to testicles; of mumps to mammae testicles.

VII. Black Letter Symptoms
(Tyler-683-85)

- Vertigo, as from intoxication.
- Vertigo Especially when sitting.
- Heaviness of head.
- Transient obscuration of sight.
- Itching burning in eyes, compels scratching and rubbing.
- Smarting itching on hairy scalp.
- A tension of face, as if parts would swell.
- Alaenasi ulcerated externally and exude watery fluid.
- Spistaxis. Flow of blood from nose with stuffed coryza.
- Gums painful as if excoriated.
- Tongue covered with viscid mucus, as with a skin.
- Middle of tongue, even when moistened, a sensation

as if it were burnt and insensible, at night and in the morning.

- Throat painful as if raw. Sore throat : scratchy : dry.
- Dryness of throat in the morning.
- Taste as of putrid flesh, with inclination to vomit.
- A burnt taste in the mouth.
- Bitter beer has to him a disgustingly sweetish taste.
- After drinking beer, a bitter taste remains in mouth.
- Dislike to butter.
- Bilious eructations in the evening.
- Diminished taste of all food.
- Adipsia.
- Frequent eruciations with the taste of what has been eaten.
- Sensation of sickness in epigastric region, especially after eating and drinking.
- Inclination to vomit, with grumbling and rumbling in subcostal region.
- Hiccough when smoking tobacco.
- In the morning in the scorbiculus cordis, aching and drawing pain.
- Immediately after supper flatulent colic: flatulence rumbles about painfully, especially in upper part of abdomen.
- The flatus is discharged with cutting pain in the abdomen in the morning.
- Bellyache as if diarrhoea must ensue, and yet there only occurs a good natural stool.
- Bellyache after the stool.
- Frequent urging to go to stool.
- Frequent soft stool mingled with mucus.
- Stools consisting of nothing but yellowish-white mucus, mingled with a little blood.
- Quite white stool.
- Frequent call to urinate.
- The urine dribbles away when sitting and walking.
- Itching, smarting inner and upper part of prepuce.
- In the morning on awaking excitement of the genitals and desire for coitus.
- Sneezing. Coryza.
- Nocturnal dry cough, which goes off by sitting up

in bed, but returns on lying down (Hyos). Expectoration of blood.

- Shooting pain in nape.
- Heaviness of legs by day.
- Hemoves about in his sleep. Sleeplessness from ebullition of blood.
- He starts up in affright in his sleep.
- At night he wakes up frightened and confused, not knowing where he is, and cannot rightly collect himself. Chattering in his sleep.
- At night he wakes up frightened and confused, not knowing where he is, and cannot rightly collect himself. Chattering in his sleep.
- Yawning.
- Chilly feeling with trembling, which recurs after some minutes, with little heat thereafter and no sweat.
- External warmth is intolerable to him, the veins are distended.
- Anxious heat as if hot water were thrown over him, with cold forehead.
- Palpitation of the heat with great anxiety so that he must throw off the clothes.
- Hypochondriacal moroseness: takes everything in bad part.
- Everything disgusts, is repugnanttohim. Breaks out into weeping.
- Fretful: irresolute: trembling anxiety, relieved by motion.
- Morose: ill-humoured: discontented: fretful.

RHEUM

I. Introduction (Cow.-653)

Synonym: Rheum Officinale.
Natural Order: Polygonaceae.
Common Name: Rhubarb.
Habitat: A native plant of China.
Preparation: Tincture from the dried root.

II. General Analysis (Cow.)

Acts upon liver, intestinal canal, increased bile secretion, purging faecal matter. Diarrhoea with excessive foul smelling stool.

III. Suited to (Allen-243)

Children, especially during dentition. Sour smell of the whole body, even after washing or bathing (Hep. s., Mag. c). Screaming of children with urging and sour stool, child impatient, desires many things and cries, dislikes even favourite playthings (Cina., Staph.). Sweat of scalp, constant and profuse, may or may not be sour. Difficult dentition, child restless, irritable, peevish, with pale face and sour smell (Calc. c., Sanic.).

IV. Clinical (Clarke-III-973)

Ardor Urinae, Breath offensive, Constipation, Deafness, Dentition difficult, Diarrhoea, Duodenum-catarrh of, Dysentery, Ears-thickening in, Frowning, Headache, Jaundice, Kidney-affections of, Meniere's disease, Milk abnormal, Mouth-mucous in, Nipples painful, Nose-pain in, Nurselings-affections of, Oesophagus-constriction of, Rheumatism, Salivation, Screaming of children, Snoring, Stomach disordered, Taste bad, Tongue-numbness of, Urination-difficult; of childbed, Urine red.

V. **Symptoms-Particular** (Nash-438)

1. Sour stools. They may be brown mixed with mucous or thin and pasty.
2. Pain before stool, of colicky nature, and may be tenesmus after the stool.
3. Not only stools, whole body smells sour, no matter how much it is bathed.
4. During dentition, in colic and diarrhoea it resembles Mag. c.

RHODODENDRON

I. Introduction (Cow.-655)

Synonym: Rhododendron Chrysanthemum.
Natural Order: Ericaceae.
Common Name: Dwarf Rose bag.
Habitat: Evergreen shrub of Siberia, growing on mountain heights.
Preparation: Tincture from the dried leaves.

It was proved by Dr. Seidel in Germany (Pierce-693).

II. General Analysis (Cow.)

Acts upon muscular and fibrous tissues, producing arthritic and rheumatic conditions (small joints). Chief expression-aggravation of all symptoms in cold stormy weather, before and during a thunder storm. Rheumatic pains.

III. Suited to (Allen-243)

Nervous persons who dread a storm and are particularly afraid of thunder; < before the storm, esp. electric storm (Nat. c., Psor., Sil.). Toothache, every spring and fall, sharp east winds < change of weather, thunderstorm, windy weather. Acute inflammatory swelling of joints, wandering from one joint to another < night < in rest and in stormy weather (Kalm.).

IV. Clinical (Clarke-III-980)

Amenorrhoea, Asthenopia, Bones-pain in, Bunions, Chorea, Ciliary neuralgia, Coryza, Delirium, Diarrhoea, Diphtheritic paralysis, Earache, Epistaxis, Eye affections, Fever, Flatus incarcerated, Gums-itching of, Hydrocele, Lienteria, Lumbago, Memory weak, Neuralgia, Nightmare, Ovary-cyst of, Rheumatism, Spleen-pain in, Sprain, Stiff-neck, Testicles-affections of, Tinnitus, Toothache, Vagina-cysts in,Wrists-pain in.

V. **Symptoms-Particular** (Nash-362)

1. Aggravation in wet stormy weather. (like Dulc.).
   < before storm (thunder)-Phos., Nat. c., Sil.
   < during rest > during motion-Rhus t..
   < during damp weather-Rhus t..
2. Marked wet weather remedies-(Rho., Rhus t., Nux. m.).
   Calc. phos. < wet cold, especially melting snow.
3. Testicles-swollen, with drawing, contusive pains, which sometimes extend to abdomen and thighs, and very sensitive to touch (Aur. m., Puls., Arg. m., Spon.).
   If the affection is of Syphilitic origin, or abuse of Mercury-Aur. m..
   If suppressed Gonorrhoea-Clem. or Puls.
   If rheumatic origin-Rho.

RHUS TOXICODENDRON

I. Introduction (Cow.-658)

Synonym: Rhus Humile
Natural Order: Anacardiaceae.
Common Name: Poison Oak, Poison Ivy.
Habitat: A shrub growing in fields, woods and along fences all over North America.
Preparation: Tincture from the fresh leaves.

It was first proved by Hahnamann (Pierce-696).

II. General Analysis (Cow.)

Acts prominently upon organs of animal life, mucous membranes, lymphatic glands, skin, muscular tissues, and the tissues which compose joints. Primarily it produces irritation, leading to inflammation. Irritation is most visible on the skin. In mucous membranes (especially conjunctiva), it causes exematous and vesicular eruption. In joints and muscles, the irritation develops into rheumatoid inflammation; in lymphatic glands it causes enlargement and inflammation. Secondarily, on organs of animal life, it produces dullness of senses and conditions of cerebral system resembling that of low fever. Its chief characteristic is aggravation of its symptoms during repose and amelioration by motion.

III. Suited to (Allen-244)

To persons of rheumatic diathesis; bad effects of getting wet, especially after over-heated. Ailments from spraining/ straining a single part, muscle or tendons (Calc. c., Nux. v.); over lifting, particularly from stretching high up to reach things, lying on damp grounds, too much summer bathing in lake or river. Pains as if strained < midnight, wet weather; lameness, stiffness and pain on first moving after rest or getting up in the morning > by walking or continued motion. Great restlessness, anxiety, apprehension (Acon., Ars.).

IV. **Clinical** (Clarke-III-991)

Abortion, Acne rosacea, After-pains, Amenor-rhoea, Anus-fissure of, Appendicitis, Appetite lost, Beri-beri, Bones-pain in, Caecum-inflammation of, Chilblains, Circulation feeble, Cyanosis, Dengue fever, Diarrhoea-chronic, Diphtheria, Dysentery, Dysmenorrhoea, Dyspepsia, Ear-eczema of, Ecthyma, Enteric fever, Erysipelas, Erythema nodosum, Exostosis, Eyes-inflammation of; choroiditis; sight weak, Feet-pain in, Gastroenteritis, Glands inflamed, Gout, Haemorrhage, Haemorrhoids, Hands-pains in, Hernia, Herpes, Herpes zoster, Housemaid's knee, Hydrocele, Influenza, Intermittents, Jaw-cracking in, Liver-abscess of, Lumbago, Measles, Menorrhagia, Metrorrhagia, Neuralgia, Ovary-tumour of, Paralysis, Paraphimosis, Pemphigus, Periosteum-pains in, Pleurisy, Pleurodynia, Pneumonia-typhoid, Ptosis, Pyaemia, Red-gum, Relapsing fever, Rheumatism, Scarlatina, Sciatica, Sleep-restless, Small-pox, Spine-diseases of, Sprain, Stricture, Tongue-affections of, Typhus fever, Urticaria, Warts, Wens, Yawning.

V. **Symptoms-General** (Nash-94-95)

1. Dry or coated tongue with a triangular red tip.
2. Great restlessness, cannot lie long in one position, changes often with temporary relief, tosses about continually.
3. Lameness and stiffness on beginning to move after rest; on getting up in the AM > by continued motion.
4. Erysipelas/scarlatina with vesicular eruption and characteristic restlessness.
5. All diseases that put on the typhoid form with the characteristic, triangular red-tip tongue and restlessness.
6. Stupor and mild, persistent delirium; continually tossing about, with laborious dreams.

7. Modalities: < when quietly sitting or lying and on beginning to move; wet, cold weather; lifting or straining; getting wet when perspiring. > by continued motion, by warmth, dry air or weather; lying on hard floor (backache). {< Excessive muscular soreness-dancing, or violent muscular exertion-Act. rac.}.
8. Muscular rheumatism, sciatica, left side (right side-Coloc..); aching in left arm, with heart disease.
9. Great sensitiveness to open air; putting the hand from under the bed cover brings on the cough (Baryt. c., Hep. s.).
10. Back; pain between the shoulders on swallowing.
11. Cough during chill; dry, teasing, fatiguing, but urticaria over body during heat.

VI. **Symptoms-Particular** (Nash-95-99)

1. Restlessness-(Acon., Ars., Rhus t.) of Rhus t. is because of aching pain and soreness, > temporarily by movement. An internal uneasiness keeps patient on the move, while there is no pain present.
2. Aggravation from rest (Bry.-reverse).

   Rhus t.—Patient tosses from side to side, which relieves pain and prostration, not so much agonizing as with Acon., Ars.

Acon. Ars.	Patient tosses from side to side without relief from pain.
Ars. Rhus t. }	-often indicated in Typhoid.

   Acon.-seldom indicated in Typhoid.

   Patient moves more and more as he feels better, until he is exhausted. But he cannot sit comfortably for long, as the aching comes and he must move for relief even if it hurts at first.
3. Very useful in Herpes zoster, eczemas of vesicular type, not relieved by scratching.
4. Stupefaction with dark or dry tongue with triangular red tip is special indication of Rhus t. Stupefaction is also found in Bap., Nux. m., Lach., Phos. ac. Stupefaction and delirium are mild, but regular and persistent.

5. Cough during chill in Intermittents.
6. Muscles are stiff and sore, may be of rheumatic character or by straining by muscular exercise of any kind or brought on by exposure to wet cold. One of the best remedies in Lumbago.
7. Its key characteristic is "lameness and stiffness and pain on first moving after rest or on getting up in the morning, relieved by continued motion".
8. Often indicated in glandular swellings of parotid or sub-maxillary glands during inflammations.
9. One of the best remedies in skin diseases. Skin Eruption are of vesicular type (Bell.-if skin is red, hot, smooth and shiny).
   (Apis., Canth., Lach., Ail.)

VII. Black Letter Symptoms
(Tyler-711-715)

- Worse in the house, relieved by walking in open air (Puls.).
- Sad, begins to weep without knowing why.
- Very restless mood.
- Great apprehension at night; cannot remain in bed.
- On rising, dizziness as if she was going to fall forward and backward.
- Inflammation of the EYES.
- Very sore around the right eye.
- The eyes are closed, or greatly swollen and inflamed.
- Great swelling of the lids.
- Left eye closed form swollen lids.
- Inflammation of the lids.
- Eyes red and agglutinated with matter in AM.
- Heaviness and stiffness of lids, like a paralysis: difficult to move the lids.
- Nasal mucous runs in profusion out of nose, as in most severe coryza in AM after rising from bed (Nux. v.). Frequent, violent, spasmodic sneezing.
- Great swelling of the FACE.
- Yawning so violent and spasmodic; causes pain in maxillary joint which is in danger of being dislocated.

- Sore sensation with redness at apex of TONGUE.
- Tongue dry. Salivation.
- THROAT much swollen externally, maxillary and parotid glands greatly enlarged.
- Parotid and sub-maxillary glands hard and swollen.
- Great thirst.
- Thirst and dryness of throat.
- Acute diseases take on a TYPHOID form-dysentery. Peritonitis, Pneumonia, Scarlatina, Diphtheria.
- Typhoid fever: mild temperament; mild delirium; at times may try to jump out of bed or try to escape. Mental and physical restlessness. Constantly tosses about bed, lies first on one side then the other, one moment sitting up, the next lying down.
- At beginning of disease wants to lie perfectly quiet on account of great weakness-prostrate-indifferent. Hallucinations: fears he will be poisoned; refuses medicine and food.
- Short COUGH, from severe tickling and irritation behind the upper part of sternum, followed the feeling of discouragement and apprehension.
- Pneumonic cough, rust-coloured sputum.
- Stiffness in small of BACK, painful on motion.
- Small of back feels bruised.
- While sitting small of back aches, as after long stooping/bending the back.
- Pain as if bruised in small of back, whenever he lies quietly upon it or sits still; on moving about he feels nothing.
- Heaviness and pressure in small of back, as if one had received a blow, while sitting.
- The LIMBS tremble after exerting them.
- All the limbs feel stiff and paralysed, during and after walking with a sensation of a hundred-weight on nape of neck.
- Sensation of stiffness on first moving the limb after rest.
- The limbs upon which he lies, especially the arm, fall asleep.
- A sensation as of trembling in arms and lower extremities even while at rest.

- Drawing in all the limbs, while lying down.
- Trembling of limbs after moderate exertion of them.
- Violent tearing pain in arm, most violent while lying still.
- Drawing and paralysed sensation left arm, at night.
- Sticking and drawing in left arm extending from above downward and out at tips of fingers.
- Pain in left upper arm as if muscles or tendons were unduly strained, when the limb is carried by them far upwards and backwards, at 2 and 3 PM.
- Jerking tearing in elbow and wrist joints, during rest, better during motion.
- Loss of power and stiffness in forearms and fingers on moving them.
- A powerless sensation in upper right forearm, on motion, and pain as if sprained in wrist, when grasping anything.
- Sensation on upper surface of left wrist on bending it, as if it were sprained.
- When grasping, feeling as if pins were pricking tips and palmar surface of first phalanges of fingers.
- Great heaviness in legs while sitting, disappeared on walking.
- Great weakness of legs while walking in open air (afternoon), hardly able to proceed, because they are so heavy and weary (Gels.): after sitting an hour, weariness disappears.
- Aching pains in legs, inability to rest in any position but for a moment.
- Pressive pain in both hip-joints on every step, and paralysed sensation in anterior muscles of thighs.
- Tension, left hip joint, while siting.
- When lying on the side the hips hurt, and when lying on the back the small of the back hurts.
- Stiffness, especially knees and feet.
- Tension left knee joint, when rising from seat.
- Tension knee, as if it were too short.
- Uneasiness in foot (from pulling and tension and tension in tendons).
- Tearing in knee and ankle, worse during rest.

- Legs heavy and weary, as if he had walked a long distance.
- Pain like a tingling in tibiae at night, when feet are crossed.
- Constantly obliged to move legs back and forth, and so unable to sleep.
- Heaviness and tension in feet while sitting, but only weariness when walking.
- Feet painful, as if sprained or wrenched on rising in AM.
- A drawing, like paralysis, in whole foot, while sitting.
- Unusual weakness of limbs, mostly during rest.
- Very great weakness, especially walking in open air.
- Weariness, worse sitting, relieved when walking; decided stiffness on rising from seat.
- Unusual RESTLESSNESS at night. Great restlessness.
- Could not sit still on account of internal uneasiness, but was obliged to turn in every direction on the chair, and move all her limbs (Pyr.).
- Great uneasiness at night.
- Stiff on rising from a seat.
- Soreness in every muscle, passes off during exercise.
- SKIN: Erysipelas, with numerous vesicles that burst, and secreted for eight days a slimy liquid.
- After 24 hours itching and burning commenced, lasting from half-an hour to two hours.
- After 36 hours, swelling of the parts, with violent itching and burning, increased on touching or moving; the parts affected as if pierced by hot needles (Ars.). White transparent vesicles appeared on the highly red and inflamed skin (Ran. b.).
- Covered from heads to foot with a fine red vesicular rash, itching and burning terribly, especially in the joints; worse at night causing constant scratching, with little or no relief, and which felt very hard when pressed with the finger; skin burning hot.
- The face became red, enormously swollen and oedematous, then also the hands and the skin of the whole body became covered with a scarlet-like

exanthema, with intolerable itching biting; on the fourth day the backs of the hands and legs became covered with blisters, which burst and slowly desquamated. Violent vesicular erysipelas of the face and hands, attended with a high state of fever.

- Burning, itching eruption.
- Urticaria from getting wet; during Rheumatism; with chills and fever. Worse in cold air.
- Eczema: raw, excoriated: thick crusts, oozing and offensive.
- Burning, itching, tingling pains. Incessant itching and scratching. The more they scratch, the greater the urgency to scratch.
- Acts on fibrous and muscular TISSUES.
- Flesh of affected parts sore to touch.
- Pain as if flesh torn loose from bones : or bones being scraped.
- Pains as if sprained; disposition to sprain a part by lifting heavy weights, or stretching up to reach things.
- Inflammation of tendons and muscles from over-exertion, or sudden wrenching as in a sprain.
- Bad effects of getting wet, especially after being heated.
- Smooth red and shining swellings, the inflamed skin being covered with small, painful, white vesicles.
- Glands swollen, hot, painful; indurated; suppurating.
- PARALYSIS: after unwanted exertion: parturition: rheumatic, from getting wet or lying on damp ground; after ague or typhoid.
- Parts painless, or painfully stiff and lame, with tearing, tingling numbness.
- Twitching of limbs and muscles.
- Restless at night, has to change position frequently.
- Bad consequences from getting wet, especially after being heated.
- FEVER. Cough during chill: dry, teasing, fatiguing.
- Slow Fever, tongue dry and brown, or red as if skinned; sordes on teeth; bowels loose; great weakness; powerlessness of lower limbs, can hardly draw them up. Great restlessness after midnight; must move often to get relief.

RUMEX CRISPUS

I. Introduction (Cow.-667)

Synonym: Rhumex Crispus.
Natural Order: Polygonaceae.
Common Name: Yellow Dock.
Habitat: Plant native of Europe.
Preparation: Tincture from the fresh root.

II. General Analysis (Cow.)

Acts upon mucous membranes, lymphatic and skin; prominent action upon mucous membranes-diminishing secretions. Excessive tea drinking. Tingling in the throat. Asthma. Catarrhal aphonia.

III. Suited to (Allen-247)

For tubular diathesis, extremely sensitive skin and mucous membranes. Extremely sensitive to open air. Dry incessant fatiguing cough < changing air or room (Phos., Spig.).; slightest inhalation of cold air; covers head with bedclothes to make air warmer; little or no expectoration.

IV. Clinical (Clarke-III-1022)

Abortion, Aphonia, Asthma, Borborygmi, Bronchitis, Catarrh, Corns, Coryza, Cough, Diarrhoea, Dyspepsia, Epistaxis, Feet tender, Gastralgia, Heart-pain in; affections of, Indigestion, Irritation, Lichen, Mouth ulcerated, Phimosis, Phthisis, Prurigo, Rheumatism, Throat-sore; ulcerated, Trachea-affections of, Urticaria.

V. Symptoms-General (Nash-383)

1. Violent, incessant dry cough, worse on inhaling the least cold air; covers the mouth to keep the cold air out with relief.

2. Brownish diarrhoea, < in morning.
3. Intense itching of the skin when undressing to go to bed.

VI. Symptoms-Particular (Nash-384-385)

1. Cough < by cold air, talking, singing. Dry, violent, incessant.
   Rum. c. +++ < warm to cold.
   Phos., < inhaling cold air, but not so.
   Spon. marked as in Rum. c.

Opposite < cold to warm.
   Bry.,
   Nat. c.

2. Sensation in cough.
   Rumex—Tingling.
   Caust.—rawness/soreness.
3. Cough with stitching pain in left lung below left nipple.
   Rum. c.,
   Nat. s.
4. Diarrhoea. < morning.
   Rum. c.—brown with cough.
   Nat.s,
   Sul.—drives out of bed early in the morning (Allen)
   Podo.
5. Itching on undressing to go to bed.
   Rumex—< warmth of bed (Merc. s., Merc. proto.).
   Olean.,
   Nat. s.—with jaundice/malaria.

RUTA GRAVEOLENS

I. Introduction (Cow.-669)

Synonym: Ruta Graveolens.
Natural Order: Rutaceae.
Common Name: Rue.
Habitat: A cultivated plant, indigenous to Southern Europe.
Preparation: Tincture from the fresh plant.

It was proved by Hahnemann (Pierce-705).

II. General Analysis (Cow.)

Acts especially upon periosteum, bones, joints and cartilage producing rheumatic symptoms-eyes, upon uterus-causing actual determination of the blood in it, and contraction of its muscular walls as an emmenagogue and abortifacient. Bruised soreness.

III. Suited to (Allen-248)

Scrofulous diathesis (swelling of the glands of the neck) and other mechanical injuries of bones and periosetum, sprain, periostitis, erysipelas. Fracture, especially dislocations (Symp.). Bruised sensation all over, as after a fall or blow; worse in limbs and joints. All parts of body on which he lies are painful as if bruised (Bap., Pyr.). Lameness after sprains, esp. of wrists and ankles (chronic sprains-Bov., Stron.). Aching in and over eyes, with blurred vision, as if they had been strained. After using eyes at fine work (Nat. m., Sen.). Prolapse of rectum, immediately on attempting a passage, from slightest stooping, frequent unsuccessful urging, after confinement,. Pressure on bladder as if full even after urinating. Scanty green urine, involuntary.

IV. Clinical (Clarke-III-1028)

Amblyopia, Anus-prolapse of, Bone-bruised; pains in, Bruises, Bursitis, Cartilages-bruises of; pains in, Chest (sternum)-pains in, Constipation, Dislocations, Dyspepsia, Enuresis, Epistaxis, Exostosis, Eyes-sight weak; pains in, Facial paralysis-from cold, Fever, Fracture, Ganglion, Haemorrhage, Hands-pains in, Paralysis, Perichondritis, Periostitis, Rectum-affections of; prolapse of, Restlessness, Rheumatism, Sciatica, Spleen-affections of, Sprain, Stammering, Tongue-cramp in; swelling of, Urination-difficulty of, Varicocele, Veins-swollen; varicose, Warts.

V. Symptoms-Particular (Nash-363-364)

1. Bruised, lame sensation all over, as after a fall (Arn.). All parts of body he lies on are painful, as if bruised < in limbs and joints.
2. Wants to change position frequently (Rhus t.).
3. Pains and lameness of Rut.. have particular liking for wrists (Eup. perf.) < in cold weather > on motion (Rhus t.).
4. Eye strain weary from close study, sewing etc.
5. Eyes weary, and ache as if strained (Nat. m., Seneg.) or they burn like ball of fire. Rut. is best remedy in eye strain.
6. Asthenopia (Poor vision).
   Rut.,
   Nat. m.,
   Seneg.
7. One of the best remedies for prolapses of the rectum.
   Rut.= Ign. Both are < on stooping, lifting or at stool (Mur. ac., Podo.).
8. Prolapsed organ is very sensitive to least touch, even the sheet he lies upon, and rectum comes down even when urinating (Aloe.). Podo.-prolapse is with characteristic diarrhoea.

VI. Black Letter Symptoms
(Tyler-720-722)

- HEAD. Shooting pain from frontal to temporal bone: from temporal bone to occiput: in the periosteum: pain as if from a fall.
- Stitches in left frontal bone, only from reading.
- Rhythmic pressive pain in head.
- Sensation of fire and heat in EYES: aching while reading, in the evening, by the light.
- Eyes feel fatigued, as after reading too long.
- Weary pain in the eyes while reading.
- Aching in and over eyes, vision blurred, after using eyes and straining them over fine work.
- Vision very weak, as if eyes were excessively strained.
- Asthenopia: irritability of every tissue of eye, from overwork, or using eyes on too fine work; heat and aching in and over eyes; eyes feel like balls of fire at night; blurring of vision; letters seem to run together; lachrymation.
- A blurring under left eye.
- Itching inner canthi and on lower lids, which smart after rubbing them, when eyes become filled with water.
- Spasm in lower eyelid; the tarsus is drawn hither and thither, and when it ceases, water runs from both eyes.
- Sensation in EAR as if a blunt piece of wood were pushed about in it: a scratching pressure.
- Cartilage of ears pain, as from a blow or fall.
- Under the mastoid process-pain as from a blow or fall.
- Tension in STOMACH > by drinking milk.
- In the HEPATIC REGION-an aching gnawing pain.
- When sitting, tearing stitches in the rectum.
- Tearing in rectum and urethra, when not urinating.
- Prolapsus of rectum. Faeces pass involuntarily while bending over. Prolapse always with and sometimes without stool.

- Protrusion of rectum after confinement. After dysentery half a year previously.
- A gnawing in left side of chest.
- In right CHEST a gnawing sensation, combined with something corrosive and burning.
- Pain, as if beaten in the SPINE.
- Itching in left upper ARM: excites scratching.
- In left elbow joint-pain as from a blow, with weakness in the arm.
- The bones of wrist and back of hand are painful, as if bruised, when at rest and when moving them.
- In the bones about the hips-pain as from a blow or fall.
- He cannot bend his body, all joints and hip bones are painful as if bruised.
- On touching the painful parts, especially hips and thigh bones, they are painful as if bruised.
- The whole anterior surface of thighs is as if bruised and painful to touch.
- If he stretches out lower extremities, even a little, the thighs are painful, as if broken through the middle.
- Posterior part of thigh and above the knee feels bruised.
- After sitting, he cannot walk immediately: falls back again.
- When walking, falls from one side to the other: his legs cannot support him ; no power and no stability in thighs.
- Difficulty in going up and down stairs, legs bend under him.
- Dare not tread strongly on feet: bones of feet painful, with feeling of heat.
- On the front of left ankle joint-a pain, throbbing and hacking, as if an ulcer were there.
- Burning and corrosive pain in bones of feet when at rest.
- Knows not where to put legs because of restlessness and heaviness, puts them first in one place and then another, and turns body from side to side.

- Lameness after sprains, especially of wrists and ankles.
- Yawning, stretching and extending the hands.
- All parts of body on which he lies, even in bed, are painful as if bruised.
- Bruises and mechanical injuries of bones and periosteum: sprains; periostitis; erysipelas.
- Bone lesions and Fracture: scrofulous exostoses.
- Coldness from the spine downwards.
- Frequent waking at night: vivid confused dreams.
- One of the peculiar sensations of Rut. is cramp in the tongue. "Spasm of tongue with difficulty of speech. Another, nausea felt in rectum.

SABADILLA

I. Introduction (Cow-672)

Synonym: Veratrum Sabadilla, Asagraea officinalis.
Natural Order: Melanthaceae.
Common Names: Indian Caustic, Barley, Cevadilla.
Habitat: A bulbous plant indigenous to Mexico.
Preparation: Tincture from seeds.

Hahnemann took part in the proving of Sabadilla (Pierce-706).

II. General Analysis (Cow.)

Through the cerebrospinal nervous system acts upon vegetative sphere, mucous surfaces, becoming more particularly involved by its action.

III. Suited to (Allen-251)

Persons of light hair, with a weak relaxed muscular system, worm affection of children (Sil., Cina., Spig.), Nervous diseases; twitching, convulsive trembling; from worms (Cina., Psor.), Sneezing paroxysm. Diphtheria, tonsilitis, can swallow warm food more easily Headache-from too much thinking (Arg. n.); from worms. Dryness of fauces and throat.

IV. Clinical (Clarke-III-1036)

Coryza, Debility, Diphtheria, Dyspepsia of pregnancy, Earache, Epistaxis, Hay-asthma, Headache, Head-lice, Imaginary diseases, Influenza, Intermittents, Mania, Melancholia, Neuralgia, Oesophagus-constriction of, Rheumatism, Tape-worm, Throat sore, Toothache, Uvula elongated, Vertigo, Worms.

SABINA

I. Introduction (Cow-674)

Synonym: Juniperus Sabina.
Natural Order: Coniferae.
Common Name: Savin.
Habitat: A woody ever green shrub in Austria and Switzerland.
Preparation: Tincture from the fresh tips of younger branches.

It was proved by Stapf, one of Hahnemann provers (Pierce-707).

II. General Analysis (Cow.)

Acts chiefly upon generative organs of female (uteric haemorrhage) and gives rise to haemorrhage and abortion; on the urinary organs causes strangury, and in the bowels purging and bloody stools. It produces in these organs congestion and inflammation.

III. Suited to (Allen-250)

Chronic ailments of women, arthritic pains/tendency to miscarriage, especially at 3rd month. Music intolerable. Ailments following abortion or premature labour/ haemorrhage Haemorrhage from uterus on least motion. Drawing pains from sacrum to pubes in nearly all diseases from back, going round to the body, to pubes (Vib. op.).

IV. Clinical (Clarke-III-1050)

Abortion-after effects of, After-pains, Boils, Condylomata, Cystitis, Dysmenorrhoea, Gonorrhoea, Gout, Inter-menstrual flow, Leucorrhoea, Menstruation profuse, Miscarriage, Mole-promotes expulsion of, Nephritis, Nymphomania, Ovaries-affections of, Penis-cartilaginous swelling on,

Phimosis, Placenta retained, Rheumatic gout, Strangury, Sycosis, Toothache, Uterus-bleeding from.

V. Symptoms-Particular (Nash-216-217)

1. "One of our best remedies for profuse flowing from female genital organs" (Nash), as in Menorrhagia, Metrorrhagia, abortions, after labour.
2. Haemorrhage apt to occur in paroxysms worse from motion (Sec.).

   Kali n. } + dark blood.
   Cycl. } +
   Sec. —dark blood.
   Croc.—dark blood but clotted.
   Caul. —after abortion with pain from back to pubes.
   Ferr. —partly clotted and partly watery.
3. Threatened abortion at the third month, esp. when the characteristic pain from back to pubes is present, if the pains begin in the back, go around and in uterus, then Vib. op.
4. Aggravation from warm room warm air and better from open air open area (a symptom of Puls., but Puls. can't be given in profuse menstrual flow, here Sabin. proves useful).
5. Arthritic swelling of wrist joint-With profuse flow from genitals-Sabin.

   (Caul. in some cases)
6. Where Puls. can't be given then Sabin. comes in. Cases of too profuse menses, because Puls. can't be given as it increases their already too profuse flow.

SAMBUCUS NIGRA

I. Introduction (Cow.-677)

Synonym: Sambucus Nigra.
Natural Order: Caprifoliaceae.
Common Name: Black elder. European elder.
Habitat: An indigenous shrub common in thickets and waste grounds.
Preparation: Tincture from fresh leaves and flowers.

It was proved by Hahnemann first (Pierce-709).

II. General Analysis (Cow.)

Acts especially upon respiratory organs, mucous membranes and the skin, causing in the mucous membranes obstructive catarrh and in skin debilitating perspiration.

III. Suited to (Allen-252)

Disease of scrofulous (tuberculous) children affecting air passages, Persons formerly robust and fleshy suddenly emaciated (Iod., Tuberc.), Bad effects of-violent mental emotions; sexual indulgence (Phos. ac., Kali p.) Dry Coryza of infants. Child inspires but can't expire (Chlorine., Mephitis.).

IV. Clinical (Clarke-III-1072)

Angina pectoris, Asthma, Chest-oppression of, Coryza-dry, Cough, Croup, Emaciation, Headaches-catarrhal, Hoarseness, Hydrocele, Ileus, Laryngismus, Perspiration, Phthisis, Scurf, "Snuffles", Starting, Whooping-cough.

V. Symptoms-Particular (Nash-460)

1. Snuffles in small children-of dry variety completely obstructing the nose, child breaths through mouth.

2. Asthma milleri. Attack suddenly in the night-child turns blue, gasps for air-seems as if almost dying-then goes to sleep and wakens with another attack again.
3. Dry heat when asleep-profuse sweat when awake. *No other remedy has this symptom.*
   Con. -Sweats as soon as he closes his eyes to sleep.
   Thuj. -Sweats on uncovered parts.
   Bell. -Sweats on covered parts.
   Puls. -Sweats one sided.
7. Nash says that many of best characteristics of the medicine are found under the so called fever symptoms including chill, heat, and sweat (Nash-461).

SANGUINARIA

I. Introduction (Cow.-678)

Synonym: Sanguinaria canadensis.
Common Name: Bloodroot.
Natural Order: Papaveraceae.
Habitat: A perennial indigenous plant (USA).
Preparation: Tincture from the fresh root.

It was first proved by Dr. G. Bute of USA. (Pierce-710).

II. General Analysis (Cow.)

Acts chiefly upon the respiratory mucous organs producing irritation and catarrhal irritation. Has decided influence upon pneumo-gastric nerve and through it causes degeneration of liver and digestive tract. Chief use-Respiratory diseases and various forms of headaches.

III. Suited to (Allen-253)

Young women with eruption on face, especially during scanty menses. Persons suffering from periodic sick headache beginning in the morning until evening, > perfect quiet in dark Room. "Tired Headache" > pressure, rubbing circumscribed cheeks. Cough returns at every cold. Headache at climacteric, every 7th day.

IV. Clinical (Clarke-III-1076)

Alcoholism, Aphonia, Asthma, Breast-tumour of, Bronchitis, Cancer, Catarrh, Chest-pains in, Climaxis, Colds, Croup, Deafness, Diphtheria, Dysmenorrhoea, Dyspepsia, Ear-polypi of, Climacteric flushes, Gleet, Granular lids, Haemoptysis, Headache, Influenza, Keratitis, Liver-cough, Menstruation-breasts painful during, Nails-ulceration of, Neuralgia, Oedema glottidis, Ophthalmia, Pharyngitis, Phthisis florida, Physometra, Pneumonia acute, Polypi,

Pregnancy-affections of, Pyrosis, Quinsy, Rheumatism, Rhus poisoning, Shoulder-rheumatism of, Smell-illusions of; loss of; Stomach-neurosis of, Syphilis, Tinnitus, Tumours, Vomiting, Whitlow, Whooping-cough.

V. Symptoms-General (Nash-239)

1. Pain beginning in occiput; spreads over the head and settles over the right eye, with nausea and vomiting, sensitive to noise and light.
2. Loose cough with badly smelling sputa; the breath and sputa smell badly to the patient himself.
3. Pain in right arm and shoulder; worse at night in bed; can't raise the arm. Also pain in places where the bones are the least covered.
4. Heat and tension behind sternum. Cough day and night with great emaciation.
5. Burning and pressing in breast, followed by heat throughout abdomen and diarrhoea. Acts intensely on right lung and chest.

VI. Symptoms-Particular (Nash-239-240)

1. Pain Behind sternum (breast bone). Cough after bronchitis or pneumonia.
   Sang., Kali hydro.
2. Circumscribed redness of checks, flushes of fever with.
   Sang.,
   Sul.,
   Lach.
3. Rheumatic pains in Right arm and shoulder < Night
   Flashes of heat at soles and palms of hand.
4. Sick headache with nausea and vomiting, settles over right eye-Sang.
   Left eye-Spig.

VII. Black Letter Symptoms (Tyler-728-729)

- Determination of blood to head, with whizzing in the ears and transitory feeling of heat, then a sensation as if vomiting was about to take place.

- Headache begins in occiput, spreads upwards and settles over right eye.
- Periodical sick headache; begins in the morning, increases during the day, lasts until evening. Head feels as if it must burst, or as if eyes would be pressed out. Throbbing, lancinating pains through brain, worse on right side, esp. in forehead and vertex; followed by chills, nausea, vomiting of food or bile; must be down and remain quiet; relieved by sleep.
- Paroxysmal headache. Headache, with nausea and chilliness, followed by flushes of heat, extending from the head to the stomach.
- Neuralgia in and over left Eye.
- Nasal polypi.
- Red Cheeks with burning in ears, with cough.
- Burning in PHARYNX and OESOPHAGUS.
- VOMITING of bitter water; of sour acrid fluids; of ingesta; or worms; preceded by anxiety; with headache and burning in stomach; head better afterwards; with prostration.
- Dry Cough, with considerable tickling in throat-pit and a crawling sensation, extending down beneath the sternum. Teasing, dry, hacking cough, with dryness in the throat. Hacking cough, caused by ticking in the throat, several evenings after lying down. Ticking cough with very dry throat.
- Severe cough occurring after whooping-cough, when patient takes cold, which partakes of the spasmodic nature of Whooping cough.
- Catarrhal irritation in chest; night sweats; after a cold, several months previously.
- RHEUMATIC PAIN in right arm and shoulder; worse at night; on turning in bed; cannot raise arm.
- Lassitude, torpor, languor, not disposed to move or make any mental exertion. Worse in damp weather.
- Lameness of right arm.

SANICULA

I. Introduction (Clarke-III-1090)

Synonym: Sanicula Acqua.
Common Name: Mineral water of O'Hawa spring (USA).
Preparation: Dilution of mineral spring water. Triturations of evaporated salts.

II. Suited to (Allen-255)

Dread of downward motion, child headstrong, cries and kicks, cross, irritable, but quickly alternates with laughter, does not want to be touched (Ant. c., rev. Cham.). Progressive emaciation like Sul. Odour of stool persists even after bathing; as if contents of pelvis will escape. Walk-must support parts by hand against vulva (Lil. t., Mur. p.). Foot-Burning of soles of feet (Lach., Medo., Sang., Sul.). Profuse dandruff in scalp, eye brows, beard etc. Constipation-Stool large, hard impossible to evacuate (Thuj., Op., Sil., Nat. m). Profuse sweats-on head and neck of children when asleep.

III. Clinical (Clarke-III-1090)

Amenorrhoea, Anterior crural neuralgia, Asthma, Bee-stings, Boils-blind, Borborygmi, Coccyx-soreness of, Condylomata, Conjunctivitis, Constipation of children, Cornea-ulceration of, Coryza, Cough, Dandruff, Debility, Diabetes, Diarrhoea, Digestion slow, Dropsy-during pregnancy, Eczema, Emaciation, Enuresis, Excoriations, Foot-sweat, Gastritis, Gum-boil, Headache, Indigestion, Influenza, Intermittents, Intestinal sand, Itch suppressed, Itching, Leucorrhoea, Liver-soreness of, Lumbago, Melancholy, Milk thin, Mouth sore, Neuralgia, Neurasthenia, Night-terrors, Nose-crusts in, Ophthalmia tarsi, Os uteri-dilated, Ossification-too early, Ozaena, Perspiration profuse, Pot-bellied children, Pregnancy-sickness of; dropsy of, Rectum-cramp in, Rheumatism, Rickets, Scurvy, Sea-sickness, Shoulder-rheumatism of, Throat sore, Tongue-ringworm of; burning, Toothache, Uterus-prolapse of; soreness of; tumour of, Vomiting-of milk; of water, Wrist-boils on.

IV. Symptoms-Particular
{Nash-pages. indicated in ()}

1. Sand in urine with much pain in the back region of kidneys (61).
2. Stools in diarrhoea-no two stools alike (24).
3. Especially suited to sweaty headed children-Calc. c. (79).
4. Stools partly protruding then slipping back-Thuj. (80).
5. Offensive foot sweats-Psor., Graph. (82).
6. Stool in constipation, of such immense size that it cannot be discharged without mechanical aid-Sel. (190).
7. In Marasmus, emaciation from above downward-Nat. m., Lyc. (316).
8. He looses flesh while eating well-Nat. m. (331).
9. Fear of falling from downward motion (412).

SARSAPARILLA

I. Introduction (Cow.-682)

Synonym: Smilax Medica, Smilax officinalis.
Natural Order: Smilaceae.
Common Name: Wild Liquorice.
Habitat: A plant indigenous to Mexico and South America.
Preparation: Triturations from the dried root bark.

II. General Analysis (Cow.)

Acts powerfully upon the blood, causing Herpes and other skin Eruption. Upon urinary symptoms produces gravel like symptoms (excellent remedy).

III. Suited to (Allen-257)

Dark-haired persons, sycotic diathesis. Great emaciation, skin becomes shrivelled and lies in folds (Abrot., Iod., Nat. m., Sanic.). In children, face like old people. Herpes on all parts of body. Urine-clear but irritating, pain at conclusion (Berb. v., Equis., Medo., Thuj.), white sand in, passed without sensation. Urine-dribbling while sitting, standing, passes freely. Itching eruption on forehead during menses (Eug. j, Sang., Psor.) Passage of small calculi, renal colic, stone in bladder.

IV. Clinical (Clarke-III-1112)

Asthma, Bladder affections, Bone affections, Breast-scirrhus of, Bright's disease, Calculi, Climaxis, Constipation, Dysmenia, Dyspepsia, Dysuria, Enuresis, Eruptions, Eye affections, Faintness, Glands enlarged, Gonorrhoea, Gout, Gravel, Hands chapped, Headache, Hernia, Herpes preputialis, Hiccough, Intermittents, Marasmus, Masturbation-effects of, Melancholia, Mercury-abuse of, Mycosis, Nipple retracted, Plica polonica, Renal colic, Rhagades,

Rheumatism-gonorrhoeal, Seborrhoea, Spermatic cords-swelling of, Spermatorrhoea, Strangury, Syphilis, Ulcer, Warts.

V. Symptoms-General (Nash-315)

1. White sand in urine; also slimy or flaky urine.
2. Much pain at the conclusion of passing urine; almost unbearable.
3. Marasmus; neck emaciates and skin lies in folds.

VI. Symptoms-Particular (Nash-315-316)

1. Excruciating Pain of Kidneys (due to stone).

   Lyc. —Red sand with clear urine.

   Sarsa. —White sand with scanty, slimy urine.

   Rheumatic trouble common to both medicines. [use in chronic Rheumatic troubles with urinary complications.]
2. Much pain at the close of Urination, almost unbearable.

   Berb. v.,
   Equis.,
   Medo.,
   Thuj.
3. Tenesmus of Bladder

   Sarsa. —no other remedy has it so strong+++.

   Puls. —in connection with enlarged prostrate.

   Nat. m.—burning and cutting after Urination in urethra.
4. Marasmus

   Sarsa. —neck emaciates and skin lies in fold.

   Iod. —general emaciation while wishes to eat all the time.

   Nat. m.—general emaciation while eats well.

   Abrot.-general marasmus, legs most.

   Sanic.
   Lyc. } (emaciation, from above to below)
   Nat. m.

   Abrot.—below to above emaciation.

   Arg. n.—All dried up, looks like mummy.

5. Headache—one of the best medicines for headache or periosteal pain due to suppressed gonorrhoea.
6. Skin—Good remedy for syphilitic eruption with emaciation, cracks on hands and feet, especially, on sides of fingers and on toes.
7. Retractions of nipples (Sil.).

SECALE CORNUTUM

I. Introduction (Cow.-684)

Synonym: Acinula clavus. Ergota.
Natural Order: Fungi.
Common Name: Spurred Rye. Ergot.
Preparation: Tincture from the fresh Fungus.

In 1865 it was fragmentally proved by Dr. Allen (Pierce-714).

II. General Analysis (Cow.)

Acts powerfully upon cerebro-spinal system and gives two distinct characteristics (i) Convulsion (ii) Gangrenous ergotism. The former resulting directly from nerve poisoning while the latter due to secondary blood disorganization leading to Ergot poisoning, convulsive form of Ergot poisoning. The powerful action of Ergot upon unstriped muscular fibre causes gravid uterus, exciting contractions of it and expelling its contents. Never to be used for hastening delivery.

III. Suited to (Allen-258)

Women of, thin, scrawny feeble, cachetic appearance, nervous temperament, sunken countenance. Very old decrepit feeble persons/women of very lax muscular fibre/ passive Haemorrhage of thin, black, watery blood. Leucorrhoea, green, brown offensive. Boils-greenish, smell, painful. Enuresis-Old people, urine suppressed, pale, watery or bloody face pale, pinched, ashen, sunken, blue rings around eyes. Boils-small, painful with green contents. Haemorrhagic diathesis-slightest wound bleeds for weeks (Lac can., Phos.). Diarrhoea-Profuse, watery, putrid, great force (Gamb., Crot. t.) exhausting, painless; anus wide open (Phos., Apis.). Skin-cold to touch, patient, but can not cover (Skin hot but can't uncover-Nux v.).

IV. Clinical (Clarke-III-1132)

Abortion threatened, After-pains, Albuminuria, Anus-incontinence of; open, Asthenopia, Bladder-paralysis of, Boils, Carbuncles, Cataract, Chilblains, Cholera infantum, Chorea, Convulsions, Cramps, Diabetes, Diaphragm-cramp in, Diarrhoea, Distortions, Dysphagia, Epilepsy, Epistaxis, Feet-cramps in; burning of; coldness of, Fibroma, Gangrene, Gastritis, Glands swollen; suppuration of, Goitre, Haematuria, Haemorrhage, Haemorrhagic diathesis, Heart-palpitation of, Hiccough, Hysteria, Impotence, Liver enlarged, Lochia-foetid, Lumbago, Menstruation profuse, Metrorrhagia, Milk suppressed, Miscarriage, Morvan's disease, Myelitis diffusa, Nails-degeneration of, Neuralgia, Night-sweats, Numbness, Oesophagitis, Ovary-tumour of, Paralysis-post diphtheritic; spastic, Placenta retained, Post-partum haemorrhage, Pregnancy-false pains of, Purpura, Raynaud's disease, Small-pox-haemorrhagic, Spinal irritation, Stammering, Stomach-cancer of, Strabismus, Stricture-spasmodic, Thrombosis, Tongue-biting of, Typhoid, Ulcer, Uterus-inertia of; neuralgia of; prolapse of.

V. Symptoms-General (Nash-210)

1. Passive haemorrhage everything open and loose, no action, in thin, scrawny (lean, dry), cachetic women.
2. Great coldness of the surface (objective) yet patient can not bear to be covered.
3. Numbness, crawling and paralysis, formication as of mice creeping there, all the parts of the body.

VI. Symptoms-Particular (Nash-210-213)

1. It has power to control haemorrhage by contracting uterus, which only few remedies can surpass (212).
2. Useful, when labour pains are weak, suppressed or distressing, in weak and cachetic women.
3. Great coldness (objective) of surface yet the patient can not bear to be covered (oftenest found in Cholera) (Camph.) for the first stage or early collapse). Feet and toes icy cold, but he is distressed when covered.

4. Sec. has burning feet (Sul.), but Sul. does not have coldness or collapse of Sec. or degree of collapse.
5. Numbness-Crawling paralysis.
6. Skin-cold (objective), dry and wrinkled, and is visensible often, or there may be much formication under, as if mice were creeping there.

SELENIUM

I. Introduction (Cow.-689)

Synonym: An element.
Preparation: Triturations.
This rare metal was first proved by Hering (Pierce-717).

II. General Analysis (Cow.)

Acts chiefly upon larynx, male sexual organs, local and general tendency to produce exhaustion and debility. In larynx inflammation. In sexual organs weakness.

III. Suited to (Allen-261)

Light complexioned, great emaciation of face, hands, legs, feet etc; very forgetful in business; but remembers in dream, Hair falls off, Headache-of drunkards, debauchery, lemonade, tea, wine, every afternoon. Aphonia-after long use of voice. Urine involuntary, dribbling while walking. Constipation, stool large, hard, requires mechanical aid (Aloe., Calc. c., Sanic., Sep., Sil.).

IV. Clinical (Clarke-III-1139)

Alcoholism, Ankle-itching eruption about, Comedo, Constipation, Debility, Enuresis, Hair falling off, Headache, Hoarseness, Impotence, Laryngitis-scrofulous; tubercular, Liver-affections of; rash over region of, Priapism, Prostatitis, Prostatorrhoea, Psoriasis palmaris, Reveries, Scabies, Scalp-eczema of, Skin unhealthy, Spermatorrhoea, Stammering, Sun-effects of, Syphilis.

V. Symptoms-Particular (Nash-189)

1. Excessive weakness-general (sexual) Sul., Acet. ac., Sanic. is of general nature unlike Stan., which is local.

2. Involuntary urination (dribbling).
   Sel. — Urine dribbles while walking.
   Sarsa. — dribble while sitting.
3. Bad effects of too much tea, all complaints.
4. Hoarseness—must clear throat at beginning of singing.
5. Very forgetful in business, but during sleep, dreams what he had forgotten.
6. Weakness–sexual (male)—Erections slow and weak, emission too rapid in coition, cross and weak afterwards. Desire strong but physically impotent. Sexual emission 2-3 times a week; weak, lame back after them. Oozing of prostratic fluid. If this continues, then emaciates in face, hands, thighs (Acet. ac.).
7. Constipation—stool of immense size removed with mechanical aids (Sanic.).

SEPIA

I. Introduction (Cow.-696)

Synonym: Sepia Octopus, Sepia Succus.
Natural Order: Dibranchiata.
Common Name: Cuttlefish. Squid.
Preparation: Triturations from inky juice of Cuttlefish {not below 3x in use (Pierce-721)}.

It was proved by Hahnemann first then further developed by Dr. Graham Bell of USA. (Pierce-720).

II. General Analysis (Cow.)

Acts mainly upon mortal, hepatic, and female sexual system and, in general, diminishes reproductive energies of vegetative system. Its action sluggish and causes torpidity and depression as general condition. Local action upon female sexual organs, weakness and irritation, and upon the skin hepatic Eruption.

III. Suited to (Allen-262)

Persons of dark hair, rigid fibre, but mild and easy disposition (Puls.), Disease of women, especially during pregnancy; childbirth and lactation or diseases attended with sudden prostration and sinking faintness (Mur. p., Nux. m.), complaints brought on after the laundry work (Washer women's remedy). Great sadness and weeping. Indifferent to one's family, Indolent, (Fluor. ac., Phos. ac.) Flashes of heat over head and face with Anxiety with Fear towards evening. Headache in terrific shocks, at menstrual nisus, scanty flow, motion, mental labour, external pressure. Pressure and bearing down, as if everything would protrude from pelvis, must cross limbs tightly or sit close to prevent it with oppression of breathing (Agar., Bell., Lil. t., Mur. p., Sanic.).

IV. Clinical (Clarke-III-1158)

Alcohol-effects of, Amenorrhoea, Anus-pressure of, Apoplexy, Appetite depraved, Ascarides, Baldness, Bladder irritable, Cancer, Change of life, Chloasma, Chorea, Condylomata, Cystitis, Dandruff, Dysmenorrhoea, Dyspepsia, Eczema, Epistaxis, Eye affections, Face yellow, Freckles, Gleet, Gonorrhoea, Gravel, Herpes circinatus, Hysteria, Irritation, Jaundice, Leucorrhoea, Liver-spots, Liver torpid, Menstruation disordered, Mind-affections of, Nails-pains under, Neuralgia, Nose-inflamed; swollen, Ozaena, Phimosis, Pityriasis versicolor, Pleurisy, Pregnancy-disorders of; vomiting of, Pruritus, Psoriasis, Ptosis, Pylorus-induration of, Quinsy, Rectum-cancer of; fissure of, Ringworm, Sacrum-pain in, Sciatica, Seborrhoea, Smell-sense of-too acute; disordered, Spermatorrhoea, Styes, Toothache, Urine-incontinence of, Uterus-bearing down in, Veins-varicose, Warts, Whooping-cough.

V. Symptoms-General (Nash-199-200)

1. Bearing down pains, must sit close and cross her legs to keep something from coming down out of the vagina.
2. Sense of fullness in the pelvic organs, and pressure down into the anus, as if a ball or weight; oozing of moisture.
3. Flushes of heat and perspiration at the climacteric.
4. Painful sense of emptiness or goneness at the pit of the stomach.
5. General relaxation, weak, faints while kneeling at church; falling womb and pelvic organs; drooping eyelids, weak back,< on walking. Cachetic, yellow face, with yellow saddle across face and nose; moth patches; ringworm.
6. Modalities; < standing, mental labour, sexual excess, jar, after sleep, laundry work; milk (diarrhoea), climacteric, kneeling at church, > Sitting with legs crossed, loosening clothes, open air.
7. Sensation of a ball in inner parts; during menses, pregnancy, lactation, great sadness and weeping.

Dread of being alone; of meeting friends, indifferent, even to one's family, to one's occupation, to those whom she loves.

8. Headache: in terrific shocks; pressing, bursting, < motion, stooping, mental labour, > by pressure, continued fast motion.
9. Urine: deposits a reddish clay sediment, which adhere to the vessel; foetid, offensive, must be removed from room.
10. Enuresis: bed wet almost as soon as the child goes to sleep; during first sleep, violent stitches upward in the vagina.
11. Dyspnoea; < sitting, after sleep, in room, > dancing or walking rapidly.

VI. Symptoms-Particular (Nash-199-206)

1. Abdomen and pelvis (especially women)-chief action upon. It produces strongest symptoms there.
2. Sensation of a ball in inner parts.
3. Rectum prolapses with sensation of fullness or of a ball etc. Oozing.
4. Flashes of heat with perspiration and faintness (Sul.).
5. Hot and cold feet and hands alternate (unlike Sul.).
   Sep. -not much burning sensation, but actual heat, congestion and throbbing.
   Sul. -is more sensational burning.
6. Urine-Sandy reddish, offensive as if burnt clay, so offensive can't be kept in room.
7. Child always wets bed during first sleep. (Adult bed wet-Caust.).
8. Bladder-Pressure on, frequent micturation with tension in lower abdomen.
9. Male organ-Chronic gleet, flacidity of organ, frequent watery seminal discharge.
   Sep. -not much discharges but persistent few drops, fluid to orifice of urethra.
   Caps. -Thick discharge with burning sensation with urinating.
   Kali i. -like Sep. (also covers cases not covered by Sep.).

10. Mental Symptoms

    Puls. = Sep. (alike), crying without reason, sad. Indifferent to her profession (Not in Puls.).

11. Headache-Comes in terrific shocks/so as to jerk the head.
12. Hemicrania of women.
13. Drooping of eyelids.

    Sep.,

    Gels.,

    Cann. sat.

14. Chronic nasal catarrh

    Sep.,

    Kali bich.-Chronic catarrh.

    Puls.-Cures catarrhal trouble but increase menstrual flow, but Sep. cures both.

15. Yellow saddle on face (abdomen) cheek and nose cure both and yellow spots on face, on abdomen. Most 'tell-tale' face.
16. Painful emptiness, goneness sensation in the stomach (205).

    Sep.-with uterine trouble.

    Ign.,

    Hydras.,

    Mur. p.,

    Stan.,

    Lil. t.

17. Vomiting of pregnancy.

    Sep.

    Colch.<smell of food.

18. Constipation—It has great straining, mechanical aid needed to accomplish stool.

    Sep. —obstinate, mostly in children.

    Sel. —like Sep. mechanical assistance required sometimes.

19. Cholera Infantum—always worse after milk-characteristic.
20. Anus-oozing moisture (Ant. c.).
21. Skin.

    Sep. compare (Sul.)-Scratching causes burning, soreness of skin, humid places, in bend of knees.

22. Brown spots-on face etc. Large suppurating pustules receiving them.

VII. Black Letter Symptoms (Tyler-740-743)

- Very irritable.
- Very indifferent towards everything and apathetic.
- Aversion to one's occupation and family.
- Great indifference to one's family-to those they love best.
- Indolent mood.
- Uneasiness in the presence of strangers.
- "So nervous that I felt unless I held on to something, I should scream".
- Headache-right side head and face, with surging sensation like waves of pain rolling up and beating against frontal bone.
- Darting pains, from left eye over side of head towards occiput.
- Tearing in left temple to upper part of left side of head.
- Headache with aversion to all kinds of food, a feeling of emptiness and goneness in stomach, very distressing.
- Headache every morning with nausea, vertigo, epistaxis.
- Headaches in women of sallow complexion, or moth-patches on forehead.
- Smell of food repulsive.
- Headache better after meals.
- Great falling out of the hair.
- Smarting right eye, evening; lids close against one's wish.
- Grain of sand sensation, especially right eye.
- Inflammatory affections of asthenic character; conjunctive dull red, some photophobia and swelling of lids, worse in a. m.
- Lachrymation morning and evening.
- Pale face. Yellowness of face and whites of eyes.

- Yellow spots on face and a yellow saddle across the upper part of the cheeks and the nose. Yellow saddle across bridge of nose.
- Large offensive-smelling plugs from nose (Ozaena.).
- Crack middle of lower lip (Nat. m., Dros., etc.).
- Dry coryza: nostrils sore, swollen, ulcerated and scabby; discharging large, green plugs.
- Nausea, morning only, passing off after eating something.
- Gnawing and weakness in stomach, which ceased at supper.
- Emptiness of stomach, with nausea as soon as she thinks of food which she would like to take, Peculiar faint, sinking emptiness.
- Nausea; after eating, also in the AM, fasting: from smell of food or cooking; when riding in a carriage: with anxiety when entering eyes: with weakness.
- Morning sickness-of pregnancy. Toothache, esp. of pregnancy.
- Vomiting: of food and bile in AM: frequently strains her so that blood comes up: of mucous, after taking the simplest food.
- Burning in pit of stomach. Stitches in pit of stomach. Canine hunger, or no appetite.
- "Sepia creates an aversion to drinking beer".
- Feeling of bearing down of all pelvic organs.
- Pot-belliedness of mothers.
- Many brown spots on abdomen: chloasma.
- Weight in abdomen: distension: rumbling and grunting.
- Sensation of emptiness in abdomen.
- Pain and weight in abdomen, on rising in AM.
- Pain, tenderness; heaviness, load during motion in abdomen.
- Sensation of bearing down in pelvic organs, with slow gragging pain from sacrum.
- Pressure in abdomen as through the contents would issue through the genital organs. Pressure in uterus, as if every-thing would issue through vulva. Feeling of crowding and pressing downwards.

- Rolling in abdomen, as if something alive were there (Croc., Thuj.) then rises up towards her throat.
- Constipation: during pregnancy: slow and difficult discharge even of soft stool: excessive straining.
- Sensation of weight, or ball, in anus, not > by stool.
- Pressure on bladder and frequent micturition with tension and painful bearing down in pelvis.
- Involuntary discharge of urine at night, especially during first sleep. The bed is wet almost as soon as the child goes to sleep, or passed within two hours after going to bed.
- Urine clear like water; thick, slimy and very offensive, depositing a pasty sediment next morning. Sediment adheres like cement.
- Turbid, clay-coloured urine, with reddish sediment in the chamber.
- Uterus congested, and a yellowish leucorrhoea pouring from it; beginning to prolapse. Slightly displaced.
- Great dryness of vulva and vagina, causing a very disagreeable sensation when walking, after cessation of menses.
- Pressure in uterus, as if everything would issue through vulva.
- Sensation in rectum not > by an evacuation: sensation that limbs must be crossed to prevent everything being pressed out of vagina. (Lil. t.).
- Pain in uterus, bearing down, comes from back to abdomen: crosses limbs to prevent protrusion of parts.
- Prolapsus of uterus, of vagina with constipation.
- Pressure in uterus, causing oppression of breathing; the pressure downwards is as if everything would fall out, with pain in abdomen. She must cross her limbs in order to prevent the protrusion of the vagina, yet nothing protruded, but there was an increase of gelatinous leucorrhoea. Yellowish leucorrhoeal discharge.
- Leucorrhoea like milk, only by day, with burning and excoriation between thighs.
- Before menses acrid leucorrhoea, with soreness of the pudendum.

- Metrorrhagia, during climacteric or pregnancy, esp. 5th and 7th months.
- Menses: too late: too early: causing faintness, chilliness, shuddering.
- Amenorrhoea: at puberty: from a cold: in feeble women with delicate skin.
- Sudden hot flushes at climacteric with momentary sweat, weakness and tendency to faint.
- Short, hacking cough, in the evening, on lying down.
- Spasmodic cough.
- Cannot sleep at night on account of incessant cough.
- Short, dry cough, seems to come out of stomach.
- Oppression of the chest morning and evening.
- Pain in back across hips.
- When stooping sudden pain in back as if struck by a hammer: > by pressing back against something hard.
- Pain in small of back: pain and weakness: weakness when walking: pain as if sprained. Pain with stiffness, better by walking.
- A short walk fatigues much.
- Sudden prostration and sinking faintness.
- Great faintness with heat, then coldness.
- Faintness while kneeling in church: at trifles.
- Great exhaustion in a. m. during menses.
- Hands generally cold, but moist with perspiration.
- Very cold feet with headache (feeling as if they stood in cold water up to the ankles).
- Attacks of flushes of heat, as if hot water were poured over one with redness of face, sweat of whole body and anxiety, without thirst.
- Profuse night sweats. Cold night sweats, chest, back and thighs.

SILICEA

I. Introduction (Cow.-704)

Synonym: Acidum Silicum., Silex.
Common Names: Flint, Silica.
Preparation: Triturations from pure silica.
First proved by Hahnemann (Pierce-726).

II. General Analysis (Cow.)

Acts powerfully upon vegetative system, especially mucous surfaces glandular structures, bones and joints. The chief property of it, is to produce a suppurative process either in soft tissues periosteum or bones themselves, secondary action is the morbid processes set up by SIL.-erethesim with exhaustion resulting in various nervous disorders, exalted activity of senses, then depression and paralysis.

III. Suited to (Allen-266)

Nervous, irritable, sanguine, dry skin, pale face, lax muscle Deficient nutrition in assimilation not in quality or quantity (Baryt. c., Calc. c.). Over sensitive, physically mentally; weariness and debility wants to lie down. Nervous Debility overcome by will. Mental labour difficult. Ailments caused by-suppressed foot sweat (Cupr., Graph., Psor.), bad effects of vaccination (Thuj.). Blood from vagina-every time child takes to breast (Crotal. h.+). Night walking (Kali bich.), every little injury Suppurates (Graph., Hep. s., Merc. c., Petr.). Open fontanelles and sutures. Vertigo-as if would fall forward, from looking up (Puls.-looking down, Kalm., Spig.).

IV. Clinical (Clarke-III-1175)

Abdomen distended, Abscess, Acne, Anaemia, Ankles weak, Anus-fistula of; fissure of, Appetite depraved, Back-weakness of, Boils, Bones-necrosis of, Brain-concussion of, Brain-fag, Breast-sinuses in, Bunions, Cancer, Carbuncles, Cataract, Cellulitis, Cheloid, Chin-eruption on, Cicatrix, Circulation feeble, Coccygodynia, Conjunctivitis phlyctenular, Constipation, Coryza, Cough, Debility, Dentition, Diabetes, Ear affections, Elephantiasis, Enchrodroma, Enuresis, Epilepsy, Eruptions, Excrescences, Eye affections, Feet burning; Feet perspiring, Fester, Fibroma, Fistula, Fistula lachrymalis, Foot-sweat suppressed, Foreign bodies-expulsion of, Fracture, Ganglion, Gastric catarrh, Glandular swellings, Headache, Hernia, Hip-joint disease, Homesickness, Housemaid's knee, Hydrocele, Hypopion, Irritation, Jaw-carries of, Joint-synovitis of, Lactation, Locomotor ataxy, Mania, Meningitis, Metrorrhagia, Miscarriage, Molluscum contagiosum, Molluscum fibrosum, Morphoea, Morvan's disease, Nails diseased, Necrosis, Neuralgia, Nodes, Nose-tip-redness of, Panaritium, Parametritis, Perspiration offensive, Phimosis, Pleurisy, Prepuce-eruption on, Psoas abscess, Pylorus-suppuration of, Rheumatism-chronic; hereditary, Rickets, Sinuses, Somnambulism, Spermatorrhoea, Spinal irritation, Strains, Strangury, Suppuration, Teeth carious, Tenesmus, Trachea, Tumours, Ulcer, Urethra-stricture of, Urine-incontinence of, Vaccination, Vagina-spasm of, Vertigo, Walking-delay in, Whitlow, Worms, Writer's cramp.

V. Symptoms-General (Nash-78-79)

1. Weak, puny children; not from want of nourishment taken, but defective assimilation.
2. Inflammations tending to end suppuration or refusing to heal; becoming chronic.
3. Coldness, lack of vital warmth, even when taking exercise; must be wrapped up, especially the head, which >.
4. Suppressed sweat, especially of feet, which is profuse and offensive.
5. Weak, nervous, easily irritated, faint-hearted; yielding, giving up disposition, "grit all gone".
6. Constipation; stool protrudes and then slips back again, again and again; weak expulsive power.

7. Modalities: < from cold or draft, motion, open air, at new moon; > in warm room, wrapping up head; magnetism and electricity.
8. Scrofulous, rachitic children with large heads; open fontanelles and sutures; much sweating about head which must be kept warm by external covering; large bellies; weak ankles, slow in learning to walk.
9. Diseases, caused by suppressed foot-sweat; exposing the head or back to any slight draft of air; from vaccination (Thuj.); dust complaints of stone cutters, with total loss of strength.
10. Vertigo; spinal headache ascending from nape of neck to head, as if one would fall forward; worse looking upwards.
11. Unhealthy skin; every little injury suppurates.
12. Promotes expulsion of foreign bodies from the tissues, fish bones needles, bone splinters.

VI. Symptoms-Particular (Nash-79-82)

Constitutional remedy over sensitive and imperfectly nourished.

1. Sweaty headed child with defective assimilation.
   Sul. —big belly　　Calc. c.—big head
   Sanic.,
   Sil. —big belly, limbs shrunken, eyes sunken, face pinched and old looking.
2. Constipation—Stool partly coming out then slipping back (Sanic., Thuj.). Changeable stools (Puls.).
   Sil. —Constipation before and during menses (Sanic.—Faeces remain long time in Anus. (Thuj.).
3. Inflammation ending in suppuration-Bone or of soft Part.
   I. stage-Hep. s., Calc. s., for discharge of pus already formed.
   II. Stage-Sil. for healing after pus discharge has taken place.

   Sil.-3x for pus forming (Comp. Mat. Med.-Ghosh, N.C. [Hindi])–786).
4. Headache—nervous, beginning in nape of neck to the eyes-(Morning to Sunset).

Right sided migraine-Sil.,
Left sided migraine-Spig.,
Right brow-Sang., Nit. } Dr. GN Chauhan
Left brow- Sep. } (Sachitra Materia
Both-Stict., Puls. } Medica-P-65, 63)

5. Vertigo-from the nape to head looking up (Spig.-looking down).
6. Better wrapping up head, want of vital warmth, even when exercising.
   Sil.,
   Mag. m.—Wrapping up head like Sil.
7. Epileptic form of spasm new moon (Sil. 200-few doses).
8. Offensive foot sweats-Suppressed by getting cold feet.
   Sanic.,
   Psor.,
   Graph.,
   Baryt. c.,

   Sil. is chronic of Puls.

VII. Black Letter Symptoms (Tyler752-755)

- Sensitive to noise.
- *Most excessive scruples of conscience, about trifles frequently.*
- *Great difficulty in fixing the attention. Thought difficult.*
- Headache rising from nape of neck to vertex.
- *The most violent headache.*
- Tearing in the whole of the head, starting from the occipital protu-berances and extending upward and forward over both sides of the head.
- *As if head would burst, relieved by binding the head tightly.* Pressive pain in occiput, relieved by warm wrapping of the head-soon followed by stitches in the forehead, with chilliness nape of neck and back.
- The head was sore to touch externally.
- The itching spots on head are painful, as if sore after scratching.

- Swelling in the region of the right lachrymal gland and sac.
- Painful sensitiveness of the ear to loud sounds.
- The gum is painfully sensitive on taking cold water into the mouth.
- Sensation of a hair lying on forepart of tongue.
- Inflammation and suppuration of salivary glands.
- Abdomen hard, tense.
- Very offensive flatus.
- Moisture in the Anus.
- Haemorrhoids painfully sensitive.
- STOOL remains a long time in rectum.
- Cutting in rectum. Stinging in rectum.
- Tension in the anus.
- Pain in the anus as if constricted during stool.
- Burning in anus after a hard, dry stool.
- Frequent desire for stool, but discharge of only mucous, with chilliness of the body.
- Constant but ineffectual desire for stool.
- Horribly offensive stools.
- Stool of hard lumps evacuated only with great effort.
- Stool scanty, difficult; after great urging and straining until the abdominal walls are sore, the stool that has already protruded slips back again.
- Very hard stool, followed by burning in anus.
- Very hard, nodular stool, like clay-stones, evacuated only with great effort.
- Very hard, unsatisfactory stools, with very great effort.
- Fistula ani and fistula in ano.
- Expectoration thick, yellow, lumpy.
- Purulent expectoration when coughing.
- The right Breast is hard, painful and swollen at the nipple-it feels as if it were "gathering".
- Darting and burning pain in left nipple.
- Aversion to mother's milk: if child nurses, it vomits.
- Stiffness nape of neck, with headache.
- The Coccyx is painful, as after a long carriage ride.
- Stinging in the os coccyx, which is also painful to pressure.

- Weakness of all the LIMBS.
- Falling asleep of the hands at night.
- Finger nails rough and yellow.
- Sensation as if the tips of the fingers were suppuration.
- Pain in the left index finger as if a panaritium would form.
- Whitlow extending to tendons and bone.
- Weakness of lower extremities.
- Pain in hips.
- The knee is painful, as if too tightly bound.
- Intolerably bad, carrion like odour of the feet, without perspiration, every evening.
- Offensive perspiration on the soles and between the toes; they became quite sore while walking.
- Offensive perspiration on the feet.
- Every morning perspiration which sometimes was very profuse.
- Sense of great debility; she wants always to be lying down.
- Great weariness. Great weakness.
- Internal restlessness and excitement.
- Sensitiveness to cold air.
- He took cold very easily.
- Takes cold easily and has a cough.
- Bruised feeling over the whole body after coition.
- The whole side of the body on which he is lying is painful, as if ulcerating, with constant chilliness on the slightest uncovering: with intolerable thirst, and frequent flushes of heat in the head.
- The whole body is painful as if beaten.
- Most of the symptoms of Sil. occur at the new moon.
- Pain aggravated by motion.
- Small wounds in the SKIN heal with difficulty and easily suppurate.
- Variola-like pustules on forehead, occiput, sternum and spine: they are extremely painful, and at last form suppurating ulcers.
- Several boils come out on different parts of the body: with stinging pain when touched.

- A boil on the nape of the neck.
- Some boils on the posterior portions of the thighs.
- Frequent ulcers about the nails.
- A large corrosive ulcer, with violent itching, on the heel.
- Sore, painful scabs below the septum of the nose, with sticking pain when touched.
- Itching suppurating scabs upon the toes.
- Pressive stinging pain in the ulcerating part of the leg.
- Sticking in an ulcer on the leg.
- Restless sleep.
- Frightful dreams.
- Dreams of his youth.
- Very Chilly all day.
- Chilliness on every movement.
- Chilliness in the evening.
- Distressing sensation of chilliness in the afternoon-in a warm room. He feels very chilly even in a warm room.
- Cramp-like chill in the evening in bed, so that he shivered.
- Icy-cold shivering frequently creeps over the whole body.
- Coldness of the legs, as far as knees, in a room.
- Icy-cold feet in the evening, even in bed.
- Icy-cold feet during the menses.
- Cold feet in the evening in bed, preventing sleep.
- Fever with violent heat in the head.
- Febrile heat all night, with violent thirst and catching respiration.
- Heat of the head.
- General sweat at night.
- Profuse Perspiration every night, towards morning.
- Profuse general night sweat.
- Profuse perspiration every night, with loss of appetite and prostration, as if he would go into a decline.
- Perspiration of a strong odour.
- Sweat on the head.
- Sweat only on the head, running down the face.

- Offensive perspiration on the soles and between the toes; they become quite sore while walking.
- Offensive perspiration on the feet.
- Remedy of anticipation(Ars., Carb. v., Gels., Lyc., Medo., Plumb., Phos. ac., Arg. n., Thuj., Sil.) (p.-759).
- Complaints from anticipation-Arg. n., Ars., Gels., Lyc., Medo., Phos. ac.
- Anxiety anticipating an engagement-Arg. n., Gels., Medo.
- Anxiety when something is expected of him-Ars.
- Timidity appearing in public-Carb. v., Gels., Plumb., Sil.,
- Diarrhoea after anticipation-Arg. n., Gels., Phos. ac.
- Diarrhoea from excitement as before a Theatre-Arg. n..
- Diarrhoea from excitement-Arg. n., Gels., Phos. ac., Thuj.

SPIGELIA

I. Introduction (Cow.-713)

Synonym: Spigelia Anthelmia.
Natural Order: Loganaceae.
Common Name: Pink root.
Habitat: Annual plant in West Indies and South America.
Preparation: Tincture from freshly dried herb.
Proved by Hahnemann (Pierce-731).

II. General Analysis (Cow.)

Acts especially on the nerves on animal life and of special senses and upon fibrous and muscular tissues of eye and the heart. Sphere is usually limited to the neuralgic pains and rheumatic conditions of head, eye and heart, left sided medicine.

III. Suited to (Allen-269)

Adopted to anaemic, debilitated persons of rheumatic diathesis; scrofulous children with ascarides and lumbrici, (China, Stan.). With light hair, pale, thin afraid of sharp objects, Nervous headache left sided, at sun rise declines till sunset (Nat. m., Tab.), Pressive pain in eye balls, Mucous drops into throat.

IV. Clinical (Clarke-III-1223)

Adenoids, Amaurosis, Angina pectoris, Ciliary neuralgia, Colds, Constipation, Depression of spirits, Diaphragm-stitches in, Goitre-exophthalmic, Eyes-pains in, Gastric catarrh, Glaucoma, Headache, Heart affections, Hernia-inguinal, Iritis, Jaw-joint painful, Neuralgia, Otalgia, Post-nasal cattarh, Prostatorrhoea, Pterygium, Rectum-cancer of, Rheumatism, Scarlatina, Sigmoid flexure-cancer of, Stammering, Strabismus, Tinnitus, Tobacco-habit, Toothache, Worms.

V. **Symptoms-General** (Nash-225)

1. Violent beating of the heart, shakes the chest; sometimes audible several inches away.
2. Left side neuralgias of head, face and eyes; pains increase and decrease with the rising and setting sun; watering of the eye, on affected side.
3. Modalities: < from motion, noise, inspiration, moving eyes, cold, damp, rainy weather; rising sun; > quiet; dry air, setting sun.

VI. **Symptoms-Particular** (Nash-226-227)

1. Violent Heart action-Valuable heart remedy. (Cact., Dig.)Heart action visible through cloth and audible from few inches away (so violent).
2. Violent palpitation-can only lie on right side-(Phos., Nat. m.) or with head very high.
3. Headache-one sided generally settles in right eye-Sang., Sil.

   Left eye-Spig.
4. Headache-with rising Sun, better with sunset, clear water from eye of effected side. (Chel., right side, water gushes out).

   Spig.,
   Nat. m.,
   Tab.
5. Patient< motion, noise, inspiration or moving the eyes, esp. in cold damp rainy weather.

   Bry.,
   Kalm.,
   Nat. m.,
   Act. rac. (motion),
   Bell.-(noise),
   China. (Touch, esp., light touch).
6. Ciliary Neuralgia-Pain being same as headache.

   Act. rac.-pain presses out wards as if eye balls too short for sockets (Como.).

SPONGIA TOSTA

I. Introduction (Cow.-717)

Synonym: Spongia officinalis, Spongia Tosta.
Natural Order: Ceratos pongiae.
Common Name: Sponge.
Preparation: Tincture or Triturations from Turkey sponge.

Proved by Hahnemann who almost called it specific for goitre (Pierce-733).

II. General Analysis (Cow.)

Acts mainly upon larynx, Trachea, Thyroid gland, heart and testicles, producing irritation, inflammation, swelling and fibrous exudation. Resembles Iodine in its action on the above. (Croup-dry, barking anxious and wheezing, *Sawing* respiration with suffocative attacks).

III. Suited to (Allen-271)

Diseases of children and women with light hair, lax fibre, fair complexion (Brom.). Tubercular diathesis. Cough, dry, sibilant, like a saw driven to pine board. Mental excitement < cough: sleeps into < headache (Lach.). Croup < inspiration, anxious, wheezing < midnight (< before morning-Hep. s.).

IV. Clinical (Clarke-III-1237)

Aneurism, Angina pectoris, Asthma, Catalepsy, Chin-affections of, Clumsiness, Constipation, Cough, Croup, Diplopia, Exophthalmos, Fainting, Goitre-exophthalmic, Heart-hypertrophy of, Hernia, Jaw-joint painful, Laryngismus, Laryngitis, Myopia, Rheumatic fever, Rheumatism, Testicles inflamed, Tuberculosis, Varicosis, Whooping-cough, Worms.

V. Symptoms-General (Nash-419)

1. Croupy cough; sounds like a saw driven through a board; < on awakening out of sleep.
2. Awakens out of sleep with a sense of suffocation, with violent loud cough, great alarm, agitation, anxiety and difficult respiration.
3. Cough < talking, reading, singing, swallowing, lying with head low.

VI. Symptoms-Particular (Nash-419-421)

1. Sore: Raw: Heavy chest; action upon respiratory organs. Larynx to air cells of the lungs.
2. Cough-Awakening out of sleep, dry, sibilant, like a saw driven sound. Talking, reading, singing, lying head low evening cold air, after Acon.
3. Croup-Often after exposure to dry cold wind; in the evening with high fever, excitement, fearfulness (Acon.). When croup becomes loose, if it becomes worse after mid night-Hep. s.
4. Hoarseness in croup, soreness.
   Bell.,
   Spon.-After Bell. has acted.
5. More croupy every evening.
   Phos.
7. Chronic respiratory affections (may lead to consumption) with soreness, burning, rawness and heaviness in chest.Cough < evening, cold air, talking, singing.
   Spon.,
   Sang.,
   Sul.,
   Spon.
8. Valvular disease.
   Awakes out of sleep from a sense of suffocation with violent loud cough, great alarm, agitation, anxiety and difficult respiration (Key note 421), sleeps into paroxysm.
9. Can't lie with head low.
10. Dry, chronic, sympathetic cough of organic heart (Better than Naja).
11. Good remedy for Goitre, with sense of suffocation after sleep.

STANNUM

I. Introduction (Cow-722)

Synonym: Stannum Metallicum.
Common Name: Tin.
Preparation: Triturations. (Use not below 3x).
Proved by Hahnemann (Pierce-735).

II. General Analysis (Cow.)

Acts prominently upon cerebrospinal system giving rise in the motor sphere to profound prostration (Neurasthenia). Acts upon respiratory tract prominently, causing catarrhal inflammation and muco-purulent expectoration. Effective as vermicide or for symptoms of worms present or not.

III. Suited to (Allen-272)

Extreme exhaustion of mind and body. Sad, despondent, feels crying all times. Worse-going down stairs (Reverse-Calc. c.). Pain (headache) begins slowly subsides slowly (Plat.). Empty gone feeling in stomach. Great weakness in chest talking, laughing etc. So weak, can't talk.

IV. Clinical (Clarke-III-1244)

Anaemia, Asthma, Bronchitis, Chilblains, Colic, Consumption, Convulsions, Cramps, Debility, Dentition, Diaphragm-pains in, Dyspepsia, Ears-ring holes-ulceration of, Epilepsy, Epistaxis, Fistula lachrymalis, Gastralgia, Haematemesis, Haemoptysis, Headache, Hectic fever, Hemiplegia, Hypochondriasis, Hysteria, Lachrymal sac-suppuration of, Milk abnormal, Nails splitting, Neuralgia, Neurasthenia, Opisthotonos, Paralysis, Phthisis pituitosa, Ptosis, Sleeplessness, Styes, Tape-worm, Trachea-affections of, Uterus-prolapse of, Vagina-prolapse of, Worms.

V. **Symptoms-General** (Nash-185)

1. Sinking, empty, all-gone sensation in stomach (Chel., Phos., Sep.).
2. Sad, despondent, feels like crying all the time, but crying makes her worse; faint and weak, especially when going downstairs; can go up well enough.
3. Colic better by hard pressure, or by laying abdomen across knee or on shoulder (Coloc.); lumbrici; passes worms.
4. Leucorrhoea; great debility; weakness seems to proceed from chest.
5. Prolapsus, worse during stool, so weak she drops into a chair instead of sitting down. While dressing in the morning has to sit down several times to rest.
6. Great weakness in chest, can hardly talk, with general debility, which centers in the chest.
7. Loose cough; with heavy, green, sweet expectoration.
8. Pains gradually increase to a great height, and as gradually subside.

VI. **Symptoms-Particular** (Nash-186)

1. Weakness in the chest (Arg. m.)-so weak, can't talk. No other remedy has it so strongly. + + +
2. So weak, drops into a chair going down stairs (Bor.) > going up < going down. Brilliant cures in uterine displacements and leucorrhoea of their, debilitated subjects. Very prominent in lung, bronchial, laryngeal affection with profuse sweat.
3. Pains gradually increase and their gradually decrease (Plat.)-neuralgic pain, may be anywhere in the tract of a nerve, but often found in Prosopoplagia, abdominal colic. pains > pressure.
   Coloc.,
   Bry.
4. Feels, despondent, sad, feels like crying.
   Nat. m.,
   Puls.,
   Sep.

5. Expectoration, profuse with cough, very sweet or exceptionally salty.

   Salty expectoration -Kali i.,
   -Sep.

   Expectoration thick, heavy and green or yellow in colour-
   -Stan.,
   -Kali i.,
   -Sep.

6. Profuse night sweat.

   Stan.,

   Kali i..-but Stan. is very weak in the chest (cannot talk).

7. Another metallic remedy. The leading characteristic is great weakness in the chest (Arg. m.); so weak cannot talk. No remedy has this symptom so strongly as Stan. It is present, not only in the laryngeal and lung troubles for which Stan. is such a great remedy, but in great debility.

STAPHISAGRIA

I. Introduction (Cow.-726)

Synonym: Delphinium Staphisagria.
Natural Order: Ranuculaceae.
Common Name: Larkspur, Staves Acre.
Habitat: A plant in poor soil in South Europe.
Preparation: Tincture from ripe seeds.

It was first proved by Hahnemann (Pierce-738).

II. General Analysis (Cow.)

Acts chiefly upon genito-urinary organs, affecting especially the prostatic portion. Also affects cerebrum, digestive tract and skin. Is of great value in spermatorrhoea.

III. Suited to (Allen-274)

Mental effects of Onanism, sexual excess. Very sensitive to slightest mental exertions, least action/words offend (Ign.). Weak memory from sexual excess. Styes on eyelids, Ailments from pride and chagrin. Mechanical injuries from sharp cutting instruments.

IV. Clinical (Clarke-III-1252)

Adenoids, Anger-fits of, Anus-itching of, Backache, Bashfulness, Blepharitis, Bone disease, Cauliflower excrescences, Chalazion, Condylomata, Cough, Cysts, Dentition, Dysentery, Dyspareunia in newly married women, Eczema, Eye-tumours of, Fistula dentalis, Gastralgia, Glands-affections of, Hip-joint disease, Hypochondriasis, Impotence, Iritis-syphilitic, Jaw-easily dislocated, Lumbar abscess, Mania, Masturbation-effects of, Neuralgia, Night-sweats, Nymphomania, Ovaries-affections of, Pediculosis, Perspiration offensive, Pregnancy-nausea of, Prostate-affections of, Psoas abscess, Ranula, Rheumatism, Sciatica, Scurvy,

Sea-sickness, Seborrhoea, Self-abuse, Spermatic cords-affections of, Spermatorrhoea, Steatoma; Stiff-neck, Styes, Swallowing-constant while talking, Teeth carious, Testicles-affections of, Tibia-pains in, Tobacco-effect of, Toe-nail-ingrowing, Tonsilitis, Toothache, Tumours-tarsal, Voice-nasal; Voice-hoarse, Warts.

V. **Symptoms-General** (Nash-403)

1. Cross, ugly, scrawny, pot-bellied children; subject to colic; < after food or drink, extreme hunger even when stomach is full of food.
2. Styes, nodosities, chalazae, (a cyst on edge of eye lids), on eyelids one after another. Sometimes ulcerating.
3. Burning in the urethra when not urinating; very sensitive to slightest mental impressions; least action or harmless word offends.
4. Bad effects from sexual abuse; mind dwelling continually on sexual subjects. Teeth decay early in children; cannot be kept clean.
5. Sensation as if stomach and abdomen were hanging down, relaxed; craving for tobacco.

VI. **Symptoms-Particular** (Nash-404-406)

Leading mind remedy.

1. Mental-Very sensitive, easily offended.
   Cham.,
   Nux. v.,
   Staph.
2. Cross, ugly, irritable.
3. Affections of anger.
   Cham.,
   Coloc.,
   Staph.
4. Onanism.
   Staph.,
   Phos. ac.
5. Hypochondriacal (excessive worry).
   Anac.,
   Aur. m.,

Staph.,
Phos. ac.,
Nat. m.

6. Stomach-hanging down, relaxed as if. (Sinking) sensation.
   Staph.,
   Tab.,
   Ipec.
7. Habitual colic in scrawny, ugly, pot bellied children especially with teeth troubles and spongy gums (sensitive, painful).
8. Dysentery after least food or drink.
9. Burning in urethra when not urinating.
   (Only in this medicine, this symptom is found).
10. Backache in bed and before rising.
11. Skin very efficauous in both dry and moist Eruption.

(a) Eczema (general)-on head, sides around ears, Oozes an acrid moisture from under the scabs, new vesicles form from the contact of exudation, which itches severely, when itching is relieved by scratching then, it appears at once in another place.

(b) Eczema of eyelids.
   Graph.,
   Staph.,
   Bor.

12. Condylomata (dry warts)-cauliflower like excrescences.
13. Chronic Blepharites (Bor.).
14. Styes, nodosities, chalazae on eyelids one after another, sometimes ulcerating.
15. Incised wounds.
   Staph.-Best in surgical.
   Calend.-lacerated.
   Arn., Led., Ham. } - for bruises.
   Sul. ac., Rhus t., Calc. c. } - for strain.
   Nux. v., Calc. phos., Symp. } - for Fracture.

VII. Black Letter Symptoms

(Tyler-761-765)

- Weakness of memory; when he has read something, after a few minutes he remembers it only dimly and when he thought about anything for himself, it soon after escaped him, and after long reflection he could hardly recall it.
- Indifference, low-spirited, dullness of mind.
- Children are ill-humoured and cry for things, which after getting they petulantly push or throw away (Cham.): worse early morning.
- Great indignation about things done by others, or by himself; grieves about consequences.
- Ailments from indignation and vexation, or reserved displeasure; sleeplessness.
- Aching, stupefying pain, in Head especially in fore-head.
- As if brain compressed, especially forehead, with roaring in ears which goes off sooner than headache.
- Feels as if occiput were compressed inwardly and outwardly.
- Heaviness of head, hard pressure in head, right temporal bone and vertex.
- Pressive pain in left temple outwardly and inwardly, as if the finger were strongly pressed on it.
- Pressive boring stitch, left forehead, from within outwards, its violence wakes him from sleep in the morning.
- Sharp, burning needle-pricks in left temple.
- Obtuse shooting in right temple, outwardly and inwardly, as if the bone would be pressed out: more violent when touched.
- Painful drawing externally on several parts of head, more violent when touched.
- Itching papules on nape.
- Eyes, very dilated pupils for many hours.
- Blepharites, margins of lids dry, with hardened styes or tarsal tumours.
- Styes, nodosities, chalazae on eyelids, one after another, sometimes ulcerating.

- Pressure on upper lid: smarting sore pain in the inner canthi. (Hahnemann adds footnote—*in a man who never had anything the matter with his eyes in his life.*).
- Inflammation of white of eye with pain.
- The eyes are excessively, deeply sunk, with blue raised borders-as after great excesses.
- Tensive stich in left ear.
- Tearing and tugging from head down through cheeks into Teeth.
- Burning, sharp shooting in left cheek: must scratch.
- Teeth turn black, or show dark streaks. Gums ache.
- Gums bleed when pressed, or when brushing teeth.
- While eating, tearing in gums and in the roots of lower molars.
- Much toothache:—in decayed teeth: in a whole row of teeth; during menses, shooting into ear, worse cold drinks and touch, not from biting; from drawing in cold air; after eating.
- Toothache when eating; teeth are not firm, but when touched waggle; when eating, feels as if teeth were pressed deeper into gums-and the same when the two rows of teeth only touch one another; but the gums are white.
- Tickling pricking in right lower molars.
- Rough throat.
- Constant accumulation of mucus in mouth, without bad taste..
- Frequent hiccough.
- Adipsia; drinks less than usual.
- After indignation, cardialgia.
- Colic, after indignation; after lithotomy; with urging to stool; or urging to urinate and squeamishness < food and drink.
- Flatulence becomes displaced in hypogastrium.
- Hard painful pressure in right Abdomen below navel.
- Pinching stitch in abdominal viscera.
- Violent, twisting about, pinching pain in whole abdomen, now in one part, now in another. Hot flatus; much flatus is developed.

- Itching needle-pricks in renal region.
- Costiveness.
- The feeling as if flatus would be discharged-thin unnoticed stool occurs.
- Itching in anus while sitting, independent of stool.
- Frequent call to Urinate, when very little dark urine is discharged.
- Call to urinate; scarcely a spoonful passes, mostly reddish or dark yellow in a thin stream, or drops, and after he has passed it always feels as if the bladder were not empty, for some urine continues to dribble away.
- On awaking from sleep, pressure on the bladder.
- Every time water is passed, burning in the whole urethra.
- Violent drawing burning stitches out of whole urethra.
- Violent drawing burning stitches out of right inguinal ring, as if in the spermatic cord as far as right testicle.
- Aching pain in left testicle, when walking, and whenever rubbed; the pain is more violent on touching it.
- Effects of onanism or sexual excesses. Seminal emissions followed by great chagrin and mortification: prostration; dyspnoea.
- Frequent sneezing without coryza-or with.
- Coryza: at first blows only thick mucus from nose, afterwards thin discharge.
- Adhesive mucus lies in his Chest.
- At top of sternum, immediately below pit of throat, itching, fine sharp pricks; must scratch.
- Tightness in chest at end of coitus.
- Pricking itching between the cartilage of the ribs.
- Sharp stitches in region of fourth costal cartilage of right and left sides, intermitting-they penetrate slowly from within outwards, without relation to respiration.
- Itching pricks in both axillae.
- Pains like dislocation in right shoulder joint, only on moving.

- Obtuse shooting pains, shoulder-joint, moving and touched.
- Violent aching pain in left joint not > motion.
- Paralytic drawing pain left upper arm < touch and motion-arms weakened. Paralytic pressure on both upper and forearms, < motion and touch.
- Paralytic drawing pain in proximal joints of fingers: < by movement.
- Fine twitching tearing in muscles of thumb, and several fingers; especially in their tips.
- Deep, itching, burning, sharp needle-pricks in thumb, must scratch.
- Feeling of a hard skin drawn over finger-tips left hand: little feeling in them, and loss of sense of touch.
- Prickling itching muscles of buttocks: on inner sides of thighs.
- When walking, pain in thighs.
- Drawing shooting, or obtuse stitches in knee joint < movement.
- On touching, stitches change into an aching pain.
- Burning shooting under left knee, outer side: in paroxysms.
- Boring stitches in right tibia, when at rest.
- Tearing in muscles of one or other leg: shooting under and in right calf and above left heel.
- Pricking itching just above right outer ankle. Must scratch.
- Drawing pains here and there in the muscles of the whole body.
- Itching, sharp pricks on various parts of the body.
- Weak in body, especially knees when walking.
- Pain in all bones.
- Violent yawning, so that tears come into eyes.
- Drowsiness in afternoon, so that eyes close.
- Amorous dreams and seminal emissions.
- In the night often wakes with chilly feeling, but cannot properly collect himself.
- Shivering and chilly feeling when eating, without thirst.

- Indisposed for serious work.
- Incised wounds.
- And stretched sphincters should be added.

STICTA PULMONARIA

I. Introduction (Cow.-731)

Synonym: Lichen Pulmonarius.
Natural order: Lichenes.
Common Name: Lung wort. Lung Moss.
Habitat: Grows on trunks of large trees in mountainous counties of UK etc.
Preparation: Tincture from fresh Lichen, grown on sugar maple.

It was first proved by Dr. SP Burdick of USA in 1864 (Pierce-741).

II. General Analysis (Cow.)

Acts upon mucous lining of respiratory tract and produces symptoms of catarrhal character.

III. Clinical (Clarke-III-1265)

Angina pectoris, Anus-pain in, Asthma, Bronchitis, Catarrh, Clergyman's sore throat, Colds, Cough, Diabetes, Diaphragm-rheumatism of, Diarrhoea, Glands swollen, Hay-fever, Headache, Housemaids' knee, Hysteria, Influenza, Laryngitis, Levitation, Measles-cough of, Migraine, Milk scanty, Neuralgia, Ozaena, Phthisis, Post-nasal catarrh, Pott's disease, Rheumatism, Seminal emissions, Sick headache, Sleeplessness, Syphilis.

IV. Symptoms-General (Nash-381)

1. Heavy full feeling, and pain and pressure in forehead and foot of the nose > by discharge.
2. Secretions in the nose dry up and form crusts; constant inclination to blow the nose, without result, on account of the excessive dryness.
3. Dry night cough; can't sleep or lie down; must sit up; cough after measles (Coff.).

V. Symptoms-Particular (Nash-381-383)

1. Acute catarrh-One of the best medicines. + + +
2. Pain and pressure in forehead and root of nose with coryza or dry clinkers.
   Stict.,
   Kali bich.-(Frontal headache).
3. Acute nasal catarrh.
   Stict.,
   Acon.,
   Amm. c.,
   Camph.,
   Nux. v.,
   Samb.,
   Amm. c.,
   Lyc.—Chronic catarrah (not as fluent watery as in Euph., Merc. c., Kali hydro.),
   Ars.—thick, bland as in-Puls., Sep., Kali s.).
4. Cough: < night keeps awake (more due to nervousness) < lying.
   Stict.,
   Coff. > Sleeplessness due to cough. (Coff.-wonderful here).
5. Inflammatory rheumatism of knee joint-Stict.
6. As if in the air, not resting on bed (hysterical).
   Stict.,
   Asar.,
   Valer.
7. Severe frontal headache at root of nose with suppressed catarrh.
   Kali bich.,
   Stict.

SULPHUR

I. Introduction (Cow.-739)

Synonym: Flores Sulphuris.
Common Name: Brimstone. Flowers of Sulphur.
Preparation: Trituration of pure sublimed Sulphur.

Hahnemann proved Sulphur for homeopathy initially with 151 symptoms and gradually added up to 1989 symptoms (Pierce-748).

II. General Analysis (Cow.)

Acts especially upon ganglionic nervous system and through it, entire vegetative sphere penetrating deeply every recess of human body. Chief local action is upon the skin, producing various forms of eruption, most noted being an itching, vesicular formation resembling scabies or itch and other kindred affections of the skin. It affects lymphatic or glandular system, mucous membranes especially of eye, bronchi, urethra, rectum, and the portal system. Allen says (Pierce) "since Sul. is an integral part of every form of protoplasm, all tissues become affected by its abnormal exhibition, and no particular limit or clear action can be assigned to it". Sul. may be indicated in any disease regardless of its character or the tissue involved. Its chief use is in chronic disease. It can be prescribed as an inter current medicine many times, even when its main symptoms are absent, both in acute and chronic diseases, to arouse the reactive energies of the system, when carefully selected medicines fail to produce favourable effect. This power of Sul. depends upon its relation to Hahnemann's *Psora*-one of the three miasmas identified by Hahnemann standing between carefully selected medicine and its favourable effect (Cow.-749).

III. Suited to (Allen-279)

Nervous temperament, quick motioned and quick tempered, plethoric. Skin very sensitive to atmospheric changes (Hep. s., Kali c., Psor.) Lean, stoop shouldered persons who walk and sit stoop, standing worst position. Dirty filthy people, prone to skin affections. Aversion to bath, after bath child kicks cloths in the night. Can't be washed (Cold water-Ant. c.). Standing is the worst position. Complaints return annually or continually relapsing. Suppressed eruption-result of when carefully selected medicine fail, complaints continually return. Constant heat on vertex-with feet cold in daytime-burning in sole in night (Medo.). sensation of burning. Diarrhoea-painless after midnight, drives out of bed every early morning (Aloe., Psor.).

IV. Clinical (Clarke-III-1299)

Acne, Adenoids, Ague, Alcohol habit, Amaurosis, Amenorrhoea, Anaemia, Anus-prolapse of, Asthma, Atelectasis, Bed-sores, Biliousness, Boils, Brain-congestion of, Breasts-affection of, Bright's disease, Bronchitis, Cataract, Catarrh, Chagres fever, Chancre, Cheloid, Chest-pains in, Chilblains, Chloasma, Climaxis-sufferings of, Colds, Constipation, Consumption, Corns, Cough, Crusta serpiginosa, Diabetes, Diarrhoea, Dysentery, Dysmeno-rrhoea, Ear affections, Eczema, Emaciation, Enuresis, Epilepsy, Eructations, Eruptions, Eye affections, Faintness, Feet burning; perspiring, Fever, Fistula dentalis, Freckles, Ganglion, Glands-affections of, Gleet, Globus hystericus, Gonorrhoea , Gout, Haemorrhoids, Headache, Head-rush of blood to, Herpes, Hip-joint disease, Hydrocele, Hydrocephalus, Hydrothorax, Hypochondriasis, Impotence, Influenza, Intermittents, Irritation, Itch, Jaundice, Laryngitis, Leucorrhoea, Lichen, Liver disorder, Lumbago, Lung affections, Lupus, Mania, Measles, Memory weak, Meningitis, Menstruation disordered, Miscarriage, Molluscum, Nettlerash, Neuralgia, Nipple sore, Nose-bleeding of; inflammation of, Oesophagus-constriction of, Ophthalmia-acute; scrofulous; rheumatic, Pelvic haematoccle, Phimosis, Phlegmasia albs dolens, Peritonitis, Pleurisy, Pneumonia, Pregnancy-affections of, Prostatorrhoea, Rectum-affections of, Rheumatic fever, Rheumatism-acute; chronic; gonorrhoeal, Ringworm, Sciatica, Self-abuse, Sinking, Skin-affections of, Sleep disordered, Smell-illusions of, Spinal irritation, Spine-curvature of, Spleen-pain in, Starting, Stomatitis, Taste-illusions of, Tenesmus, Thirst, Throat-mucus in, Tongue coated, Tonsilitis, Toothache, Trachea-irritation in, Ulcer, Urticaria, Uterus-prolapse of, Vaccination, Varicocele, Varicosis, Vertigo, Warts, White swelling, Worms, Worry, Yawning.

V. **Symptoms-General** (Nash-64)

1. Hahnemann's king of anti-psorics; combating all psoric manifestations, as described in Hahnemann's chronic diseases.
2. Itching eruption on skin everywhere; scratching is followed by burning.
3. Burning everywhere, general and local, especially feet; has to stick them out of bed to cool them.
4. Redness of all orifices, as if pressed full of blood (lips, ears, nostrils, eyelids, anus, urethra etc.).
5. Exudations into serious sacs following acute inflammations.
6. Weak, faint, after hot flashes, followed by sweat, especially at 11 AM.
7. Modalities: < 5 AM. (diarrhoea), standing; 11 AM. close room. open Air, bathing, cold damp weather > doors and windows open, sitting or lying.

VI. **Symptoms-Particular** (Nash-64-71)

1. King of anti Psorics, (Psor., Caust., Graph., etc.).
2. ITCHING, BURNING, REDNESS-lips, ears, nostrils, eyelids, arms, urethra etc.
3. < 11 AM.
4. When best selected medicines fail then Sul. (Psor.)
5. Burning—Everywhere and anywhere:

   Ars., Phos., Sul.—lead burners in Homeopathy.
   Sul.—leader in chronic affections.
   Ars.—Leader in acute affections.

(*Others are: Acon., Canth., Agar., Caps., Apis., Bell., Phos. ac.*).

6. Local or chronic congestions (local) (action upon circulation) Boils, swellings, felons, abdominal or portal congestions/inflamations. "Feels so oppressed that he wants all doors etc. open" (chest congestion).
7. All orifices are Red as if full of blood (lips vermilion red such as) esp. after suppression or retrocession of skin eruption or trouble.
8. Power of absorption, after the stage of effusion has set in or results of inflammatory process are to be gotten rid of.

   Bry.—one of the best remedies.
   Kali m.,
   Sul.—when Psora. has intervened.
9. Skin—most positive and persistent action. Voluptuous Itching with or without eruption, burning.—Pushes everything internal on the surface.
10. "Dirty, filthy people, prone to skin affections".
11. "Children can't bear to be washed or bathed".
12. "Voluptuous itching; scratching relieves; after it, burning".
13. "Complaints continually relapsing".
14. "Congestion to single parts".
15. "Pain in heart, extending to back".
16. "Scrofulous(Psoric) chronic disease that result from suppressed Eruption".
17. "Discharges from every outlet acrid, excoriating and reddening".
18. "Offensive odour of body despite frequent bathing".
19. "Hot flushes with spells of faintness, or debility passing off with a little moisture, faintness or debility".
20. "Weak, faint spells frequently during the day".
21. "Burning in feet, wants to find a cool place for them; puts them out of bed to cool them off". (Cham., Medo., Sanic.).
22. "Feels suffocated; wants doors and windows open, particularly at night".
23. "Diarrhoea after midnight; painless, driving out of bed early in the morning, as if the bowels were too weak to retain their contents".

24. "Weak, empty, gone or faint feeling in stomach about 11 AM".
25. "White tongue with very red tip and borders".
26. "Bright redness of lips as if the blood would burst through". (Tuberc.).
27. "Heat on crown of head; cold feet; frequent flushing".
28. Particularly efficacious with lean stoop shouldered persons, who walk or sit stooped-standing is the most uncomfortable position.

VII. Black Letter Symptoms (Tyler-786-792)

- Foolish happiness and pride, thinks himself in possession of beautiful things; even rags seem beautiful.
- Indisposed to everything, work, pleasure, talking or motion; indolence of mind and body.
- Melancholy mood; dwelling on religious or philosophic speculations; anxiety about soul's salvation; indifference about lot of others.
- Too lazy to rouse himself up, and too unhappy to live.
- Hypochondriasis after suppression of eruption.
- Dread of being washed (in children).
- Heat on crown of Head; cold feet; frequent flushing.
- Brain affections in children who do not like to be washed, have pimples, boils and other Eruption on head, face and everywhere, pick at nose, have red lips, crave sour things, feel faint in forenoon, may have diarrhoea early in morning; sleep restless, start when falling asleep, cry out during sleep, or murmur, whine, moan or snore; feet cold in morning, hot in evening; they run about but do not like to stand, sit hunched and walk stooping.
- Severe itching on forehead and scalp.
- Itching pimples on forehead; inflamed, painful to touch.
- Inflamed and suppurating pimples on hairy scalp.
- Humid, offensive eruption on top of head, filled with pus, drying up into honey-like scabs.

- Dry, offensive, easily bleeding, burning eruption, begins on back of head and behind ears; pains and cracks; > from scratching.
- Humid, offensive eruption, with thick pus, yellow crusts, bleeding and burning.
- Dimness of vision; as of a veil or gauze before Eyes; as from a fog; with headache; as if cornea had lost its transparency; sudden paroxysms of nyctalopia; while reading; objects seem more distant; for near and distant objects; with weakness of eyes, blindness, cataract, glaucoma; with innumerable, confused, dark spots floating before eyes.
- Keratitis parenchymatosa in a scrofulous subject, cornea like ground glass, photo phobia, lids swollen and bleed easily.
- Burning heat in eyes; painful smarting.
- Lachrymation; in morning, followed by dryness; and burning in morning; profuse and burning from acrid, excoriating tears; in open air, dry in room; itching and biting in eyes.
- Deafness; preceded by over-sensitiveness of hearing; especially for human voice; from disposition to catarrhs; < after eating or blowing nose.
- Otitis; in psoric patients with tendency to skin Eruption, coryzas, and cerebral congestion; from a furuncle in meatus; in children who suddenly cry out in pain, while they appear listless and unobservant and where it seems doubtful whether irritation is in brain or in intestinal canal; in complication with meningitis or eruptive Fever; lancinating, stinging, tearing in ear, extending to head and throat, < by disturbance, musical sounds, and all noises and human voice is heard imperfectly; chronic with a purulent discharge.
- Smell before nose as an old catarrh; as of old offensive mucus.
- Frequent sneezing.
- Swelling and inflammation in nose; red nose.
- Face: painful eruption about chin.
- Bright redness of lips, particularly with children, complexion sallow.

- Lips dry, rough and cracked.
- Toothache: coming on in open air; from least draught, at night in bed; from washing with cold water; with congestion to head, or stitches in ear.
- Stomacace; aphtha.
- Dryness of Throat; exciting cough; at night; constant desire to swallow saliva in order to moisten affected parts.
- Stitches in throat on swallowing; painful contraction.
- Swelling of palate and tonsils, elongation of palate.
- Appetite: excessive; canine; ravenous, obliged to eat frequently, if he does not he has a headache and great lassitude, and has to lie down; feeling of faintness with strong craving for food at 11 AM ; voracious children put everything they see into mouth, swallow everything, watch everyone eating.
- Drinks much, but eats little.
- Desire for sweets; diseases from eating sweet things, candy, etc.
- Desire to imbibe alcoholic drinks, from morning until night.
- Drinks much, eats but little.
- Weak, empty, gone or faint feeling in stomach about 11 AM.
- Heaviness in stomach; feeling of weight.
- Inflation of Abdomen with wind; rumbling and gurgling in bowels.
- Emission of flatus; especially in evening and night; having odour of bad eggs, or sulphurated hydrogen; inodorous.
- Rumbling and gurgling in bowels; painless diarrhoea, driving patient out of bed at 5 AM.
- Big belly and emaciated limbs; children disliked to be washed.
- Portal stasis; haemorrhoids, congestions; with indigestion,constipation etc.
- Sudden call to Stool on walking in morning.
- Desire to stool, with colic, awakes him about 5 AM.
- Thin stool every morning, with cutting in lower abdomen.

- Diarrhoea after midnight; painless, driving out of early in morning; as if bowels were too weak to retain their contents.
- Dysentery: child was faint regularly at 11 AM; early morning aggravation.
- Cholera asiatica; as a prophylactic, a pinch of the powdered milk of sulphur worn in stockings in contact with soles of feet; diarrhoea commence between midnight and morning, with or without pain, with or without vomiting, ineffectual desire to evacuate; diarrhoea and vomiting at same time; numbness of limbs; cramp in soles of feet and calves; blueness under eyes; coldness of skin; indifference of mind; during convalescence, red spots, furuncles, etc.; susceptibility to temperature, warm things feel hot; nerve symptoms.
- Burning and pressure in rectum.
- Itching in rectum.
- Increased congestion of haemorrhoidal vessels.
- Haemorrhoids, moist, blind, or flowing dark blood, with violent bearing-down pains from small of back towards anus.
- Suppressed haemorrhoids, with colic, palpitation, congestion to lungs, back feels stiff as if bruised.
- Large haemorrhoids, violent burning and sticking in anus; pressing in rectum during and after stool; it feels full.
- Burning in anus; after sitting a while; after soft stools in evening.
- Constant bearing down towards anus; forcing down after sitting.
- Itching in anus. Bleeding from anus.
- Excoriation about *URETHRA*.
- Itching in urethra.
- Both flow of urine and discharge of faeces are painful to parts over which they pass.
- Involuntary discharge of semen, with burning in urethra.
- Testicles relaxed, hanging down; soreness and moisture of scrotum, or offensive sweat of genitals.

- Itching on glans penis.
- Discharge of prostatic fluid after micturition and stool.
- Soreness and moisture of scrotum; soreness between thighs when walking.
- Foetid perspiration on genital organs, with soreness and excoriation destroying most of hair, painful in walking, with thickening and induration of scrotum.
- Hot flushes at climacteric period, with hot head, hands and feet and a great goneness in stomach.
- Burning in vagina, scarcely able to keep still.
- Troublesome itching of vulva with pimples.
- Feels hungry and Faint about 11 AM ; cannot wait for dinner.
- Shortness of breath; and oppression on bending arms backward; from talking too much; when walking in open air; in evening in bed.
- Feels suffocated; wants doors and windows wide open; particularly in night.
- Oppression, heaviness and pressure and pressure in Chest.
- Burning in chest, rising to face.
- Shooting in left side of chest through to back.
- Stitches through chest, extending into left scapula; < lying on back and during least motion.
- Congestion of blood to chest.
- Pleurisy: (after Acon.) acute, plastic form.
- Rush of blood to Heart.
- Palpitation: anxious; in evening in bed; and fluttering of heart; without anxiety, at any time of day; during stool; violent at night, on turning in bed; violent and rapid on falling asleep; when going upstairs or when climbing a hill; visible.
- Sensation as if heart were enlarged.
- Sharp stitches in pericordial region.
- Sharp pain at heart going through chest, to between shoulders; especially with dyspeptic symptoms.
- Great orgasm of blood, with violent burning in hands.

- Pain in small of Back; could not walk erect, was obliged to walk bent over; violent only on stooping, tensive as if everything were too short; on rising from a seat; gnawing; after heavy lifting and taking cold at same time; violent, as if bruised, also in coccyx; tiresome feeling as if bruised; stitches.
- Curvature of spine, vertebra softened.
- Rheumatic pains in Shoulder, especially in left.
- Perspiration in armpits, smelling like garlic; offensive to patient.
- Tremulous sensation in Hands when writing; cold trembling hands.
- Burning of hands.
- Rhagades on hands, esp. between fingers, on finger joints and in palms.
- Stiffness in Knees and cracking.
- Cramp in calves and soles, particularly at night; looseness of bowels.
- Stiffness of ankle joints.
- Burning in feet, wants to find a cool place for them; puts them out of bed to cool them off.
- Burning in soles; on stepping after sitting a long time; and itching, especially on walking; wishes to find a cool place for them, puts them out of bed; wants them uncovered.
- Weak, fainting spells frequently during day; feels very faint and weak, with a strong craving for food, from 11 to 12 every morning.
- Excessively sensitive to open air and will not be washed; very much inclined to take cold.
- Chorea; in chronic disease, particularly after suppressed Eruption; frequent spasmodic jerking of whole body; tremor of hands; unsteady walk; peevish, irritable, obstinate; faint and hungry spells at 10 AM ; soles of feet burn.
- Irresistible drowsiness in day time, wakefulness at night.
- Wakes up at 3, 4 or 5 AM and cannot sleep again.
- Heavy, un-refreshing sleep.
- Finds himself at night lying on his back.

- Nightmare.
- Dreams: vivid, anxious, as if pursued by wild beasts; vivid, comic, with loud laughter, continued for some time after walking; vivid, believing she sits on chamber causes her to wet bed; horrible, with great palpitation, that he has bitten by a dog; that he is falling.
- Wants doors and windows open.
- Orgasm of blood; frequent flushes of Heat.
- Flushing heat in face, with febrile shivering over whole body.
- Heat in head; prevents falling asleep; in morning; in evening with cold feet.
- Hot flushes, with spells of faintness, or passing off with a little moisture, faintness or debility.
- Complaints continually relapsing.
- Alternate: pale and red cheeks; diarrhoea and constipation; asthma or gout and skin Eruption.
- Offensive odour of body despite frequent washing; averse to washing.
- Does not walk erect; stoops or bends over forward in walking or sitting; standing is most disagreeable position.
- Scrofulous chronic disease that result from suppressed eruption.
- Discharges in every outlet of body acrid, excoriating skin wherever they come in contract.
- Congestion to single parts; eyes, nose, chest, abdomen, arms, legs, etc.
- Complaints are continually relapsing; seems to get almost well when disease returns.
- Itching: all over body; spots painful after scratching; itching spots bleed & bite after scratching; in various parts, disappearing after scratching; at times followed by sticking or burning; over whole body, recurring every night in bed; and biting on nates; violent on thighs and legs, at night; about knees; on toes; of toes that had been frozen; at night, in heat of bed, now in one place, now in another, especially on nape of neck; in palms of hands, sometimes sticking, burning; is obliged to rub them,

after which they burn; on backs of hands; in eyebrows; on abdomen, at night; in scrotum; on inside of thighs; in axillae and hollows of knees; as if she were alive beneath skin; as if vermin were running about; < at night, and in morning, in bed after waking; above left eyebrow; in ears externally; of nose externally; about chin; on neck; on chest; of old tetter, is obliged to scratch until it bleeds.

- Burning in skin of whole body.
- Formication of skin over whole body.
- Voluptuous itching; scratching relieves after it; burning; some times little vesicles.
- After violent scratching aching, numbness of skin, swelling of skin, even ulceration.
- Nettle rash; with fever; on face, arms, neck and lower extremities on back of hand.
- Itching hives over whole body, hands and feet.
- Boils.
- Skin rough, scaly, scabby.
- Soreness in folds of skin.
- Comedoes; black pores of skin, particularly in face.
- Lean, Stoop-shouldered persons who walk and sit stooped; standing is the most uncomfortable position.
- Persons of nervous temperament, quick-motioned, quick-tempered, ple-thoric, skin excessively sensitive to atmospheric changes.
- Dirty, filthy people, prone to skin affections.
- Children; cannot bear to be washed or bathed; emaciated, big bellied; rest-less, hot, kick off clothes at night; have worms.
- Adapted to persons of scrofulous diathesis, subject to venous congestion, especially of portal system.

SULPHURIC ACID

I. Introduction (Cow.-751)

Synonym: Hydrogen sulphate.
Common Name: Sulphuric Acid.
Preparation: Diluted in water for 1x and 2x; 3x and above with dilution in Alcohol.

It was first proved by Hahnemann (Pierce-748).

II. General Analysis (Cow.)

Acts upon mucous tissue, especially of alimentary canal, respiratory tract and upon skin.

III. Suited to (Allen-282)

Light haired, old people, especially women, flushes of heat in climacteric years, not willing to answer because of inaptness rather than obstinacy. Always in hurry (Ars.). Pain builds up gradually ceases suddenly. Child sour smelling. (Hep. s., Mag. c, Rhe.); Black blood from all outlets of body (Croc., Mur. ac., Nit. ac., Tereb.).

IV. Clinical (Clarke-III-1327-1328)

Acidity, Alcoholism-chronic, Aphthae, Back-stiffness of, Bowels-looseness of, Brain-concussion of, Breath offensive, Cancer, Cancrum oris, Chafing, Chilblains, Climaxis-sufferings of, Constipation, Corns, Diabetes, Diarrhoea, Diphtheria, Dyspepsia, Erythema nodosum, Flushing, Gangrene, Gastralgia, Glossitis, Hair-grey; falling out, Heartburn, Hernia-inguinal, Hiccough, Impotence, Intermittents, Irritation, Liver-affections of, Menorrhagia, Metrorrhagia, Myopia, Nightmare, Oesophagitis, Paralysis-lead, Perspiration profuse, Phthisis, Pneumonia, Pregnancy-sickness of, Purpura, Rheumatism, Scurvy, Spleen-affections of, Sterility, Ulcer, Uterus-prolapse of, Vagina-prolapse of, Varicosis, Warts.

V. **Symptoms-General** (Nash-248-249)

1. Extreme weakness, with sense of internal trembling, which is not observable to others.
2. Haemorrhage from every outlet of the body, with ecchymosed spots under the skin.
3. Child smells sour all over, despite actual cleanliness, sour, acid vomiting.
4. Adopted to the light haired, old people, especially women; flushes of heat in climacteric years.
5. Aphthae, of mouth, gums, or entire buccal cavity, gums bleed readily; ulcers painful; offensive breath. Bad effects from mechanical injuries, with bruises, chafing and livid skin; prostration.
6. Sensation as if the brain was loose in forehead and falling from side to side (Bell., Bry., Rhus t., Spig.). Often very useful in the stomach troubles of old whiskey topers.

VI. **Symptoms-Particular** (Nash-249-250)

1. Sour vomit, stool and smell, with aphthous mouth.
2. Sour vomit and sour Eructation, sour stomach.
   Sul. ac.,
   Iris v.,
   Rob.
3. Sour smell despite greatest of cleanliness.
   Sul. ac.,
   Rhe.,
   Hep. s.,
   Mag. c.
4. Sense of internal trembling (not observable) often found in old topors.
   Sul. ac.-subjective, very distressing.
   Ran. b.
5. Black and Blue spots (ecchymosis) of the skin.
   Sul. ac.,
   Led.,
   Amm. c.
6. Haemorrhage from every outlet (Purpura Haemorrhagica) of the body, blood also settles in ecchymosed under the skin.

Crotal. h.,

Sul. ac.-Hence useful in Black and blue spots in the skin.

Acet. ac.,

Thlaspi.,

7. Flashes of heat due to Sulphur, useful when Sul. fails in flushes of heat at the climacteric.
8. Follows well Arn., Led., for ecchymosis "black-eye" from injury.

   (Rut.-for bruises of periosetum).

TABACUM

I. Introduction (Cow.-754)

Synonym: Nicotiana Tabacum.
Natural Order: Solanaeae.
Common Name: Tobacco.
Habitat: Native of Central America but cultivated widely.
Preparation: Tincture from dried leaves of the genuine Havana tobacco.

Proved by Nening, one of Hahnemann's provers (Pierce-761).

II. General Analysis (Cow.)

Acts especially upon pneumogastric nerve and medulla oblongata, producing complete relaxation and paralysis of involuntary muscular system causing nausea, vomiting, vertigo etc. secretions of intestinal mucous membrane increased. Its chief expression is deathly nausea accompanied by pallor, vertigo, cold sweat and intermittent pulse.

III. Suited to (Allen-287)

Dim-sighted, sees as through a veil, face pale, blue, pinched sunken; collapsed icy coldness of surface, covered with cold sweat (on forehead-Verat.). Symptoms occur in paroxysm, asthma, sick headache, vertigo on opening eyes, sneezing, sudden pain on right side of head. Violent vomiting with cold sweat. Vomiting, violent, on beginning to move, during pregnancy (Lactic. ac., Psor.) Seasickness < by least motion, > on deck in fresh cold air.

IV. Clinical (Clarke-III-1356)

Amaurosis, Anaemia, Angina pectoris, Anus-prolapse of, Apoplexy, Asthma, Backache, Brain-anaemia of, Brain-fag,

Catalepsy, Cholera, Cholera infantum, Colour-blindness, Constipation, Diarrhoea, Epilepsy, Freckles, Glands enlarged, Heart intermittent, Hernia, Hiccough, Idiocy, Leg-jerking of, Lip-cancer of, Masturbation-effects of, Meniere's disease, Oesophagus-constriction of, Optic neuritis, Pregnancy-pruritus of; sickness of; toothache of, Prostatorrhoea, Pruritus, Pyrosis, Rectum-paralysis of; stricture of, Sea-sickness, Speech embarrassed, Strabismus, Tetanus, Toothache, Varicocele.

V. **Symptom–Particular** (Nash)

1. Vertigo with nausea, esp., on opening the eyes. (153).
   —Vertigo on closing eye-lach, thrya.
   —Vertigo on looking of word (Pul, Sil)
2. Headache—One Sides, < with riesing. of sun, > with its going down (Tab, Nat. m)— (226)
3. Icy coldmen of surface, covered with cold sweat (Tab, Hell. n.) (264)
4. Stomach–Searation as if it were hauging down relaxed. (404)

TARENTULA

I. Introduction (Cow.-758)

Synonym: Lycosa Tarentula.
Natural Order: Araneideae.
Common Name: Tarentula
Preparation: Triturations of the live spider.

II. General Analysis (Cow.)

Acts especially upon cerebrospinal system, causing restlessness and great mental and physical depression. Choreic phenomena more prominent than sexual excitement. Used in nymphomania, dysmenorrhoea, menstrual irregularities. Chief use is in Chorea, hysteria, hystero-epilepsy; diseases of female sexual organs.

III. Suited to (Allen-289)

Highly nervous organism, especially Choleric (emotional hostess), affections where whole body or right arm and left leg are affected (left arm, right leg-Agar.). Constant movement of the legs, arms, trunk with inability to do anything. Cannot keep quite in any position, restless. Through walking < all symptoms (Reverse of Rhus t., Rut.).

IV. Clinical (Clarke-III-1372)

Angina pectoris, Callosities, Chorea, Coccygodynia, Cornea-opacity of, Cystitis, Depression of spirits, Diphtheria, Dysmenorrhoea, Epistaxis, Erotomania, Fibroma, Headache, Hiccough, Hysteria, Intermittents, Kleptomania, Levitation, Locomotor ataxy, Mania, Meniere's disease, Migraine, Onanism, Ovaries-enlargement of, Paralysis agitans, Physomet, Proctalgia, Pruritus pudendi, Quinsy, Septic diseases, Spinal irritation, Spinal sclerosis, Tumours, Uterus-cancer of; neuralgia of, Vertebrae-tumours of.

V. Black Letter Symptoms

(Tyler-800-802)

- Great excitement caused by music; one hour after it, general and copious perspiration.
- Paroxysms of insanity; strikes head, pulls hair, complains; threatens, scratches herself, restlessness, her clothes annoy her; restless legs, threatening words of destruction and death: comes out of attack with severe headache, eyes wide and staring.
- Sees small fingers hovering before her eyes.
- Hysteria with bitter belching.
- They sing, dance, cry, extreme gaiety.
- Ludicrous and lascivious hysteria; had to be restrained by force.
- Vision of monsters, animals, frighten him; of different things not present, faces, insects, ghosts.
- Feigned paroxysms; feigns fainting and insensibility; looks sideways to observe the effect on those around her.
- Taciturn, irritable, desire to strike himself and others.
- Extreme disposition to laugh and joke.
- Laughs, runs, dances, gesticulates, sings till hoarse and exhausted.
- Sadness, grief, moral depression are not only the almost constant symptoms of the sting, but are present, in a striking manner, during different provings of the medicine.
- Fear which could not be stopped; tried to find a cause and leaves others to think there is one; really there was none.
- Constant fear that something would happen to prevent my finishing a thing; would start and hastily change my position, through fear that something would fall on me; walking, would stop and throw head to one side, through fear of striking against some imaginary object suspended a few inches above my head.
- Great desire to be alone, with fear of being alone.
- Changeable mood; from gaiety to sadness; from fixed ideas to uneasiness of mind.

- Does not understand questions; does not know the persons she sees every day: can't say her prayers.
- Fits of nervous laughter; desire to joke, play, laugh.
- Extreme gaiety.
- Great excitement caused by music; later general, copious sweat.
- Sudden fox-like destructive efforts, requiring utmost vigilance to prevent damage; followed by laughter and apologies.
- Threatening words of destruction and death.
- Suddenly sprang away from attendants, swept ornaments from mantel-piece; said she was sorry but could not help it.
- Very mischievous and destructive, amusing and cheerful.
- Attacks of hystero-mania daily about the same hour: first quarrelsome and despondent, suddenly a state of great exaltation hits and abuses everyone, destroys whatever she can lay hold of, tears her cloths, laughs and sings; mocks aged people with their age; if restrained becomes violent; attacks and in a comatose sleep.
- Jumps form bed, destroying whatever she could get hold of; so quickly that she could not be prevented.
- Headache as if a quantity of cold water were poured on head and body.
- Intense headache, as if thousands of needles were pricking brain.
- Pain in occiput, as if struck by a hammer, extends to temples.
- Burning, scorching heat in occiput.
- Pain in right maxillary nerve, with tickling sensation in stomach. It seems as if a living body were moving or tingling in the stomach, with tendency to ascend to throat.
- Diabetes—constant craving for raw articles, disgust for meat; polyuria.
- Involuntary micturition when coughing, laughing, making any effort.
- Precordial anxiety, tumultuous beating of heart.

- Pain, shooting pain in heart and arteries of left chest, extending to left arm; the contact with dress is very painful.
- Tumours about the vertebral column.
- Strange fancies in regard to colours.
- Anguish of heart if they see an unpleasant colour.
- Angina pectoris.
- Precordial anxiety; tumultuous beating of heart; trembling and thumping, as if form a right.
- Precordial anguish; movement of heart not felt. Constant want of air. heart ceases to beat and patient fears to die.
- Right pupil much dilated, left contracted. Loss of vision in right eye, till dilated, pupil contracted.
- Face expressed terror.
- Face pale earthy, contrasting with nearly purple neck.
- Burning and sweat in pelvis of hands.
- Pain in lower jaw as if all the teeth were going to fall out.
- Onanism; violent nymphomania,
- Intense, unbearable puritis vulvae.
- Terrible pruritis, as of insects creeping and crawling.
- Outer parts, as if worms or insects were boring and crawling.
- Itching, burning, formication, ecchmosed spots, Painful vesicular and especially pustular Eruption.

TEREBINTHINA

I. Introduction (Cow.-760)

Synonym: Oleum Terebinthinae.
Common Name: Oil of Turpentine.
Preparation: Dilution on decimal scale.
Proved by Dr. Scidal of Germany (Pierce-763).

II. General Analysis (Cow.)

Acts chiefly upon the kidneys, producing, irritation inflammation and congestion together with haematuria and albuminuria. It affects mucous membranes of bronchia and intestines, producing cough and loose bloody stools, but more especially of mucous lining of bladder and urethra, causing inflammation and strangury.

III. Suited to (Allen-291)

Urinary problems with urine having odour of violets. Tongue glossy, red. Haematuria-thoroughly mixed with urine. Sediments-coffee ground, cloudy albuminous, profuse, dark, painless.

IV. Clinical (Clarke-III-1393)

Albuminuria, Amblyopia potatorum, Asthma, Backache, Bladder irritable, Brachial neuralgia, Bronchitis, Chordee, Chorea, Ciliary neuralgia, Cystitis, Dentition, Dropsy, Dysentery, Dysmenorrhoea, Enteric fever, Epilepsy, Erysipelas bullosa, Erythema, Fibroma, Gall-stone colic, Glands-inguinal; swelling of, Gleet, Gonorrhoea, Haematuria, Haemorrhoids, Hernia strangulated, Herpes labialis pudendi, Hydrophobia, Hypochondriasis, Insanity, Intestines ulcerated, Iritis, Jaundice, Kidneys-congestion of; neuralgia of, Lumbago, Neuralgia-supraorbital, Ovaries-pains in; dropsy of, Pityriasis, Purpura haemorrhagica, Scabies, Scarlatina,

Sciatica, Spermatorrhoea, Strangury, Stricture, Tetanus, Tympanites, Uraemia, Urine-suppression of; retention of, Worms.

V. Symptoms-General (Nash-311-312)

1. Burning and smarting on passing urine; urine red, brown, black or smoky in appearance.
2. Tongue smooth, glossy, red, with excessive Tympanites (typhoid).
3. Haemorrhage from all outlets, especially in connection with urinary or kidney trouble.

VI. Symptoms-Particular (Nash-312)

1. Urinary-more strangury and blood in urine than Berb. v.
2. First stage of albuminuria-burning, smarting in passing Urine
   Canth.,
   Cann. sat.,
   Tereb.,
   Berb. v. (Second stage-Merc. c..)
3. Anti Haemorrhagic remedy, especially in typhoid, purpura haemorrhagica.
4. Smoky Urine
   Hell. n.,
   Colch.,
   Lach.,
   Apis.
   Dropsy after scarlatina with.
5. With glossy red tongue.
   Crotal. h.,
   Pyr.,
   Tereb.
6. Haematuria, haemaptysis and haemorrhage from bowels, especially in typhoid. (acts splendid).

VII. Black Letter Symptoms (Tyler-811-812)

- Tongue remains dry, with abdominal tension; after cleansing becomes dry again with increase of Tympanites (Inflammation of eardrum).

- Tongue does not clean gradually but rapidly and in large flakes first form middle, leaving tongue smooth and glossy.
- Distension of abdomen: feeling of, as from flatus.
- Meteorism, excessive Tympanites, abdomen sensitive.
- Haemorrhage from bowels with ulceration;epithelial degeneration passive.
- Violent drawing pains in the region of kidneys.
- Albuminuria; early stages when blood and albumen abound more than casts and epithelium.
- Sensitiveness of hypogastrium, tenesmus of bladder.
- Violent burning and cutting in bladder, alternating with a similar pain in umbilicus; < at rest; > when walking in open air.
- Urine scanty and bloody, burning in urethra.
- Strangury; spasmodic retention of urine.
- Frequent urination at night, with intense burning and pain in small of back.
- Urine cloudy and smoky, bloody; clear, watery, profuse.
- Haematuria. Urine black, with coffee-ground sediment.
- After scarlatina; passes small quantities of dark, sweet smelling urine, turbid and having a sediment like coffee-grounds; sometimes mind dull, or patient drowsy, even in a stupor; dropsy; urine though rich in albumen and flood, contains few if any casts.
- Metritis and peritonitis puerperalis, with tendency to mortification; lochia checked, terrible burning in uterus, abdomen fuller than usual; headache with thirst; brown dry tongue, nausea and vomiting; distended abdomen, sore to touch: pulse smell, frequent.
- Bronchial catarrh and pneumonia in typhus.
- Haemorrhage from lungs.
- Malarial and African Fever.-Prostration.-Purpura haemorrhagica.
- Congestion and inflammation of viscera; kidneys, bladder, lungs, intestines and uterus.

- Ascites with Anasarca.
- Scarlatina, esp. when kidneys are involved, with stupor, bloody, smoky urine.

THERIDION CURASSAVICUM

I. Introduction (Cow.-764)

Synonym: Theridon Curassevicum. Aranya,
Class: Araneideae.
Natural Order: Araneideae.
Common Name: Orange Spider, Black Spider of Curacoa.
Preparation: Tincture from live spider.

II. General Analysis (Cow.)

Acts upon cerebrospinal system, giving rise to headaches, vertigo, neuralgia, accompanied by gastric disorders, due to reflex action.

III. Suited to (Allen-292)

Persons whose time passes too quickly (too slowly-Arg. n., Cann. ind., Nux. m.), Vertigo-on closing eyes. (Lach., Thuj. on opening them)-from least noise. Headache-dull behind eyes, least motion. Every sound seems to penetrate the whole body, causing nausea and vertigo.

IV. Clinical (Clarke-III-1410)

Angina pectoris, Anthrax of sheep, Bone affections, Caries, Climaxis, Cough, Dysmenorrhoea, Eye-teeth-pains in, Fainting, Headache, Hysteria, Liver-disorder of; abscess of, Meniere's disease, Nausea, Necrosis, Nose-cattarrh of, Ozaena, Photophobia, Phthisis florida, Pregnancy-sickness of, Rickets, Scrofulosis, Sea-sickness, Spinal irritation, Tetanus, Toothache, Vertigo.

V. Symptoms-General (Nash-153)

1. Vertigo, with nausea, on closing the eyes, or the least noise.

2. Over-sensitiveness of nerves; scratching on linen or silk, or paper is unbearable.
3. Pain running through upper left chest to shoulder.

VI. Symptoms-Particular (Nash-153-154)

1. Vertigo with nausea esp. on closing eyes-Lach., Thuj.
   -on opening-Tab.
   -on looking upward-Puls., Sil.
   -from least noise. Every Sound seems to penetrate through whole body, causing nausea and vertigo-Asar.
2. Over sensitiveness of nerves-even scratching of linen, crackling of paper.
   Ferr.,
   Tarax.
3. Vertigo occurs in different affections of head or stomach, and cures thewhole trouble when present, vertigo on looking up (Puls., Sil.); on lying down turning head (Con.)
4. One of the best medicines in Rachitis, Caries, Necrosis.

THUJA OCCIDENTALIS

I. Introduction (Cow.-766)

Synonym: Thuja Occidentalis.
Natural Order: Coniferae.
Common Name: Arbor Vitae
Habitat: An indigenous evergreen tree in North USA and Canada.
Preparation: Tincture from the fresh leaves.
Proved by Hahnemann (Pierce-765).

II. General Analysis (Cow.)

Acts chiefly upon genito-urinary organs, anus, and the skin, producing irritation, changing secretions to acid corroding character and destruction of tissues. Chief action is—wart like excresences upon mucous and cutaneous surfaces, resembling fig warts and condylomata which characterize the sycotic poison.

III. Suited to (Allen-294)

Hydrogenoid constitution of Gramuogl, related to sycosis. Ailments: bad effects of vaccine from (Ant. tar., Sil.); from suppressed and mal-treated Gonorrhoea (Medo.). Strange ideas as if a person were at his side. Vertigo when closing eyes (Lach., Tereb.). White scaly dandruff, hair dry, falling out. Headache: as if a nail driven into parietal bone (Coff., Ign.). Fig warts, Condylomata, wart like excrescences.

IV. Clinical (Clarke-III-1419)

Abdomen distended, Abortion, Angina pectoris, Anus-fistula of; fissure of, Asthma, Balanitis, Cancer, Catalepsy, Chorea, Clavus, Condylomata, Constipation, Convulsions, Coxalgia, Diarrhoea, Dyspareunia, Dysmenorrhoea, Ear-polypi of, Enuresis, Epilepsy, Epulis, Eyes-tumours of;

granular inflammation of, Fatty tumours, Feet foetid, Flatus incarcerated, Frontal sinuses-catarrh of, Ganglion, Gleet, Gonorrhoea, Haemorrhage, Haemorrhoids, Hair-affections of, Headache, Hernia, Herpes zoster, Ichthyosis, Intussusception, Jaw-growth on, Joints-cracking in, Levitation, Morvan's disease, Mucous patches, Muscoe volitantes, Myopia, Naevus, Neck-cracking in, Onanism, Ovary-left-pain in, Ozaena, Neuralgia, Nose-chronic catarrah of; polypi of, Paralysis, Pemphigus, Polypi, Post-nasal catarrh, Pregnancy-imaginary, Prostate-disease of, Ptosis, Ranula, Rheumatism-gonorrhoeal, Rickets, Sciatica, Seminal emissions-nocturnal, Sycosis, Syphilis, Tea-effects of, Teeth carious, Tongue-ulcers of; biting of, Toothache, Tumours, Vaccination, Vaccinosis, Vaginismus, Warts, Whooping-cough.

V. **Symptoms-General** (Nash-400)

1. Hahnemann's chief anti-sycotic.
2. Proliferations or pathological vegetations; condylomata, polypi, warts, sycotic excrescences, etc.
3. Bad effects following vaccination; never well since.
4. Especially suited to the treatment of ailments following suppressed gonorrhoea.
5. Urethritis in sycotic patients which Cann. sat. does not relieve; stream split, cutting after urination; discharge thick.
6. Sweat only on uncovered parts.
7. Modalities: < cold, damp air (Hydrogenoid); after vaccination excessive, tea drinking, extension of limbs; > drawing up limbs.

VI. **Symptoms-Particular** (Nash-400-403)

1. Chief anti sycotic miasma medicine (Sulphur-chief anti-psoric) (Nit. ac., Staph., Sabin., Cinnab. etc.-other medicines).
2. Anti syphilitic-Mercury.
3. Nose discharge-Thick green (Puls.).
4. Stool recedes after partial expulsion.

Sanic.,
Sil.,
Thuj.

5. Anus fissured. Condylomata (dry warts)
   Ant. c.,
   Graph.,
   Sil.,
   Thuj.
6. Peculiar mental symptom—fixed ideas as if some other person were at his side, as if limbs were made of glass, as if a living animal in the abdomen.
7. Headaches of sycotic origin, with various symptoms; white dandruff, hair falling off or grow slowly and splits; eyelids bear styes, chalazae, tarsal tumours, or condylomata; ears inflame, discharge pus, or grow polypi, Nose discharges thick, green mucous like Puls., or scabs are formed in it; warts on outside of nose or eruption on its wings; face has greasy or shiny look; teeth begin to decay at roots as soon as they come, the crowns remaining sound. Ranula under the tongue, or varicosities in the mouth or throat; a great deal of croaking, rumbling and grumbling in the abdomen, as if of an animal crying; abdomen puffed and big, protruding here and there as if from the arm of a foetus, or of something alive; constipation of hard black balls; chronic; stools large; and stool recedes after being partially expelled (Sanic., Sil.); or diarrhoea forcibly expelled, copious gurgling like water from a bung hole of a barrel; diarrhoea, especially from the effects of vaccination; anus fissured or surrounded with condylomata (Ant. c., Graph. and Sil.); ovarian troubles; asthma; nails brittle, distorted, crumbling, misshapen or soft; warts, condylomata, bleeding fungous growths; noevi; epithilioma, and many other affections in sycotic subjects.

VII. Black Letter Symptoms (Tyler-828-829)

- Nervous, sycotic or syphilitic headaches.
- White, scaly dandruff; hair dry and falling out.

- Ophthalmia neonatorum.
- Condylomata at *Anus.*
- Anus fissured, painful to touch, often with warts, sometimes immense numbers of flat, most, mucous tubercles or condylomata surround anus, especially in syphilitic subjects.
- Prostatic affections form suppressed or badly treated gonorrhoea.
- Gonorrhoea: scalding when urinating, urethra swollen; urinal stream forked; discharge yellow, green, watery; with warts, red erosions on glans; sub acute and chronic cases, especially when injections have been used and prostate is involved.
- Condylomata, mucous tubercles, sycotic cauliflower excrescences; fig-warts, smelling like old cheese or herring brine.
- Warts, condylomata and other excrescences about vulva.
- Condylomata moist, suppurating, stinging and bleeding.
- *Sleeplessness*; sees apparitions on closing eyes; parts lain on painful, from heat and restlessness; from mental depression; after re-vaccination.
- Wart-like excrescences on back of hand, on chin and on other places.
- Warts and condylomata, large, seedy and pedunculated; sometimes oozing moisture and bleeding readily.

TRILLIUM PENDULUM

I. Introduction (Cow.-771)

Synonym: Trillium Pendulum.
Natural Order: Trilliaceae.
Habitat: An indigenous plant growing in rich soils, damp, rocky and shady woods, in USA. (Middle, Western states).
Preparation: Tincture from fresh roots.
Proved by Hahnemann.

II. General Analysis (Cow.)

Acts upon the mucous membrance of capillary blood vessels, especially of uterus causing both active and passive haemorrhage. (From Nose, bleeding gums, stools with pure blood, cough with bloody sputum. Bright red haemorrhage. (Hoering in Pierce).

III. Suited to (Allen-297)

Women especially at climacteric, menses profuse, *every too weeks*, lasting a week or longer, haemorrhage both active and passive, usually bright red-from nose, lungs, kidneys and uterus (Ipec., Mill.).

IV. Clinical (Clarke-III-1452)

Bladder—catarrh of, Climaxis, Diabetes, Dysentery, Fainting-with flooding, Fibroma- Haemorrhage from, Haemorrhage- post-partum; ante-partum, Menorrhagia, metrorrhagia, Writer's cramp.

TUBERCULINUM BACILLINUM

(Nosode) (a disease product)

A glycerine extract of a pure cultivation of tubacle bacilli (human) (Clarke-III-1460).

I. **Suited to** (Allen-298)

Persons of light complexion, blue eyes, tall, slim, flat chest, active and precocious mentally, physically weak, tubercular diathesis when best selected medicines fail with tuberculosis family history. Takes cold easily without knowing how and where, losing flesh while eating well (Abrot., Calc. c., Con., Iod., Nat. m.). Symptoms ever changing. Emaciation rapid and pronounced. Melancholia. Ailments affecting one organ then another; beginning suddenly ceasing suddenly.

II. **Clinical** (Clarke-III-1460)

Acne, Albuminuria, Appendicitis, Asthma, Bones-caries of, Bronchitis, Catarrhal pneumonia, Chilblains, Corneaopacity of; ulceration of, Dentition, Erysipelas, Erythema, Haematuria, Haemoptysis, Headache, Heart-affections of; palpitation of, Influenza, Leprosy, Leucorrhoea, Lungs-oedema of, Lupus, Mania, Menses too early, Nephritis, Night-terrors, Oedema glottidis, Paralysis, Phthisis, Pleurisy, Pneumonia acute, Tuberculosis.

III. **Symptoms-General** (Nash-425)

1. Cosmopolitan; never satisfied to remain in one place long; wants to travel.
2. Wandering pains in limbs and joints; stiff when beginning to move; < standing, > continued motion.
3. Longs for open air, wants doors and windows open, or to ride in strong wind.

4. Takes fresh cold on least exposure, can't get rid of one before another comes.
5. Emaciation even while being well, and so hungry must get up nights to eat.
6. Pain through left upper lung to back, tubercular deposit begins there.
7. Persons with a history of tuberculosis in the family.
8. Symptoms ever changing, begin suddenly, ceasing suddenly.

IV. Symptoms-Particular (Nash-425-426)

1. Late menses with Tuberculosis history when Puls. fails, then Tuberc.
2. Hydrocephalus (water in brain) with TB history in family-Tuberc.
3. Symptoms ever changing from one organs to other (Allen-299)
4. Symptoms begin suddenly, cease suddenly.
5. Takes cold easily.
   Hep. s.,
   Tuberc.
6. Suited to both incipient as well as advanced cases of Phthisis.
7. Tuberc. ranks with Psor. in chronic diseases.
8. Ailments with history of Tuberculosis.

VALERIANA

I. Introduction (Cow.-776)

Synonym: Valerina officinalis.
Natural order: Valerianaceae.
Common Names: Valerian. All heal.
Habitat: A herbaceous plant of Europe and Asia.
Preparation: Tincture from the dried root.

Proved by Hahnemann but his followers developed it. (Pierce-774)

II. General Analysis (Cow.)

Through cerebrospinal system it affects directly the nervous centres, producing a high degree of irritation, pain and spasm resembling hysterical character, most important feature of this remedy. Sciatica pain: < standing, > walking.

III. Suited to (Allen-300)

Excessive nervous excitability, hysterical nervous temperament (Ign., Puls.), persons with predominant intellectual faculties. Changeable disposition. As if floating in the air (Asar., Lac can., Stict.). Red parts become white (Ferr.).

IV. Clinical (Clarke-III-1496)

Asthma-spasmodic; nervous, Bed-sores, Change of life, Clairvoyance, Coxalgia, Headache, Heart-palpitation of, Heels-pain in, Hypochondriasis, Hysteria, Levitation, Neuralgia, Sciatica, Sleeplessness, Toothache.

V. Symptoms-Particular (Nash-458)

1. General nervous irritation.
2. Can't keep still, tearing pains and cramp in different places.

3. Feels as if floating in air (Stict.-legs floating).
4. Sensation of a thread hanging down throat.
5. Sciatica-pain < standing and letting foot rest on floor.
6. Over-sensitiveness of all senses.

VERATRUM ALBUM

I. Introduction (Cow.-778)

Synonym: Helleborus Albus.
Natural Order: Melanthaceae (Liliaceæ).
Common Name: White Hellebore. European Hellebore.
Habitat: Perennial herbaceous plant of Europe, and of Asiatic Russia.
Preparation: Tincture from dried root.
Proved by Hahnemann (Pierce-776).

II. General Analysis (Cow.)

Through cerebrospinal nervous system, it acts upon the nutrition system affecting entire vegetative sphere, giving rise to choleric conditions, general coldness, prostration, collapse, copious watery vomiting and purging, spasmodic colic, cramp, rigid contraction of muscles, cold clammy profuse perspiration. It also affects sensorium but to a less degree choleric condition as above is the chief feature of this remedy.

III. Suited to (Allen-302)

For children and old people who are habitually deficient in vital heat and are habitually cold. Young people of a nervous, sanguine temperament. Diseases with rapid sinking of vital forces complete prostration, collapse. Cold perspiration on forehead (entire body-Tab.) nearly in all complaints.

IV. Clinical (Clarke-III-1507)

Amenorrhoea, Anaemia, Anasarca, Angina pectoris, Apoplexy, Asthma, Bronchitis, Cholera asiatica, Cholerine, Colic, Collapse, Constipation, Coprophagia, Cramps, Debility, Diaphragm-affections of, Diarrhoea, Dysmenorrhoea,

Emphysema, Epilepsy, Fainting, Gastric catarrh, General paralysis, Headache-sick, nervous, Hernia, Hydrocephaloid, Hysteria, Influenza, Intermittent fever, Intussusception, Labour-constipation after, Lips cracked, Liver-hyperaemia of, Lockjaw, Lungs-oedema of, Mania, Measles, Mendacity, Melancholia, Meningitis, Menstruation-nausea before; diarrhoea before, Neuralgia palpebralis, Nyctalopia, Oesophagus-constriction of, Peritonitis, Pernicious fevers, Plica polonica, Pneumonia, Pregnancy-imaginary, Ptosis, Pyaemia, Rheumatism, Salivation, Scarlatina, Sleep-whining in, Spleen swollen, Sternum, Throat, Toothache, Typhoid fever, Vertigo, Water-brash, Whooping-cough, Yellow fever.

V. Symptoms-General (Nash-262)

1. Collapse, with general coldness and cold sweat, especially on forehead; hippocratic face.
2. Mania, with desire to cut and tear things, with lewdness, lascivious talk, religious or amorous.
3. Disposed to silence, but if irritated gets mad, scolds, calls names and talks of faults of others.
4. Rice water stools, profuse, exhausting, cramp in calves, coldness collapse.
5. Rheumatic affection, < in damp weather, drives patent out of bed.
6. The pains are maddening, driving the patient to delirium.
7. Copiousness of discharges: stools, vomiting, urine, saliva, sweat; craving for acids or refreshing things.

VI. Symptoms-Particular (Nash-262-264)

1. Strong mental mania.
2. Cold sweat on Forehead (key) skin, hand, feet, back, whole body.
3. Cholera asiatica.
   - Camph.,
   - Cupr.,
   - Verat.
4. Silent, but violent when provoked-Cupr.

5. Collapse—"Rapid sinking of forces, complete prostration, cold sweat and cold breath".
   —"Skin blue, purple, cold, wrinkled, remaining in folds, when pinched".
   —"Face hypocratic (Sunken); nose pointed".
   —"Whole body icy cold".
   (Icy coldness of body covered with cold sweat-Tab.)
6. Cramp in calves.
7. Grand key-note: "Cold sweat on face and forehead".
8. Stools-Profuse in Verat.. (scanty in Camph.)
9. Face-Bloated, very red-Stram. } Both very loquacious and religious
   -Sunken, pale -Verat. } and also at times violent.

VII. Black Letter Symptoms

(Tyler-853-856)

- Persistent raging.
- Inconsolable over a fancied misfortune, runs about the room howling and screaming, looking upon the ground, or sits brooding in a corner, wailing and weeping in an inconsolable manner.
- Taciturnity.
- Crossness, when cause given.
- Attacks of pain with delirium, driving to madness.
- Mania with desire to cut and tear everything, especially clothes with lewdness and lascivious talk: religious or amorous.
- Delusions of grandeur.
- Cold sweat on forehead with anguish and fear of death.
- Despair of salvation with suppressed catamenia.
- His consciousness is as if in a dream.
- Flat-pressing headache, vertex: which became throbbing when moving.
- Sensation of a lump of ice in vertex.
- Cold sweat on forehead.
- Pale face: sunken: with anxious expression.
- He became pale in the face with frequent stools.

- He can't speak.
- Saliva runs incessantly out of mouth like water brash.
- Tasteless saliva want of taste in mouth.
- Taste and coolness in mouth, as from peppermint.
- Pungent peppermint taste in throat: sensation of heat rises into the mouth.
- Thirst for coldest drinks, craves ice; fruit.
- Violent hunger, excessive thirst during perspiration.
- Great thirst with hunger.
- Great nausea before vomiting.
- Violent vomiting of slimy, acid liquid, with food.
- Forcible, excessive vomiting.
- Vomiting and diarrhoea as many as ten times, with pale sunken face, covered with cold seat.
- Vomiting of green mucous.
- Gastric catarrh, great weakness; cold, sudden sinking.
- Colic, as if intestines twisting into a knot.
- Cold feeling in abdomen.
- Colic with burning, as if intestines twisted into a knot, with cold sweat.
- Cutting pains; flatulent colic, which attacks the lower bowels here and there and the whole abdomen: the longer the flatus is retained the more difficult it is to be expelled.
- Diarrhoea with profuse perspiration.
- Frequent and violent diarrhoea: very profuse and painful.
- Excessive evacuations; copious evacuations.
- Constipation on account of the hardness and size of the evacuations.
- Cholera morbus: worse at night: cold sweat on forehead; vomiting and purging at the same time, after fruits; profuse brownish discharges; thirst: Cramp prostration: cold sweats: great weakness after stool.
- Cholera asiatica—violent evacuations upwards and downwards: icy coldness of body; cramp in caves. Vomiting with constant desire for cold drinks: face

colourless or bluish: blue margins round eyes: deathly anguish in features: cold tongue and breath: great oppressive anguish in chest, with desire to escape from bed: violent colic, especially about umbilicus, as if abdomen would be torn open. Sensitive to contact, drawing and cramp, wrinkled skin in palms, retention of urine.

- Palpitation of heart with great anxiety and quickened audible respiration.
- Excessive anxiety that takes away the breath.
- Spasmodic constriction of larynx with contracted pupils.
- Suffocative attacks of constriction in larynx.
- Deep hollow cough in three or four shocks.
- Seems in danger of suffocation, the respiration is so restricted.
- Cold breath (in cholera).
- Hands icy cold, blue, blue nails.
- Rheumatic pain, felt when moving.
- Very great difficulty of walking, like paralysis, first right then left hip-joint.
- Pain under knee, as if bone had been broken and was not quite firm.
- Heavy pain of legs, as from fatigue.
- Prostration and weakness of the whole body: extreme weakness.
- Syncope, yawning, paralytic sinking of strength.
- Whole body and face pale.
- Chill and shivering with frequent stools.
- Febrile chill with coldness and thirst.
- Creeping coldness through whole body.
- Cold skin.
- Creeping coldness over head, especially vertex. "Lump of ice" sensation, vertex.
- Face cold, collapsed.
- Coldness back: extremities cold, Great coldness of hands.
- Cold sweat, cold sweat on forehead. Profuse perspiration on forehead with the evacuation.
- Cold perspiration over whole body.

- Typhoid forms of fever when vital forces sink: cold sweat: coma.
- Vomiting and watery diarrhoea: bluish face: pointed nose: wrinkled skin.
- Internal chill ran through him from head to toes of feet with thirst.
- Heat and redness of face.

VERATRUM VIRIDE

I. Introduction (Cow.-784)

Synonym: Helonias Viridis.
Natural Order: Melanthaceae (Liliaceae)
Common Names: American white Hellebore, Indian Poke, Swamp Hellebore.
Habitat: A coarse plant in wet meadows and swamps in Canada to Georgia.
Preparation: Tincture from fresh root.

Proved by Dr. Bort and by Dr. Hale (Pierce-779).

II. General Analysis (Cow.)

Acts upon cerebro-spinal system especially pneumogastric nerve, producing profound paralysis of cerebro-spinal nerve and other nerve centres, causing congestion of brain and other organs like stomach and lungs. Thus it differs from Bell. and other congestants by exciting nerve centres rather than by paralysis. Chief action upon heart and circulation indicated by loud strong heart beat, quick pulse.

III. Suited to (Allen-305)

Full blooded plethoric persons. congestion especially to base of brain. Violent pains, attending inflammation. Cerebro-spinal diseases, convulsion-dim vision, child on verge of spasm.

IV. Clinical (Clarke-III-1520)

Amaurosis, Amenorrhoea, Apoplexy, Asthma, Bunions, Caecum-inflammation of, Chilblains, Chorea, Congestion, Convulsions, Diplopia, Diaphragmitis, Dysmenorrhoea, Erysipelas, Headache-nervous; sick, Heart affections, Hiccough, Hyperpyrexia, Influenza, Malarial fever, Measles,

Meningitis, Menses suppressed, Myalgia, Oesophagus-spasm of, Orchitis, Pneumonia, Proctalgia, Puerperal convulsions, Puerperal mania, Sleep dreamful, Spine-congestion of, Spleen congested, Sunstroke, Typhoid fever, Uterus-congestion of.

V. Symptoms-General (Nash-260)

1. A narrow, well developed red streak right through middle of the tongue.
2. Intense fever, with twitching and tendency to spasms.

VI. Symptoms-Particular (Nash 260-262)

1. It should not be used to control or depress the pulse as it can have bad effects injurious to patient. Quick pulse. Slows down (Dig.).
2. Peculiar symptom is a narrow well defined red streak right through middle of the tongue (characteristic).
3. One of the best medicines for spasm, twitching and convulsions.

VII. Black Letter Symptoms (Tyler-861)

- Quarrelsome and delirious.
- Dilated pupils.
- Face flushed. Dry mouth, and lips, dry all day.
- Tongue somewhat red in centre.
- Tongue (coated yellow) with red streak in centre.
- Tongue: white or yellow, with red streak down middle; dry or moist, with white or yellow coating or no coating on either side.
- Feels scalded.
- Vomiting.
- Menstrual colic, with dysmenorrhoea; much nausea and vomiting; plethora; cerebral congestion.
- Pneumonia, pulse hard, strong, quick, engorgement of lungs, with faint feeling in stomach, nausea, vomiting: or slow or intermittent pulse.
- Congestion, especially to base of brain, chest, spine and stomach.
- Pain and soreness just above the pelvis.

VIBURNUM OPULUS

I. Introduction (Cow.-789)

Synonym: Viburnum Edule.
Natural Order: Caprifoliaceae.
Common Name: Cranberry tree. Sheep's Berry. Snowball, High Cranberry.
Habitat: A shrub growing in low grounds along streams in the USA.
Preparation: Tincture from the fresh bark of the root.
First provings made by Dr. H. C. Allan (Pierce-783).

II. General Analysis (Cow.)

Through cerebro-spinal system its main action is upon female generative organs.-Congestive neuralgic dysmenorrhoea.

III. Clinical (Clarke-II-1535)

After-pains, Cough-of pregnancy, Cramps, Dysmenorrhoea-spasmodic; neuralgic; membranous, Ears painful, Epididymitis, Headache, Hysteria, Labour-false pains of, Lumbago, Menstruation painful, Miscarriage, Ovaries-pain in, Paralysis, Uterus-cramps in; bearing down in.

IV. Symptoms-Particular (Nash-209-210)

1. Pain beginning in the back, going around in the locus and to the uterus, ending in Cramp there, a sign of impending abortion.
2. Neuralgic dysmenorrhoea:
   Act. rac. (back),
   Cham. (unbearable),
   Caul. (intermittent, spasmodic),
   Mag. phos. > (hot applications to hypogastruim).
3. Medicine of undoubted value in painful womb troubles.

V. Black Letter Symptoms
(Tyler-864-865)

- Dull frontal headache.
- She has cramping colic pains in lower abdomen, almost unbearable.
- Pains come suddenly and with terrible severity.
- Before menses: severe bearing down; drawing in anterior muscles of thigh; heavy aching in sacral region and over pubes; occasional sharp, shooting pains in ovaries; they make her so nervous that she can't sit still, excruciating, cramping, colicky pains in lower abdomen and through womb. Pains begin in back and go around, ending in cramp in uterus.
- During menses: nausea; cramping pain and great nervous restlessness, flow ceases for several hours, then returns in clots.
- Menstrual flow scanty, thin, light-coloured, with sensation of lightness of head, faint when trying to sit up. Spasmodic, or membranous dysmenorrhoea.
- Leucorrhoea thin, yellow-white or colourless, except with stool, when it is thick white, blood-streaked.
- Neuralgic and spasmodic dysmenorrhoea.
- Pain beginning in back and going round to loins and across pubic like labour pains.
- Cramp like colic pain in lower abdomen (during menses).
- Irritable ovaries, with dysmenorrhoea.
- Cramp-like pains and spasms of stomach, bowels, bladder or other organs, when reflex from uterine irritation.
- Cramp in abdomen and legs of pregnant women.
- Will prevent miscarriage if given before the membranes are injured, and when the pains are spasmodic and threatening.
- General irritation of nervous system.
- Cramp and contractions of extremities, especially during pregnancy.
- Hysterical Convulsion from uterine irritation.

ZINCUM

I. Introduction (Cow-795)

Synonym: Zincum Metallicum.
Common Names: Zinc, Spelter.
Preparation: Triturations.

Franz, a follower of Hahnemann, proved this remedy (Pierce-786).

II. General Analysis (Cow.)

Acts prominently upon cerebro-spinal system producing erethism in the brain, medulla oblongata and spinal cord; marked by delirium, spasms, neuralgia tremors and cerebral depression and exhaustion of nerve centres (Paralysis most important characteristic of this drug). In blood it produces anaemia.

III. Suited to (Allen-306)

Cerebral and nervous exhaustion nerve power wanting. Must move lower limbs to avoid fidgety feeling. Menses; with flow all complaints cease, but return after flow ceases. Child cries during sleep whole body jerks during sleep wakes up frightened, starts, rolls head from side to side. Repeats everything said to him.

IV Clinical (Clarke-III-1583)

Alcoholism, Amblyopia, Asthma, Brain-fag, Brain-paralysis of, Breasts-affection of, Cataract, Chilblains, Chin-eruption on, Chlorosis, Cholera, Chorea, Constipation, Cracks, Dentition, Diarrhoea-nervous; with stupor, Diphtheria, Dysentery, Dysuria, Earache, Eczema, Enuresis, Eruptions suppressed, Eyes-affections of; granular lids, Fag, Foot-sweat suppressed, Gastralgia, Headache-nervous; chlorotic, Heels-pain in, Hernia-inguinal, Hiccough, Hydrocephalus,

Hyperpyrexia-nervous, Hypochondriasis, Hysteria, Inflammatory pain, Joints-creaking in, Lips-affections of, Lochia suppressed, Malar bones-neuralgia in, Masturbation, Memory weak, Meningitis, Mind-weakness of, Milk-defective; suppressed, Neuralgia-intercostal; subcostal, Neurasthenia, Nipple sore, Nose-redness of, Nymphomania, Oesophagus-spasm of, Otorrhoea, Photopsia, Prostatorrhoea, Ptosis, Reaction defective, Rheumatism, Screaming, Sleepiness, Somnambulism, Spermatorrhoea, Spinal irritation, Spinal affections, Spleen-neuralgia of, Strabismus, Suppressions, Tarsal tumours, Throat sore, Tibia-burning in, Typhoid fever, Ulcer, Urine-hysterical retention of, Varicosis-during pregnancy; of external genitals, Whooping-cough, Worms.

V. **Symptoms-General** (Nash-181)

1. Inability to develop or hold out the rash in eruptive diseases, can't expectorate or menstruate, is > if can.
2. Can't take stimulants, as they aggravate, in general.
3. Fidgety feet, must move them constantly.
4. Twitching of single muscles all over the body.
5. Violent trembling all over, so as to shake the bed; lost nerve control.
6. Weakness and weariness in nape of the neck; < holding head long in one position; backache < sitting.
7. Modalities: < from wine; > by restoration or development of eruption, during menses, resored expectoration, seminal emission, discharges generally.
8. Defective vitality, brain and nerve power wanting; to comprehend, to memorise.
9. Child cries out during sleep; rolls the head from side to side; face alternately pale and red,

VI. **Symptoms-Particular** (Nash-181-185)

1. "What iron is to the Blood, Zinc. is to the nerves".
2. Better by development of eruption.

   Zinc.—never comes to surface due to lack of vitality.

   Cupr.—has been suppressed due to some out ward cause.

3. This weakness shows else where also.
   Can't expectorate } better if can.
   Can't menstruate } (Lach. > during menses).
4. He can't take wine or stimulants.
5. If taken < all sufferings. (Glon., Led., Fluor. ac., Ant. c. etc.).
6. Aching and weariness in the nape of the neck < in one position too long.
7. Backache < sitting > moving about (Rhus t., but general aching is not relieved by motion in Zinc.).
   Puls. has it but only in menstrual irregularities. (Cobalt).
8. General nervous weakness is further reflected in the "Violent, incessant fidgety feeling in the lower limbs; must move than constantly".
9. "Burning in the whole length of spine".
10. General trembling—Zinc. is one of the best remedies.
11. Brain troubles with Zinc. symptoms.

LIST OF REMEDIES

(ABBREVIATIONS and SIGNS)

Abbreviations.	***Names of Medicines.***
Abrot.	Abrotanum
Acet. ac.	Acetinum acidum glaciale
Acon.	Aconitum napellus
Act. rac.	Actæa racemosa
Æsc. hip.	Æsculus hippocastanum
Æth. c.	Æthusa cynapium
Agar.	Agaricus muscarius
Agn. cast.	Agnus castus
Ail.	Ailanthus
All. c.	Allium cepa
Amm. c.	Ammonium carbonicum
Amyl nit.	Amyl nitrosum
Anac.	Anacardium orientale
Angust.	Angustura vera
Anthrac.	Anthracinum
Ant. c.	Antimonium crudum
Ant. tar.	Antimonium tartaricum
Apis	Apis mellifica
Apocy.	Apocynum cannabinum
Apom.	Apomorphia
Aran.	Aranea diodema
Arg. m.	Argentum metallicum
Arg. n.	Argentum nitricum
Arn.	Arnica montana
Ars.	Arsenicum album
Arum t.	Arum triphyllum
Asa.	Asafoetida
Asar.	Asarum Europeum
Ast. r.	Asterias rubens
Aur. m.	Aurum metallicum

Balsam	Balsamum Peruvianium
Bap.	Baptisia
Baryt. c.	Baryta carbonica
Bell.	Belladonna
Bellis	Bellis perennis
Benz. ac.	Benzoicum acidum
Berb. v.	Berberis vulgaris
Bism.	Bismuthum
Bor.	Borax
Bov.	Bovista
Brom.	Bromium
Bry.	Bryonia alba
Bufo	Bufo rana
Cact.	Cactus grandiflorus
Calad.	Calcadium
Calc. c.	Calcarea carbonica
Calc. phos.	Calcarea phosphorica
Calc. s.	Calcarea sulphuris
Calend.	Calendula
Camph.	Camphora
Cann. ind.	Cannabis indica
Cann. sat.	Cannabis sativa
Canth.	Cantharis
Caps.	Capsicum
Carb. a.	Carbo animilis
Carb. v.	Carbo vegetabilis
Caul.	Caulophyllum
Caust.	Causticum
Cedr.	Cedron
Cham.	Chamomilla
Chel.	Chelidonium majus
Cheno.	Chenopodium anthelminticum
Chim.	Chimaphila umbellata
China.	Cinchona officinalis
Cic. v.	Cicuta virosa
Cimicif. r.	Cimicifuga racemosa
Cinchona rub.	Cinchona rubra
Cinnab.	Cinnabaris
Cistus	Cistus canadensis

Clem.	Clematis erecta
Cobalt	Cobaltum
Coca	Erythroxylon coca
Cocc.	Cocculus Indicus
Coc. cact.	Coccus cacti
Coff.	Coffea cruda
Colch.	Colchicum
Collin.	Collinsonia
Coloc.	Colocynthis
Como.	Comocladia dentata
Con.	Conium
Cop.	Copaiva
Coral. r.	Corralium rubrum
Croc.	Crocus sativus
Crotal. h.	Crotalus horridus
Crot. t.	Croton tiglium
Cupr.	Cuprum metallicum
Cycl.	Cyclamen
Dig.	Digitalis
Diosc.	Dioscorea villosa
Diphth.	Diphtherinum
Dolichos.	Dolichos pruriens
Dros.	Drosera rotundifolia
Dulc.	Solanum dulcamara
Elap.	Elaps corallinus
Eup. perf.	Eupatorium perfoliatum
Eup. purp.	Eupatorium Purpureum
Euph.	Euphrasia
Ferr.	Ferrum
Ferr. ac.	Ferrum aceticum
Ferr. mur.	Ferrum muriaticum
Ferr. phos.	Ferrum phosphoricum
Fluor. ac.	Fluoricum acidum
Gamb.	Gambogia
Gels.	Gelsemium
Glon.	Glonoinum

Gnaf.	Gnaphalium
Graph.	Graphites
Grat.	Gratiola
Grind.	Grindelia squarrosa
Ham.	Hamamelis
Hell. n.	Helleborus niger
Helod.	Heloderma
Helon. d.	Helonius dioica
Hep. s.	Hepar sulphuris
Hydras.	Hydrastis cenadensis
Hydrocy. ac.	Hydrocyanicum acidum
Hyo.	Hyoscyamus niger
Hyper.	Hypericum perfoliatum
Ign.	Ignatia
Iod.	Iodum
Ipec.	Ipecacuanha
Iris v.	Iris versicolor
Jal.	Jalapa
Jatr.	Jatropha curcas
Kali bich.	Kali bichromicum
Kali brom.	Kali bromatum
Kali c.	Kali carbonicum
Kali chlor.	Kali chloricum
Kali i.	Kali iodatum
Kali m.	Kali muriaticum
Kali n.	Kali nitricum or Nitrum
Kali s.	Kali sulph
Kalm.	Kalmia latifolia
Kreoas.	Kreoasotum
Lac can.	Lac caninum
Lac def.	Lac defloratum
Lach.	Lachesis
Led.	Ledum palustre
Lil. t.	Lilium tigrinum
Lith. c.	Lithium carbonicum

Lobel.	Lobelia inflata
Lyc.	Lycopodium clavatum
Lyss.	Lyssin (Hydrophobinum)
Mag. a.	Magnesia acetica
Mag. c.	Magnesia carbonica
Mag. m.	Magnesia muriatica
Mag. phos.	Magnesia phosphorica
Mag. s.	Magnesia sulphurica
Mang.	Manganum metallicum
Medo.	Medorrhinum
Meli.	Melilotus alba
Merc. c.	Mercurius corosivus
Merc. i. fl.	Mercurius iodatus flavus
Merc. proto.	Mercurius protoiodide
Merc. s.	Mercurius solubilis Hahnemanni
Merc. v.	Mercurius vivus
Mez.	Daphne mezereum
Mill.	Millefolium
Mur. ac.	Muriaticum acidum
Mur. p.	Murex purpurea
Naja	Naja tripudians
Nat. ars.	Natrum arsenicicum
Nat. c.	Natrum carbonicum
Nat. m.	Natrum muriaticum
Nat. phos.	Natrum phosphoricum
Nat. s.	Natrum sulphuricum
Nit. ac.	Nitricum acidum
Nux m.	Nux moschata
Nux v.	Nux vomica
Olean.	Oleander
Op.	Opium
Oxal. ac.	Oxalicum acidum
Petr.	Petroleum
Petrosel.	Petroselinum
Phos.	Phosphorus

Phos. ac.	Phosphoricum acidum
Phyt.	Phytolacca
Pic. ac.	Picricum acidum
Plat.	Platina
Plumb.	Plumbum
Plumb. ac.	Plumbum aceticum
Podo.	Podophyllum peltatum
Psor.	Psorinum
Ptelea.	Ptelea trifoliata
Puls.	Pulsatilla nigricans
Pyr.	Pyrogen (also called Sepsin)
Ran. b.	Ranunculus bulbosus
Ratan.	Ratanhia
Rhe.	Rheum
Rho.	Rhododendron
Rhus t.	Rhus toxicodendron
Rob.	Robinia
Rum. c.	Rumex crispus
Rut.	Ruta graviolens
Saba.	Sabadilla
Sabin.	Sabina
Samb.	Sambucus nigra
Sang.	Sanguinaria canadensis
Sanic.	Sanicula
Sarsa.	Sarsaparilla
Sec.	Secale cornatum
Sel.	Selenium
Seneg.	Senega
Sep.	Sepia
Sil.	Silicia
Spig.	Spigelia
Spon.	Spongia
Squil.	Squilla
Stan.	Stannum
Staph.	Delphinium staphisagria
Stict.	Sticta pulmonaria
Stram.	Stramonium
Stron.	Strontium

Strych.	Strychnia
Sul. ac.	Sulphuricum acidum
Sul.	Sulphur
Symp.	Symphytum officinale
Syph.	Syphilinum
Tab.	Tabacum
Tarax.	Taraxacum
Tarent. cub.	Tarentula Cubensis
Tereb.	Terebinthina
Ther.	Theridion curassavicum
Thlaspi.	Thlaspi bursa pastoris
Thuj.	Thuja Occidentalis
Tuberc. k.	Tuberculinum Kochii
Valer.	Valeriana
Verat.	Varatrum album
Verat. v.	Veratrum viride
Verb.	Verbascum
Vib. op.	Viburnum opulus
Xanth.	Xanthoxylum
Zinc.	Zincum
<	Worse, or aggravation
>	Better, or amelioration
=	Compare
Gb. gb	Great
Esply.	Especially
M.M.P.	Materia Medica Pura
+ + + }	One of the best, provenfully
+ + + }	Excellent
+ +	Very Good
+	Good

GLOSSARY OF MEDICAL TERMS

Term	*Meaning*
Abscess	A localised collection of pus in a cavity formed by disintegration of tissue.
Acetonaemia	Acetone bodies in the blood.
Achromegaly	Abnormal enlargement of the extremities of the skeleton.
Acidemia	Increased acidity of blood.
Acne	A skin condition in adolescence with a papular and pustular eruption on face, neck etc.
Acne rosacea	Disorder of skin of face involving red pimples and small suppurating blisters.
Actinomycosis	Ray fungus affecting lungs, jaws and intestine.
Addison's disease	Lowered blood pressure, marked anaemia, great muscular weakness.
Adenitis	Inflammation of gland.
Adenoids	Over growth of lymphoid tissue.
Adhesions	Abnormal union of two parts, often after inflammation.
Agalactia	Non secretion of milk after childbirth.
Ague	Malaria or remittent fever, chill.
Ala	A wing-like process.
Albuminaria	The presence of albumin in urine.
-algia	A suffix (word-ending) meaning pain.
Alopecia	Baldness.
Amaurosis	Partial or total blindness.
Amblyopia	Irreversible decline in vision approaching blindness.
Amenorrhoea	Absence of menses.
Anæmia	Condition of blood caused by lack of red corpuscles.

Anæsthesia	State of being unable to feel pain, heat, cold etc.
Anasarca	Dropsy.
Aneurism	Local dilation of blood vessels.
Angina	Sense of suffocation or constriction.
Angina pectoris	Pain in the chest caused by inadequate supply of oxygen to the heart muscle.
Anidrosis	Deficient sweat secretion.
Anorexia	Loss of appetite for food.
Anosmia	Absence of sense of smell.
Ante-partum	Before expulsion of placenta (afterbirth).
Anterior crural	Paroxysmal pain extending along the course of nerve of front neuralgia part of leg
Anthax of Sheep	A contagious disease of cattle.
Antrum of Highmore	A cavity in a bone.
Aortitis	Inflammation of the aorta (major artery).
Aphasia	Disorder of speech due to brain lesion.
Aphonia	Loss of voice.
Aphthae	Small grey areas surrounded by a ring of erythema (reddening of skin).
Apoplexy	Sudden unconsciousness usually caused by cerebral embolism (obstruction of blood vessel).
Appendicitis	Inflammation of appendix.
Arachnitis	Inflammation of the delicate arachnoid membrame.
Arachnoid	Delicate membrane interposed between dura mater (outer most) and pia mater (inner most) membrane covering the brain and spinal cord.
Ardor Urinae	Abnormal effort required for urination.
Arthritis	Inflammation of a joint.
Arthritis deformans	Rheumatoid Arthritis. A chronic, systemic disease primarily of the joints, marked by inflammatory changes in synovial membranes and articular structures and by atrophy and rarefaction of bones. In late stages deformity and ankylosis develop.

Articular	Pertaining to a joint.
Ascarides	Worm in the intestine.
Ascites	Accumulation of fluid causing abdominal dropsy (swelling).
-asis	A suffix (word-ending) meaning 'state' or 'condition'.
Asphyxia	Suffocation-cessation of breathing.
Asphyxia neonatorium	Respiratory failure in the newborn.
Asthenia	Weakness, debility.
Asthenopia	Poor vision.
Asthma	Attacks of tightness of chest causing difficulty in breathing.
Astigmatism	Defective vision due to irregular curvature of cornea or lens.
Atelectasis	Collapse of part of the lung.
Atheroma	Fatty deposit on walls of artery.
Atony	Lack of normal tone or strength.
Atrophy	Degeneration, wasting, emaciation in size & function.
Aural	Pertaining to ear.
Axilla	Armpit-nerves, blood and lymphatic vessels of.
Balanitis	Inflammation of glans penis and prepuce.
Balanorrhoea	Discharge of mucous from glans penis.
Barber's itch	Chronic skin condition in the beard area of face.
Bazin's disease	A chronic recurrent disorder in skin of legs of young women.
Beri Beri	A deficiency disease caused by lack of vitamin B.
Bile	A bitter, alkaline, greenish yellow fluid secreted by the liver.
Blenorrhagia	A copious mucous discharge. Gonorrhoea.
Blepharitis	Inflammation of eyelids.
Blepharo-	Eyelids. Eyelashes. Prefix (word-beginning) for ailments of the eyelids or eyelashes.

Blepharospasm	Spasm of muscles in the eyelids.
Borborygmi	Rumbling noises in intestines caused by flatus.
Brachial	Pertaining to arm, vessels in this region.
Brachialgia	Pain in arm.
Brain fag	Fatigue of brain.
Bright's disease	Inflammation of kidneys. Nephritis.
Bronchia	Two tubes into which windpipe divides at its lower end.
Bronchitis	Inflammation of bronchia.
Bronchorrhoea	Excessive discharge of mucous from windpipe.
Brow ague	Malaria type fever.
Brown-ague	Ague with reddish or brownish appearance of skin.
Bubo	Enlargement of lymphatic glands, esp. in groin.
Bulimy (Bulimia)	Excessive appetite.
Bullae	Large watery blisters.
Bunion	Prominent bone with its Bursa containing a small quantity of synovial (membrane lining a joint cavity) fluid.
Bursa	Membranous sac or cavity filled with viscid fluid.
Bursitis	Inflammation of a Bursa.
Cachexia	State of constitutional disorder with emaciated, sallow, unhealthy skin and lustreless eyes.
Caecum	Blind pouch-like commencement of the colon.
Calculi	Small stones.
Callosities	Hardening of skin, common on feet and palms.
Cancer	Malignant growth in any part of the body.
Cancrum oris	Gangrenous stomatitis (inflammation of mouth).
Canthus	Angle at either end of the fissure between eyelids.
Carbuncles	Inflammation involving several hair follicles.

Carcinoma	Tumour.
Cardia	Oesophagal opening into the stomach.
Cardiac	Pertaining to the heart.
Cardialgia	Pain in the heart (often used for heart burns).
Caries	Inflammatory decay of bone or teeth.
Carious	Affected by caries.
Cartilage	Specialised, fibrous connective tissue in adults. Soft bone.
Caruncle	Small piece of flesh, often abnormal. Red fleshy projection.
Catalepsy	Sustained immobility, trance-like state, rigidity of muscles, diminished responsiveness.
Cataract	Opacity of crystalline lens of eye or its capsule.
Catarrh	Inflammation of a mucous membrane with constant flow of mucus.
Catheter	A hollow tube of variable length and bore.
Cellulitis	Inflammation of small cell.
Cerebellum	Part of brain which lies behind and below cerebrum.
Cerebral	Pertaining to cerebellum (largest & uppermost part of brain).
Cervix uteri	Neck of the uterus.
Chafing	Sore by rubbing.
Chalazion	A cyst on the edge of eyelid.
Chancre	Syphilitic ulcer with swelling of local lymph glands.
Chancroid	Venereal disease. Multiple painful ulcers on penis or vulva.
Chaps	Skin cracked, rough or sore.
Chemosis	Swelling of conjunctiva of eye.
Chilblains	Congestion and swelling attended with itching and burning.
Chloasma	Harmless, light brown patches of irregular size.
Chlorosis	A disorder of pubescent females, with greenish yellow discoloration of the skin.

Cholera	Acute contagious intestinal disorder with violent diarrhoea, vomiting, muscle cramps & prostration.
Cholera asiatica	See Cholera.
Cholera infantum	Cholera of infants. See Cholera.
Cholera morbus	See Cholera. Morbus means disease.
Cholerine	Mild form of Cholera.
Chordee	Painful erection of the penis due to urethritis.
Chorea	Irregular, spasmodic movements beyond control.
Choroiditis	Inflammation of Choroid (outer membrane of eyeball).
Chyle	An alkaline milky fluid from small intestine.
Chyluria	Chyle in urine, giving it a milky appearance.
Cicatrix	A scar. Fibrous tissue left after healing of a wound.
Cilia	Eyelids or their outer edges. Eye-lashes. Minute hair like projections from certain epithelial cells.
Ciliary	Pertaining to or resembling cilia. Of the eye.
Cirrhosis	Widespread cell death and hardening of an organ, esp. liver.
Clairaudience	Extra-sensory perception (sound).
Clairvoyance	Extra-sensory perception (vision).
Clavus	A corn.
Clergyman's - sore throat	Sore throat due to excessive speaking.
Climacteric	The menopause.
Clonic spasm	Alternate involuntary muscular contraction and relaxation.
Coccygodynia	Pain in region of Coccyx.
Coccyx	Last bone of vertebral column.
Colic	Severe pain in an abdominal organ.
Coma	Unconsciousness from which patient cannot be roused.

Coma vigil	Locked-in syndrome.
Comedo	Black-head.
Commissures	Union between two parts.
Concussion	Result of a violent jar or shock.
Condylomata	Pointed dry warts in moist areas of the body.
Congenital	Existing from birth or before.
Conjunctivitis	Inflammation of conjunctiva (membrane covering the surface of eyes and the underside of eyelids).
Consumption	Pulmonary tuberculosis.
Constipation	Lack of bowel movement for several days associated with hard, dry faeces.
Contraction	Shortening, esp. of muscle of fibre.
Convulsions	Sudden involuntary movements due to abnormal stimulation of brain.
Coprophagia	Eating of filth or faeces.
Cornea	The transparent membrane in front of the eyeball.
Corns	Highly localised callous formation on skin forming a horn-like piece of tissue.
Corpulency	Fatness, stoutness, obesity.
Coryza	Running at nose, brief upper respiratory tract infection.
Costiveness	Constipation.
Coxalgia	Pain in hip-joint.
Cramp	Involuntary, powerful, painful contraction of muscle(s), often due to poor blood supply to it.
Cretinism	Congenital thyroid deficiency.
Croup	Condition of infants & children, due to obstruction of the larynx by allergy, foreign body, infection, growth etc., marked by a resonant barking cough and hoarseness.
Crusta lactea	A crust formed by drying of secreted milk.
Crusta serpiginosa	A crust having a much wavy or indented border.
Cyanosis	Bluish condition of skin and mucous membranes due to oxygen shortage.

Cyst	A sac enclosing semi-fluid or semi-solid matter.
Cystitis	Inflammation of urinary bladder.
Dandruff	Abnormal scaliness of skin of head which shows as small white flecks in hair and on shoulders.
Decubitus	Lying down.
Delirium	Condition of lowered consciousness associated with disorientation, confusion, hallucinations, & often great fear.
Delirium tremens	Delirium from alcoholic intoxication.
Term	Meaning
Deltoid	Triangular. The deltoid muscle.
Delusions	A false idea of reality.
Dementia	Deterioration of mental faculties due to decay of brain cells.
Dengue	Fever and skin eruptions with rheumatic pains, caused by a mosquito.
Diabetes mellitus	Metabolic disorder in which body is unable to control levels of blood sugar (glucose).
Diaphragm	A membrane separating the chest and abdominal regions.
Diaphragmitis	Inflammation of diaphragm.
Diarrhoea	Deviation from established bowel rhythm with increase in frequency and fluidity.
Diathesis	Unusual constitutional susceptibility or predispo-sition to a particular disease.
Diphtheria	An acute, infectious disease of upper respiratory tract.
Diplopia	Double vision because the vision of one eye is not co-ordinated with that of the other eye.
Dyspareunia	Painful sexual intercourse.
Dropsy	Sweeling (see Anasarca, Ascites, Oedema).
Duodenum	First portion of small intestine.
Dupuytren's contraction	Hand condition in which fingers are forced into a claw shape and cannot be used.

Dyscrasia	Disease or pathological condition.
Dysentery	Inflammation of bowel, evacuation with blood mucous, tenesmus and colic.
Dysmenia	Painful menstruation.
Dysmenorrhoea	Painful menstruation.
Dysmenorrhoea-membranous	Dysmenorrhoea marked by membranous exfoliations derived from the uterus.
Dyspepsia	Indigestion.
Dysphagia	Pain during and after swallowing.
Dyspnoea	Difficulty in breathing.
Dysuria	Painful or difficult urination.
Ecchymosis	Small hamorrhagic spot in the skin or a mucous membrane, forming a rounded or irregular blue or purplish patch.
Ecthyma	Inflammatory skin disease on legs (See Impetigo).
Eczema	Non-infectious itchy inflammation of skin.
Eczema impetiginoides	Eczema with bacterial inflammation of skin.
Eczema rubrum	Eczema with scarlet / red skin.
Elephantiasis	Swelling of a limb, esp. of legs.
Emaciation	Excessive leanness.
Embolism	Obstruction of a blood vessel.
Emphysema	Gaseous distension of lung tissues.
Empyaema	Collection of pus in a cavity.
Enchrodroma	Cartilaginous tumours.
Endometritis	Inflammation of mucous lining of the uterus.
Enteralgia	Pain in gastro-intestinal tract.
Enteric fever	Typhoid or para-typhoid fever.
Enteritis	Inflammation of the intestines.
Entropion	Inward turning lower eyelid, often due to old age.
Enuresis	Incontinence of urine, esp. bed wetting.
Enuresis diurna	Enuresis during daytime.
Enuresis nocturna	Eneursis at night.
Ephelis	Freckles.

Epididymitis	Inflammation of epididymis (a tubule conveying sperms to vas deferens (excretory duct of testicles) (See Orchitis).
Epiglottis	Thin leaf shaped flap of cartilage behind tongue.
Epilepsy	Abnormal electrical activity in brain causing convulsions.
Epistaxis	Bleeding from the nose.
Epithelioma	Malignant growth in epithelial tissue, usually skin.
Epulis	A tumour on or from the gum.
Erethism	Extreme irritability or sensitivity of an organ or tissue
Erotomania	Exaggerated sexual behaviour or reaction; preoccupation with sexuality.
Eructations	Noisy expulsion of gas from the stomach.
Erysipelas	An acute specific disease of the skin (red skin) with fever and other constitutional disturbances.
Erysipelas bullosa	Erysipelas with bullous lesions. (Bullous-a fluid-containing, elevated lesion of skin)
Erythema	Reddening of skin due to toxic or allergic skin affections, or congestion of capillaries.
Erythema nodosum	An acute inflammatory skin disease marked by tender red nodules (usually on shin) due to exudation of blood & serum
Eustachian tubes	Canals which maintain air pressure on both ear-drums.
Excoriations	Superficial injury to skin or mucous membranes
Excrescences	Abnormal growths of tissue.
Exophthalmos	Abnormal protrusion of eye.
Exostosis	A benign growth of bone tissue forming a tumour.
Extravasation	Escape of a fluid from its normal enclosure into the surrounding tissue.
Exudation	Oozing out of fluid through pores of skin (sweat).

Fag	Drudgery.
Favus	A type of ring-worm.
Fester	To become inflamed, to suppurate superficially.
Fibroma	A benign tumour composed mainly of fibrous or fully developed connective tissue.
Fissures	A split or cleft or groove.
Fistula	Abnormal communication between two body surfaces or cavities.
Flatulence	Excessive formation of gas in the stomach or intestine.
Flatulent colic	Colic with or due to flatulence.
Foetus	An unborn child.
Fontanel	The large fontanel is the space between the forehead bone and the temporal bones; the small fontanel is between the bones. A fontanel consists of rigid periosteum which protects the blood vessels and brain beneath it.
Fracture	Break or split in a bone.
Frontal sinuses	Two cavities which open into the upper part of nasal cavity.
Frost-bite	Damage to skin caused by very low temperatures, mostly affecting tip of nose, fingers or toes.
Fungus	Mushroom (a low form of vegetable life).
Furuncle	A boil.
Galactorrhoea	Flow of milk outside breast-feeding period.
Gall-stones	Stones occur in gall-bladder or bile duct
Ganglion	A mass of nerve tissue forming sympathetic nervous system. Cystic tumour. Enlargement on the course of a nerve.
Gangrene	Death of tissues due to shortage of oxygen.
Gastralgia	Pain in the stomach.
Gastric	Pertaining to the stomach
Gastritis	Inflammation of mucous lining of stomach.

Gastrodynia	Pain in the stomach.
Gastro-enteralgia	Inflammation of stomach and intestines.
Gastroenteritis	Inflammation of mucous lining of stomach & small intestine.
Gastromalacia	An abnormal softening of the stomach.
German Measles	Rubella (an acute, infectious, eruptive fever with coryza, conjunctivitis and a pink rash.
Giant Urticaria	Nettle-rash. Hive. Allergic skin eruption-multiple, smooth, circumscribed, pinkish, itchy weals.
Glanders	Contagious ulcerative disease of horses, who can infect man.
Glaucoma	Abnormally high fluid pressure within eyeball.
Gleet	A chronic urethral discharge usually in males.
Globus hystericus	Feeling of a lump in the throat. Can also include difficulty in swallowing. (Hysteria, anxiety, depression)
Glossitis	Inflammation of the tongue.
Glossopharyngeal	Pertaining to the tongue and pharynx.
Glottis	Part of larynx associated with voice production.
Goitre	An enlargement of the thyroid gland.
Gonorrhoea	An infectious disease of venereal origin in adults, with urethritis and dysuria.
Gout	Metabolic disorder in which uric acid crystals accumulate in joints which may become painful and swollen.
Granular conjunctivitis	Grain-like out-growth of new capillaries and connective tissue cells. See Conjunctivitis
Gravel	A sandy deposit in bladder, may pass with urine.
Groin	Junction of the thigh with the abdomen.
Gum-boil	Abscess on the root of a tooth.
Gumma	A soft gummy tumour. Late benign syphilis.

Haematemesis	Vomiting of blood.
Haematocele	A swelling filled with blood.
Haematuria	Blood in urine.
Haemoglobin	Respiratory pigment in red blood corpuscles.
Haemoglobinuria	Haemoglobin in urine.
Haemophilia	Prolonged bleeding even from minor injuries.
Haemoptysis	Coughing of blood.
Haemorrhage	Bleeding from a vessel.
Haemorrhagic diathesis	Bleeding tendency.
Haemorrhoids	Varicosity (dilated vein) around the anus. Piles.
Hallucination	Sensory perception of thing that does not exist.
Hang-nails	Narrow strip of skin partly detached from nail fold.
Hay-asthma	Allergic asthma.
Hay-fever	Allergic rhinitis with acute conjunctivitis, lachrymation, itching, nasal catarrh, sudden attacks of sneezing, and often asthmatic symptoms.
Heartburn	Pyrosis. Acidity. Sharp burning feeling behind breastbone when mucous membrane of oesophagus comes in contact with gastric juices from stomach.
Hemicrania	Unilateral headache. Migraine.
Hemiopia	Loss of half the field of vision.
Hemiplegia	Paralysis of one side of body.
Hepatisation	Transformation into a liver-like mass, esp. the solidified state of the lung in lobar pneumonia.
Hepatitis	Inflammation of liver.
Hernia	Abnormal protrusion of tissue through an abnormal, hitherto non-existing opening.
Herpes	Inflammatory skin disease marked by formation of small vesicles in clusters; vesicular blister due to a virus infection.

Herpes circinatis	Herpes resembling a ring.
Herpes facialis	Herpes of face
Herpes labialis pudendi	Herpes of lips of vagina.
Herpes preputialis	Herpes of prepuce of penis.
Herpes zoster	Shingles. An acute, unilateral, self-limited inflammatory disease of cerebral ganglia and peripheral nerves, caused by chicken-pox virus, associated with neuralgic pain.
Hiccough (Hiccup)	Sudden closure of glottis producing a characteristic sound.
Hives	Nettle-rash, Urticaria (an allergic skin eruption).
Hodgkin's disease	Enlargement of lymphatic glands with fever and anaemia, with occasional skin manifestations.
Housemaid's knee	Inflammation of the bursa of the patella (knee-bone), with fluid accumulating within it.
Hydraemia	Relative excess of plasma (fluid fraction of blood).
Hydroa	Inflammation of skin and intensely itching eruption of skin.
Hydrocele	A swelling due to accumulation of serous fluid in the testes.
Hydrocephalus	Accumulation of cerebrospinal fluid inside the skull (water on brain).
Hydropericardium	Water (fluid) around heart.
Hydrophobia	Fear of water. Rabies in man. See Rabies.
Hydro-salpingitis	Inflammation of fallopian tube with watery fluid.
Hydrothorax	Presence of fluid in pleural (thin membrane covering surface of lung on to chest wall) cavity.
Hydronephrosis	Distension of kidney pelvis with urine.
Hygroma	Accumulation of fluid in a sac, cyst or bursa.
Hyperaemia	Excess of blood in an area.

Hyperaesthesia	Excessive sensitiveness of a part.
Hypermetropia	Long-sightedness.
Hyperpyrexia	Body temperature above 40(-41(C (105(F)
Hypertrophy	Increase in the size of tissues or structures independent of natural growth.
Hypochondriasis	Excessive worry about one's health.
Hypocondrium	Upper latter region of the abdomen.
Hypopion	Collection of pus in the anterior chamber of eye.
Hysteria	A functional (neurotic) disorder usually arising from mental conflict with characteristic symptoms such as tics / paralysis.
Hysterical joint	A condition that resmbles arthritis but is of psychic origin.
Ichthyosis	Skin like fish-skin.
Idiocy	Most severe form of mental deficiency with IQ less than 25.
Ileum	Lower three fifths of the small intestine.
Ileus	Intestinal obstruction may cause vomiting and/or distension of abdomen.
Impetigo	An inflammatory, infectious, pustular skin disease.
Incontinence	Inability to retain urine, normal in children.
Indigestion	Slight, temporary digestive disorder. Dyspepsia.
Induration	Hardening of tissue.
Infantile	Relating to a child under one year old.
Inflammation	Infection or irritation with pain, swelling redness and heat.
Influenza	An acute viral infection of naso-pharyngeal (cavity at the back of the mouth) and respiratory tract.
Inframammary pain	Pain below breast.
Inguinal	Where the lower abdomen meets the groin.
Insomnia	Discontent with the quantity or pattern of sleep.

Intercostal	Between the ribs.
Inter-menstrual flow	Menses flow between menstrual periods.
Intermittents	Fever occurring at intervals.
Interscapular pain	Pain under scapula.
Intertrigo	Small suppurating blisters due to regular friction in moist skin folds under the breasts, the buttock cleft or the groin.
Intra-ocular	Within the globe of the eye.
Intussusception	One part of the bowel slips into lower part, causing intestinal obstruction.
Iris	Circular coloured membrane of the middle coat of eyeball.
Iritis	Inflammation of Iris.
Jaundice	Yellow colouring of skin, mucous membrane an bodily fluids due to excess in bloodstream of bilirubin, the colouring matter of bile.
Keratitis	Inflammation of the cornea.
Kerato-iritis	Inflammation of cornea and iris.
Kleptomania	Mental disturbance leading to compulsive stealing.
Labia	Lip-like folds encircling the vagina.
Lachrymal duct	Connects the lachrymal gland to the upper conjunctival sac.
Lachrymal sac	Tear sac.
Lachrymation	Out flow of tears.
Lactation	Secretion of milk.
Laryngeal	Pertaining to larynx.
Laryngismus	Attack of laryngeal spasm.
Laryngitis	Inflammation of the larynx.
Larynx	The voice box. A sphincter which closes the top of the trachea (tube leading to lungs) to prevent objects from blocking the wind-pipe. Consists of strong muscles attached to a skeleton of cartilage.

Leprosy	A progressive and contagious disease caused by a bacillus which establishes itself in the skin and nerves in particular.
Leukocythemia	See Leukemia.
Leukocytosis	Transient increase in the number of leukocytes in the blood.
Leucorrhoea	A sticky, whitish vaginal discharge.
Leukemia	Cancer which originates in white blood cells causing them to be abnormal in type or number.
Levitation	Sensation as if flying in air.
Lichen	Skin disorder causing intense itching.
Lisping	Speech disorder in which sounds "s" and "z" are pronounced as "th"; "sing" is pronounced "thing".
Liver torpid	Sluggish liver.
Liver-spot	Yellowish brown, red or black spot or patch on skin, formerly attributed to faulty functioning of the liver.
Lochia	Vaginal discharge during first week or two after child-birth.
Lockjaw	Tetanus. Trismus.
Locomotor ataxy	Failure of muscular co-ordination. Irregularity of muscular action. Paroxysms of intense pain, disturbance of sensation.
Lumbago	Pain in the lumbar (pertaining to loins) region.
Lumbar abscess	Abscess in lumbar (pertaining to loins) region.
Lungs	Organs of respiration lying, on either side of heart.
Lupus	Inflammation reactions in all parts of body, usually in women, causing fever, fatigue, weight loss, swollen joints
Lymph	A clear body fluid formed in and flowing through system of vessels called lymphatics. Assists in distribution of nutrients and plays important role in immune defence system.

Malar bones	Zygomatic bones-forming hard part of cheek and lower, lateral portion of rim of each orbit.
Malaria	Infectious disease caused by mosquito bite, associated with headache, muscular pain, loss of appetite, etc.
Malignant pustule	Pustule (small pus-containing lesion of skin) tending to become worse and end in death.
Mammae	Breasts.
Mania	Unreasonable agitation.
Marasmus	Malnutrition due to prolonged severe caloric deficit, chiefly in 1st year of life, with growth retardation and wasting of subcutaneous fat and muscle.
Mastitis	Inflammation of the breast.
Masturbation	Auto-stimulation of genitalia.
Measles	Infectious viral infection usually in children, associated with high fever, cold in nose, inflamed eyes and dry cough followed with rough round or oval red patches on body.
Melaena	Blood in the faeces.
Melancholia	A depressed and unhappy emotional state with abnormal inhibition of mental and bodily activity.
Melancholy	See Melancholia.
Melanoma	The most malignant and least common form of skin cancer.
Melanosis	Dark pigmentary deposits.
Mendacity	A lie; untruth. Tendency to lie.
Meniere's disease	Severe attacks of vertigo, associated with nausea & vomiting
Meningeal headaches	Headache caused by inflammation of meninges (three membranes covering brain and spinal cord)
Meningitis	Inflammation of the membrane surrounding the brain, often after influenza, otitis or pharyngitis.

Menopause	Change of life. Period of gradual decrease in ovulation and cessation of menstruation, marking the end of a woman's reproductive period, usually between the ages of 46 and 52.
Menorrhagia	Excessive menstruation.
Menses	Monthly flow of blood from female genital tract.
Menstruation	Flow of menses which occurs regularly every 24 to 34 days.
Menstruation-vicarious	Discharge of blood from an extra-genital source at the time menstruation is normally expected.
Mentagra	See Sycosis. Pustular inflammation of hair follicles
Mental alienation	Insanity.
Mercurial syphilis	Syphilis caused by mercurial poisoning.
Metrorrhagia	Uterine bleeding, usually of normal amount, occurring at completely irregular intervals.
Migraine	Severe headache caused by narrowing of blood vessels, usually on one side of head with nausea and vomiting.
Milia	Small creamy white spots on skin, usually on face, caused by accumulation of grease under skin
Miliaria	Heat rash. Prickly heat. Small white or red eruptions due to obstruction of the ducts of sweat glands.
Miliary eruption	Eruptions characterised or accompanied by lesions about the size of millet seeds. A form of tuberculosis in which many minute tubercles get formed.
Milk fever	A mild puerperal fever erroneously attributed to accumulation of milk in the breasts.
Milk-leg	See Phlegmasia alba dolens.
Miner's asthma	Sudden attack of difficulty in breathing, particularly of mine workers.

Miscarriage	Spontaneous abortion before sixteenth week of pregnancy.
Mole	Common skin abnormality involving local accumulation of black or brown pigment. See Naevus.
Mollities ossium	Osteomalacia. Adult equivalent of Rickets.
Molluscum contagiosum	Contagious virus infection of skin characterised by small blobs with a central indentation from which a porridge-like substance can be expressed.
Morning sickness	Vomiting during pregnancy upon waking.
Morphinomania	Morbid and habitual craving for morphine.
Morphoea	Connective tissue replacement of the skin and sometimes the subcutaneous tissues, with formation of firm ivory white or pinkish patches, bands or lines.
Mucous	Adjective for mucus (noun). A clear, viscous fluid consisting of lipids, minerals and dead cells.
Mumps	See Parotitis. Infectious viral disease associated with high fever, pain and swelling of salivary glands.
Muscoe volitantes	Specks seen as if floating before the eyes.
Myalgia	Muscular pain usually caused by strain.
Mycosis	Disease caused by fungi.
Mycosis fungoides	Chronic, malignant lymphoreticular neoplasm of skin with development of large painful ulcerating tumours
Myelin	A fatty substance enclosing nerve cells.
Myelitis	Inflammation of the spinal cord; of the bone marrow.
Myelitis diffusa	Inflammation of the spinal cord.
Myopia	Short-sightedness due to inability of eye to focus.
Naevus	Common skin abnormality involving local accumu-lation of pigment, also called a mole.

Naso-pharynx	Part of the pharynx above the soft palate.
Nausea	Feeling of being sick, preceding or accompanying vomiting.
Necrosis	Cell death.
Nephritis	Inflammation of the kidney.
Nettle-rash	See Urticaria.
Neuralgia	Paroxysmal pain extending along the course of nerve(s).
Neuralgia palpebralis	Neuralgia of the eyelid.
Neuralgia-consupraorbital	Neuralgia above orbit (bony cavity taining eyeball and its associated muscles, vessels and nerves.
Neurasthenia	Obsolete category of neurosis, marked by chronic weakness and easy fatigability.
Neuritis	Inflammation of a nerve with loss of function.
Night-blindness	Failure or imperfection of vision at night or in dim light.
Node	A small mss of tissue in the form of a swelling, knot or protuberance, either normal or pathological.
Noma pudendi	Gangrenous processes of the genitalia.
Nucha	The nape, or back, of the neck.
Nurselings	Infants.
Nyctalopia	Night-blindness.
Nymphomania	Insatiable sexual desire in women. .See Satyriasis.
Nystagmus	Involuntary rhythmic movement of the eyeball.
Occipital	The back part of the head. Occiput.
Occiput	See Occipital.
Oedema	Increase in quantity of fluid in the space between tissue cells due to leakage from lood vessel walls.
Oedema glottidis	Oedema of glottis.
Oesophagitis	Inflammation of the mucous membrane of the oesophagus, often due to acidity.

Oesophagus	A hollow pipe of thick muscle lined with mucous membrane that carries food from mouth to stomach
Onanism	Masturbation.
Ophthalmia	Severe inflammation of the eye.
Ophthalmia neonatorum	Ophthalmia of a new-born infant.
Ophthalmia tarsi	Severe inflammation of cartilaginous plate forming the frame of the eye.
Opisthotonos	Form of extreme hyperextension of the body in which head and heels are bent backward and the body bowed forward.
Optic	Of or pertaining to the eye.
Orbital neuralgia	Paroxysmal pain extending along course of eyeball and its associated muscles, vessels and nerves.
Orchitis	Swelling of the testicles, often as a result of mumps in young adults.
Os	(1) Any body orifice; (2) bone.
Os uteri	Orifice or mouth of the uterus.
Ossification	Formation or conversion into bone or a bony substance.
Osteoma	A benign, slow-growing tumour composed of compact bone, occurring particularly in the skull and facial bones.
Osteo-myletis	Inflammation of bone marrow.
Otalgia	Pain in the ear.
Otitis	Ear infection, usually in middle ear, often due to cold, measles, scarlet fever or sore throat.
Otorrhoea	Discharge of pus from ear due to perforation of eardrum.
Ovaries	The female gonads (sexual glands) in which ova are formed.
Ovaritis	Inflammation of ovary.
Oxaluria	Hyperoxaluria. An excess of oxalate (salt of oxalic acid) in the urine.
Ozaena	Atrophic Rhinitis marked by thick mucopurulent discharge.

Palpitation	Subjective sensation of unduly rapid or irregular heartbeat.
Palsy	Paralysis.
Pancreas	Gland producing hormones (insulin and glucagon) to regulate blood sugar levels.
Pancreatitis	Inflammation of the pancreas.
Pannus	Superficial vascularisation of the cornea with infiltration of granulation tissue.
Panophthalmitis	Inflammation of all the eye structures or tissues.
Paralysis	Loss of ability to move muscles.
Paralysis agitans	A slowly progressive form of Parkinsonism, usually seen late in life, marked by tremour of resting muscles, slowing of voluntary movements, peculiar posture, muscular weakness & sometimes excessive sweating and feelings of heat.
Parametritis	Inflammation of the parametrium, the extension of the subserous coat of the super-cervical portion of the uterus.
Paraphimosis	Obstruction of blood flow due to tight foreskin causes swelling in glans and foreskin.
Paraplegia	Paralysis of the lower part of the body including the legs.
Paresis	Slight or incomplete paralysis.
Paronychia	Inflammation in the folds of tissue around the fingernail.
Parotid gland	Gland near the ear.
Parotitis	Inflammation of the parotid gland.
Paroxysm	Sudden recurrence or intensification of symptoms. A spasm or seizure.
Pediculosis	Infestation with lice.
Pelvic cellulitis	Inflammation of the soft or connective tissue of pelvis, in which a thin, watery exudate spreads. It may lead to ulceration and abscess.
Pelvic haematoccle	A swelling caused by profusion of blood into the space between the bladder and uterus.

Pemphigus	Serious skin disorder involving formation of blisters and abrasions all over body.
Penis	The male genital organ.
Pericarditis	Inflammation of membrane enclosing heart.
Perichondritis	Inflammation of the perichondrium, the layer of fibrous connective tissue investing all cartilage except articular cartilage of synovial joints.
Perimetritis	Inflammation of the perimetrium, the serous membrane enveloping the uterus.
Periosteum	Firm mucous connective tissue lining outer surface of bone.
Periostitis	Inflammation of periosteum.
Peritonitis	Irritation of peritoneum, the membrane that lines the abdomen and encloses abdominal organs.
Perityphlitis	Inflammation of tissue around caecum.
Pertussis	Whooping-cough. An infectious disease marked by catarrh of respiratory tract and peculiar fits of cough ending in a prolonged crowing or whooping respiration.
Petit mal	Epilepsy characterised by absence seizures, usually having its onset in childhood or adolescence.
Pharyngitis	Inflammation of mucous membrane of throat and surrounding lymph nodes.
Phimosis	Opening of foreskin so narrow that foreskin cannot be pulled back over penis. See Paraphimosis-mild cases where foreskin can be partially pulled back.
Phlebitis	Inflammation of a vein.
Phlegmasia alba dolens	Inflammation of the femoral vein, with swelling of the leg, usually without redness
Phlyctenular	Associated with the formation of phlyctenules (minute vesicles; ulcerated nodules of cornea or conjunctiva) or of vesicle like prominences.

Phosphaturia	Excess of phosphates in urine.
Phobia	Severe unfounded anxiety about a certain object or situation.
Photophobia	Abnormal visual intolerance to light.
Photopsia	Appearance as of sparks or flashes, in retinal irritation.
Phthiriasis	Infestation with lice in the pubic region.
Phthisis	Wasting of the body. Tuberculosis.
Physometra	Gas in the uterine cavity.
Piles	See Haemorrhoids.
Pityriasis	Harmless, common skin condition with typical patches.
Pityriasis rubra	Pityriasis with characteristic 'medallions'-yellow on inside with red edge, usually scaly.
Pityriasis versicolor	Slightly itchy, superficial fungus infection of skin with characteristic brown patches which are dark in fair persons and lighter in dark persons.
Placenta	Tissue connecting unborn baby to womb. It carries nutrition and oxygen to the baby and waste products away from it.
Plague	Bacterial infection transmitted by ratfleabite. Plagues are pneumonic or bubonic(characterised by swollen lymph nodes [Buboes] in groin).
Plethora	An excess of blood.
Pleurisy	Inflammation of the mucous membrane surrounding the outer lung membranes (pleura).
Pleurodynia	Paroxismal pain in the inter-costal (between ribs) muscles.
Pleuro-pneumonia	Pleurisy complicated by pneumonia.
Plica polonica	A matting of hair with crusts and vermin. (Plica = a fold.)
Pneumo-gastric paralysis	Paralysis of lungs and stomach.
Pneumonia	Inflammation of the lung.
Polypi	Growth or mass protruding from a mucous membrane.

Post-partum	After expulsion of placenta (afterbirth).
Pott's curvature	See Pott's disease.
Pott's disease	Tuberculosis of spine.
Prepuce	Foreskin of penis.
Presbyopia	Worsening near-vision in older people.
Priapism	Sudden and persistent erection of penis, without previous sexual stimulation, and not resulting in ejaculation.
Prickly heat	Skin condition from exposure to excessive heat.
Proctalgia	Pain in the rectum.
Proctitis	Inflammation of rectum.
Prolapsus ani	Falling down or downward displacement of anus.
Prolapsus recti	Falling down or downward displacement of rectum.
Prosopoplagia	Facial paralysis.
Prostate	Gland below bladder, which partially encloses urethra in males, and secretes seminal fluid.
Prostatitis	Inflammation of prostate gland.
Prostatorrhoea	Catarrhal discharge from prostate.
Prurigo	Itchy skin eruption in which characteristic lesion is dome shaped, followed by crusting.
Pruritus	Itching. Unpleasant symptom of a number of skin disorders.
Pruritus ani	Itching of anus.
Pruritus mercurialis	Itching due to mercurial poisoning.
Pruritus pudendi	Itching of genital organs.
Pruritus senilis	Itching in the aged, due to dryness of skin.
Pruritus vaginae	Itching of vagina (female sex organ)
Pruritus vulvae	Itching of vulva (external female sex organ).
Pseudo-hypertrophic	Increase in size without true hypertrophy (growth).
Psoas abscess	Abscess of either of two muscles of loin that connect the spinal column and the thigh bone.

Psoriasis	Skin disorder characterised by red patches and silvery white scales on head, elbows and knees.
Psoriasis palmaris	Psoriasis of palm.
Psychosis	Mental disorder in whichperceptions and ideas cannot be related to reality.
Pterygium	Wing-like structure, esp. an abnormal triangular fold of membrane in eye.
Ptosis	Prolapse of an organ or part. Paralytic drooping of eyelid.
Ptyalism	Excessive secretion of saliva.
Puerperal	Pertaining to a woman who has just given birth.
Eclampsia	Convulsions and coma in pregnant woman.
Puerperal fever	Childbed fever. Infection of a woman's internal genital organs, in first week after having a baby, associated with fever and foul smelling discharge.
Purpura	Purplish-red haemorrhages, due to capillary inflammation destroy blood vessels and cause multiple small haemorrhages just below skin.
Purpura haemorrhagica	Disease marked by haemolytic anaemia, neuro-logical manifestations, decrease in number of platelets in circulating blood, fever and thrombosis in arterioles and capillaries.
Pustules	Small elevated circumscribed lesions of skin containing pus.
Pyaemia	Septicemia in which secondary foci of suppuration occur and multiple abscesses are formed.
Pyelitis	Inflammation of the renal pelvis and kidney tissue, usually after urinary tract infection.
Pylorus	Distal aperture of the stomach opening into the duodenum.
Pyrosis	See Heartburn.
Pyuria	Pus in urine.

Quinsy	Abscess near or around tonsils.
Rabies	See Hydrophobia. Infectious viral disease of the central nervous system of mammals, resulting from bite of a rabid animal, is marked by paralysis of muscles of deglutition and glottal spasms provoked by drinking or sight of liquids, and by maniacal behaviour, convulsions & respiratory paralysis.
Ranula	A cystic tumour beneath the tongue.
Raynaud's disease	Dead fingers. Blood vessels in fingers, mostly of young women, become constricted so that one or more fingers turn pale and 'dead'.
Relapsing fever	Alternating periods of fever and non-fever each lasting from 5 to 7 days.
Remittent fever	Fever that varies 2(or more in 24 hours but does not return to normal.
Renal calculi	Stones of the kidney
Renal colic	Colic of the kidney.
Retina	The light-sensitive hemi-circle of tissue inside eyeball at the back of the eye.
Retinitis	Inflammation of retina.
Reveries	Dreamy thinking or imagining of aggreable things; day-dreaming; fanciful musing.
Rhagades	Fissures, cracks, linear scars in the skin, especially around regions subjected to frequent movements, such as the mouth.
Rheumatic fever	Fever due to inflammation around joints and heart.
Rheumatic gout	Rheumatoid arthritis. A chronic systemic disease primarily of the joints marked by inflammatory changes, atrophy, deformity of bones etc.
Rheumatism	Disorder of movement, associated with pain and limitation of movement usually caused by inflammation of a joint.
Rhinitis	Inflammation of the nasal mucous membrane.

Rickets	Disturbed bone metabolism in children causes delayed bone formation and deficiency of vitamin 'D' and calcium.
Ringworm	Fungus infection of skin which takes the form of a ring with normal skin in the centre.
Rodent ulcer	Most common, least malignant form of skin cancer forming a glassy, greyish patch with a rim.
Roseola	Harmless viral disease of children between 6 months and 3 years of age. Starts with cold, slight temperature and loss of appetite. Soon a rash of small red spots appear on trunk and neck which fade away, along with the fever, after 2 days.
Rumination	Regurgitation of food, by infants, part being vomited and the rest being re-swallowed.
Rupia	Thick dark raised crusts on the skin.
Sacrum	Fused vertebrae constituting the posterior wall of the pelvis.
Satyriasis	Insatiable sexual desire in men. See Nymphomania
Scabies	Itch. A parasitic, highly contagious skin disease
Scapula	Shoulder blade.
Scarlatina	Scarlet fever. Acute disease marked by pharyngo-tonsilitis and a skin rash which is a bright scarlet with many points of deeper red.
Scelorsis of arteries	Hardening of arteries
Sciatica	Severe stabbing, radiating pain in one leg caused by pressure on sciatic nerve, the large nerve which runs from base of spine down the back of the leg. Pain radiates from buttock; increases if leg is bent.
Scirrhus	Hard or indurated.

Scleroderma	Persistent systemic sclerosis (hardening) of tissues.
Sclerotitis	Inflammation of the sclera (outer coat of eyeball).
Scrofula	Primary tuberculosis of cervical lymph nodes.
Scurf	Little dry scales shed by the skin as dandruff.
Scurvy	Consequence of vitamin 'C' deficiency, such as swelling and bleeding of gums, pain in joints, etc.
Sebaceous glands	Glands which secrete a waxy substance (sebum) associated with hair roots and downy hairs over skin surface. Sebaceous glands are everywhere except palms of hand & soles of feet.
Seborrhoea	Excessive secretions from sebaceous glands.
Self-abuse	See Masturbation.
Seminal emissions	Emissions of seminal fluid.
Septic diseases	Diseases marked with sepsis (presence of poisons in blood).
Serous	Producing, containing or pertaining to serum.
Sick headache	See Migraine.
Sigmoid flexure	A 'C' or 'S' shaped bend or fold.
Sinuses	Hollow air passage in bones of forehead.
Small-pox	Viral infection causing fever and skin eruptions.
Snuffles	Catarrhal discharge from nasal mucous membrane.
Somnambulism	Sleep-walking. Walking while asleep.
Somnolence	Sleepiness, unnatural drowsiness.
Spasm	Alternate involuntary muscular contraction and relaxation in succession. See Clonic spasm.
Spastic	Increased muscular tension. Muscles look well-developed but cannot exert force.
Spermatic cords	Tubes that carry sperm.

Spermatorrhoea	Involuntary escape of semen without orgasm.
Spina bifida	Congenital defect of spinal column through which meninges may protrude.
Spinal caries	Caries of the spinal bones.
Spleen	A sponge like purplish organ on left side of abdomen between stomach and left kidney.
Splenalgia	Pain in the spleen.
Sprain	Stretching and rupture of joint ligaments.
Staphyloma	Protrusion of sclera (outer coat of eyeball) or cornea due to inflammation.
Steatoma	Fatty mass retained within a sebaceous gland.
Sternum	Breastbone.
Stomatitis	Oral thrush. Inflammation of mucous membrane of mouth.
Strabismus	Squint. Both eyes do not point in the same direction.
Strangury	Slow, painful discharge ofurine.
Stricture	Abnormal narrowing of a duct or passage.
Stumps	End of a limb left after amputation.
Stuttering	Spasmodic repetition of words, especially initial consonants.
Styes	Acute inflammation of sebaceous gland at the base of an eyelash causing swelling, redness and pain.
Subcostal	Below a rib or ribs.
Subinvolution	Incomplete involution (rolling or turning inward).
Suppuration	Formation or discharge of pus.
Surgical fever	Fever due to surgery.
Sycosis	Papulopustular inflammation of hair follicles, especially of the beard.
Synovitis	Inflammation of synovial (fluid in joint cavities) membrane.
Syphilis	Hard chancre. A venereal disease.
Syringo-myelia	A central cavity surrounded by scar tissue, usually in upper part of spinal cord.

Tabes mesenterica	Tuberculosis of mesenteric (membrane attaching organs to body wall) glands in children.
Tape-worm	A parasite that lives and grows in the intestine.
Tarsal	Pertaining to bones between foot and leg, ankle or instep.
Tendo Achilles	Tendon at back of heel.
Tendons	Tough connective tissue at the end of a muscle by which it is attached to a bone.
Tenesmus	Ineffectual and painful straining at stool or in urinating.
Testicles	Organs in male scrotum which produce sperm.
Tetanus	Lockjaw. Serious wound infection causing extremely painful muscular spasms.
Tetany	Sharp flexion of the wrist and ankle joints, muscle twitching, cramps and convulsions.
Tetters	Any skin disease, such as eczema, characterised by itching.
Threadworms	Pinworm. Common intestinal parasite.
Thrombosis	Presence of blood clot in vein or artery.
Tibia	Large bone of lower leg.
Tic douloureux	Pain in the face caused by several factors. Includes hemicrania or migraine.
Tinea	Ring-worm. Superficial fungal infection of skin.
Tinea capitis	Fungal infection of scalp.
Tinea capitis faciei	Fungal infection of face other than et bearded area.
Tinea versicolor	A chronic non-inflammatory disorder marked by multiple patches.
Tinnitus	Hearing sounds in the ear or head without a source of noise.
Tinnitus aurium	Tinnitus of the ear.
Tonsil	Glands in throat behind tongue which have a protective function against bacteria and viruses.
Tonsilitis	Inflammation of the tonsils.
Trachea	Wind-pipe.

Trauma	Physical or psychic wound or injury.
Traumatic fever	Fever due to trauma.
Tremor	An involuntary trembling or quivering
Trichiasis	In-growing eyelashes or appearance of hair like filaments in urine.
Trifacial-nerve paralysis	Paralysis of the trigeminal nerve.
Trigeminal nerve	Either of the fifth pair of cranial nerves, each of which divides into three branches supplying the head and face.
Trismus	Spasm of jaw muscles. Lockjaw. Early symptom of tetanus.
Tuberculosis	An infectious disease of lung spreading to other organs.
Tumour	Swelling, a cardinal sign of inflammation. Growth of tissue in which cell-multiplication is uncontrolled and progressive.
Tympanites	Abnormal distension due to the presence of gas or air in the intestine or the peritoneal cavity.
Tympany	See Tympanites.
Typhlitis	Inflammation of tissues of caecum.
Typhoid	See Typhus.
Typhus	Group of closely related, acute diseases (including Typhoid) marked by headache, chills, fever, stupor, eruptions, etc.
Ulcer	A local defect or excavation of surface of an organ or tissue.
Ulceration	Formation or development of an ulcer.
Umbilicus	The navel. The scar marking the site of attachment of the umbilical cord in the foetus.
Uraemia	Excess of nitrogenous end products of protein and amino acid metabolism in the blood.
Urethra	Membranous canal through which urine is discharged from bladder to exterior of the body.

Urethritis	Inflammation of the urethra.
Uric-acidaemia	Hyper-uricemia. Excess of uric acid in the blood.
Urine phosphatic	Phosphaturia. Excess of phosphates in urine.
Urticaria	See Hives. A vascular reaction of the skin marked by itching and slightly elevated patches redder or paler than the surrounding skin.
Uterine atony	Loss of tone or strength of uterus.
Uterine spasm	Spasm of uterus
Uterus	A hollow muscular organ in females where the foetus is embedded.
Uvula	A pendant, fleshy mass, hanging from the soft palate above the root of the tongue.
Vaccinia	The cutaneous and sometimes systemic reactions associated with small-pox vaccination.
Vaccinosis	Disorders due to vaccination.
Vagina	The canal in the female, from the vulva to the cervix, which receives the penis in copulation.
Vaginismus	Involuntary, painful spasm of the vagina severe enough to prevent intercourse.
Varicella	Chicken-pox.
Varices	Enlarged tortuous veins, arteries or lymphatic vessels.
Varicocele	Varicosity of the spermatic cord, forming a scrotal swelling that feels like a 'bag of worms'.
Varicose	Unnaturally and permanently distended (esp. vein).
Varicosis	Condition of being varicose.
Variola	Small-pox.
Varioloid	Resembling Small-pox.
Vertebrae	The thirty-three bones of the spinal column.
Vesication	Process of blistering or a blistered spot or surface.

<table>
<tr><td>Viscera</td><td>Large interior organs, esp. those in the abdomen.</td></tr>
<tr><td>Vulva</td><td>External genital organ of the female.</td></tr>
<tr><td>Warts</td><td>A hyper-plastic epidermal lesion with a horny surface.</td></tr>
<tr><td>Water-brash</td><td>Heartburn with regurgitation of sour fluid or almost tasteless saliva into the mouth.</td></tr>
<tr><td>Wens</td><td>Sebaceous or epidermal inclusion cysts.</td></tr>
<tr><td>White leg</td><td>Inflammation of the wall of a nerve.</td></tr>
<tr><td>Whitlow</td><td>Primary herpes infection of the terminal segment of a finger with extensive tissue destruction.</td></tr>
<tr><td>Whooping-cough</td><td>See Pertussis.</td></tr>
<tr><td>Worm fever</td><td>Fever due to infection by worms.</td></tr>
<tr><td>Writer's cram</td><td>A muscle cramp in the hand caused by excessive writing.</td></tr>
<tr><td>Yellow fever</td><td>An acute, infectious mosquito borne viral disease marked by fever, jaundice and albuminuria.</td></tr>
<tr><td>Zona</td><td>See Herpes zoster.</td></tr>
<tr><td>Zoster</td><td>See Herpes zoster.</td></tr>
<tr><td><</td><td>Worse (symptom).</td></tr>
<tr><td>></td><td>Better (symptom).</td></tr>
<tr><td>=</td><td>Compare.</td></tr>
<tr><td>+</td><td>Good (effectiveness of medicine).</td></tr>
<tr><td>++</td><td>Better (effectiveness of medicine).</td></tr>
<tr><td>+++</td><td>Best (effectiveness of medicine).</td></tr>
<tr><td>||</td><td>Reverse.</td></tr>
</table>

Understanding Homeopathic Medicines

(From Farrington)

Proving of Drugs

Just as a mechanic knows how the parts are to be fitted in a machine he wants to build, a Homeopath should know his tools, i.e., Homeopathic medicines. The best way for this, indeed the only way, is to know how a medicine works on a healthy human organism. Symptoms are of two types-subjective and objective. Subjective symptoms are those which the prover himself experiences and narrates in his own language. Objective symptoms are those that appear directly before the observer.

If a medicine is given to a prover, he may feel stomach ache, but it does not apply directly to the senses of the observer. On the other hand, if there is a swelling or a boil on the skin of the prover, the observer can touch and feel it. This is an objective symptom. So when an observer proves a medicine on a prover he gets a mass of symptoms. These symptoms are to be interpreted to understand the genius of a drug.

To analyze a drug, the following schema is suggested:

1) Blood and blood vessels,
2) Lymph and its vessels,
3) Nerves, brain, spinal cord and sympathetic muscle, tendons and ligaments,
4) Connective tissue,
5) Bones, cartilage and joints,
6) Serous and synovial membranes,
7) Mucous membranes,
8) Skin,
9) Organs.

A Homeopath must study the effect of the medicine on all the above. Deviations from the normal will be noted under each of these headings. Under the blood, increase will indicate plethora or hyperaemia, decrease anaemia or ischaemia and alteration-as in Chlorosis or Pyaemia. Same is true of other headings which may show increase, decrease or change. Thus the idea of a drug as a whole or genius of the drug is understood.

The next step is to learn to differentiate one drug from the other as well as their common points. A cowherd knows each one of his cows from its distinctive features while a new person will not be able to differentiate one cow from another. This is called comparison of remedies.

Relationship of Drugs

When a drug is studied as a whole and analyzed then it appears that drugs have a relationship with each other. There are five such relationships:-

I. Family relationship-medicines which have similarity in origin. When drugs belong to the same family they have a similar action, such as Arachnid family which has Tarentula and Theridion or Rubiaceae having China, Ipecac. and Coffea. "This resemblance though relationship is sometimes so nearly identical that these drugs do not follow each other well". Ignatia and Nux Vomica belong to the same order of plants; they do not follow each other well and they do not antidote each other. Antidote is explained below.

II. Concordant relationship-drugs which present marked similarity in action, though dis-similar in origin. Such drugs may follow each other well.

III. Complementary relationship-when a drug cannot complete a cure and another medicine is required to complete it, then such medicines are called complementary. Belladonna and Calcarea have this relationship.

IV. Relationship of antidote-there are medicines which antidote each other. A patient may be too susceptible to the actions of a remedy. Then another medicine is required to modify its effects. This called antidote medicine. Nux Vomica provided for a cold may also cause headache. If Coffea which is antidote to Nux Vomica is given, then it relieves headache by modifying the action of Nux Vomica.

V. Inimical relationships-they are medicines which have strong resemblance to each other, seem as they ought to be concordant remedies, yet they are inimical. Apis. has inimical relationship with Rhus Tox, China, Psorinum, Silica and Mercury (see chart).

Action of a drug

Hahnemann in his "Organon" (Rule 63) differentiates between two actions of a drug-primary action and secondary action. Nash says in his Leaders "so called secondary action is only the reaction of the organism against the first or primary action of the drug. For instance, real action of Opium is to produce sleep or stupor, the reaction is wakefulness; of Podophyllum, Aloe etc. Catharsis, the reaction constipation......I think that truly Homeopathic curative must be in accord with primary effects of the drug in order to get the best and most radical cure..."

Broad divisions of Homeopathic medicines

Homeopathic medicines have been divided in four broad categories depending on the source from which they are derived. The families and important drugs in each category, which appear in this book, are listed ahead:

The Vegetable Kingdom

The largest number of Homeopathic medicines are derived from this kingdom:

1. Anacardiaceae - Anac., Rhus t.
2. Apocynaceae - Apocy., Olean., Vinc. m.
3. Araceae - Aur., Arum t.
4. Berberidaceae - Berb. v., Caul., Podo.
5. Boraginaceae - Symp.
6. Campanulaceae - Lobel.
7. Cananbinaceae - Can. i., Can. s.
8. Sambucaceae - Samb., Vib. op.

9. Chenopodiaceae - Cheno., Cheno. v.
10. Cistaceae - Cistus.
11. Compositae - Calend., Arn., Cham., Cina, Eup. perf., Eup. purp., Mill.
12. Cynarocephalae - Card. m.
13. Coniferae - Thuj., Sabin.
14. Covolvulaceae - Jal.
15. Cucurbitaceae - Bry., Coloc.
16. Dioscoraceae - Diosc.
17. Droseraceae - Dros.
18. Equisetaceae - Equis.
19. Ericaceae - Kalm., Led., Rho., Chim.
20. Euphorbiaceae - Crot. t., Jatr.
21. Fungi - Agar., Bov., Sec.
22. Gattiferae - Gamb.
23. Haemamalidaceae - Ham.
24. Hypericaceae - Hyper.
25. Iridaceae - Iris. v.
26. Labiatae - Collin.,
27. Lauraceae - Camph.
28. Leguminoseae - Bap., Meli., Rob., Cop.
29. Lichenes - Stict.
30. Liliaceae - All. c., Aloe, Lil. t.
31. Loganiaceae - Gels., Ign., Nux v.
32. Lycopodiaceae - Lyc.
33. Melathaceae - Colch., Hell. n., Sabad., Verat., Verat. v.
34. Menispermaceae - Cocc.
35. Myristicaceae - Nux m.
36. Palmaceae - Sabal. serr.
37. Papaveraceae - Cheli., Op., Sang.
38. Phytolaccaceae - Phyt.
39. Plantaginaceae - Plant.
40. Plumbaginaceae - Plumb.
41. Polygonaceae - Ratan., Rhe., Rum. a., Rum. c.
42. Primulaceae - Cycl.
43. Ranunculaceae - Hydras., Puls., Ran. b., Acon., Act. rac., Hell. n., Staph.
44. Rosaceae - Pru. s.

45. Rubiaceae	-	Coff., China., Ipec.
46. Rutaceae	-	Jab., Rut.
47. Sapindaceae	-	Aesc. hip.
48. Scrophulariaceae	-	Dig., Grat., Lept., Verb., Euph.
49. Simarubaceae	-	Ail.
50. Smilaceae	-	Sarsa.
51. Solanaceae	-	Bell., Dulc., Hyos., Stram., Tab.
52. Thymalaceae	-	Mez.
53. Tiliaceae	-	Til.
54. Trilliaceae	-	Trill.
55. Umbelliferae	-	Aeth. c., Asa., Cic. v., Con., Petrosel.
56. Valerianaceae	-	Valer.
57. Verbenaceae	-	Agn. cast.

The Animal Kingdom:

The second important source are animals. Medicines are derived from healthy animals:

1. Araneidea	-	Tarent. cub., Ther.
2. Cephalopoda	-	Sep.
3. Coleoptera	-	Canth.
4. Crotalidae	-	Crotal. h.
5. Elapidae	-	Naja
6. Fibrospongiae	-	Spon., Bad.
7. Gorgoniaceae	-	Coral. r.
8. Helodermidae	-	Heloderma
9. Hemiptera	-	Cimex., Cocc.
10. Hymenotera	-	Apis.
11. Lamellibranchiata	-	Cal. c.
12. Orthoptera	-	Blatta. a., Blatta. o.
13. Scorpiodae	-	Scorpio.
14. Viperidae	-	Lach.

The Mineral Kingdom

Mendeleeff has grouped various mineral sources of medicines as given below. The relationship between medicines belonging to the same origin (same mineral) is the same as in the vegetable kingdom-they do not follow one another well. For example, says Farrington (pg. 459), "if Sulphur is given for some symptom and there seems to be no improvement, then other compounds belonging to the Sulphur group should not be given. Some preparation of another element, say Calcarea, should be tried instead.

Group	***Mineral***		***Medicines***
I	Lithium	-	Lith. c.
	Kali-Potash salts	-	Nat. a., Nat. c., Nat. m., Nat. phos., Nat. s.
	Natrum	-	Kali bich., Kali brom., Kali. carb., Kali sulph.
II	Magnesium	-	Mag. c., Mag. m., Mag. p.
	Calcium	-	Calc. c., Calc. p., Calc. s.
	Barium	-	Baryta carb.
	Zincum	-	Zinc.
III	Cadmium	-	Cad. s.
	Mercurious	-	Merc. c., Merc. cya., Merc. p., Merc. s., Merc. v.
IV	Aluminium	-	Alumina
	Indium	-	Ind. met.
	Thallium	-	Thallium
V	Carbon	-	Carb. v., Carb. an., Graph., Petro.
	Silicon	-	Sil.
	Stannum	-	Stan.
	Plumbum	-	Plumb., Plumb. ac.
VI	Nitrogenium	-	Nit. ac.,
	Phosphorus	-	Phos., Phos. ac.
	Arsenicum	-	Ars.
	Antimonium	-	Ant. c., Ant. t.
	Bismuthum	-	Bism.
VII	Chromium		
	Tungsten		
	Uranium		
	Sulphur	-	Sul., Sul. ac.
	Selenium	-	Sel.
	Tellurium	-	Tell.

VIII	Manganum	-	Mang.
	Fluoricum	-	Fluor. ac.
	Bromium	-	Brom.
	Iodum	-	Iod.

Some other mineral groups are as follows

1. Aluminium	-	Alumina
2. Antimonium	-	Ant. c., Ant. t.
3. Arsenicum	-	Ars.
4. Barium	-	Baryta carb.
5. Bismuthum	-	Bism.
6. Bromium	-	Brom.
7. Cadmium	-	Cad. s.
8. Calcium	-	Calc. c., Calc. p., Calc. s.
9. Carbon	-	Carb. v., Carb. an., Graph., Petro.
10. Fluoricum	-	Fluor. ac.
11. Indium	-	Ind. met.
12. Iodum	-	Iod.
13. Kali-Potash salts	-	Nat. a., Nat. c., Nat. m., Nat. phos., Nat. s.
14. Lithium	-	Lith. c.
15. Magnesium	-	Mag. c., Mag. m., Mag. p.
16. Manganum	-	Mang.
17. Mercurious	-	Merc. c., Merc. cya., Merc. p., Merc. s., Merc. v.
18. Natrum	-	Kali bich., Kali brom., Kali. carb., Kali sulph.
19. Nitrogenium	-	Nit. ac.,
20. Phosphorus	-	Phos., Phos. ac.
21. Plumbum	-	Plumb., Plumb. ac.
22. Selenium	-	Sel.
23. Silicon	-	Sil.
24. Stannum	-	Stan.
25. Sulphur	-	Sul., Sul. ac.
26. Tellurium	-	Tell.
27. Thallium	-	Thallium
28. Zincum	-	Zinc.
29. Halogens	-	Bromine, Iodine, Chlorine, Spongia.

30. Acids - Fluoric, Sulphuric, Nitric, Hydrocyanic, Picric.
31. Mercury - Merc. v., Merc. sol., Merc. cor., Merc. acet., Merc. proto., Merc. cya., Merc. s.
32. Aurum - Aur. met., Aur. mur.
33. Silver - Arg. n., Arg. m.
34. Cuprum - Cupr. m.
35. Soda salts - Nat. c., Nat. s., Nat. hypo., Nat. m., Nat. ars., Borax.
36. Causticum - Caust.

Nosodes

They are remedies derived from mortal tissues / secretions, containing specific virus of the disease. Some important nosodes are:

1. Adrenalin (extract of suprarenal bodies).
2. Bacillinum (a maceration of a typical tuberculous lung).
3. Cholesterinum (cholesterine).
4. Lac Felinum (cat's milk).
5. Lac Vaccinum (cow' milk).
6. Malaria Officinalis.
7. Medorrhinum.
8. Psorinum.
9. Thyroidin (thyroid extract).
10. Tuberculinum.
11. Vaccininum.

INDEX OF MEDICINES

Abrot 21, 96, 335, 365, 449, 452, 453, 569, 570, 647
Acet. ac 61, 258, 283, 452, 577, 578, 627, 665
Acon 9, 11, 12, 31, 73, 74, 78, 97, 99, 121, 127, 129, 180, 189, 205, 231, 232, 247, 256, 274, 289, 295, 299, 315, 328, 329, 330, 341, 363, 364, 408, 436, 474, 489, 508, 509, 518, 542, 543, 598, 612, 616, 621, 665, 712
Act. rac 175, 203, 406, 543, 596, 659, 665, 712
Aesc. hip 44, 239, 240, 484, 713
Aeth. c 15, 713
Agar 61, 247, 329, 381, 462, 494, 579, 616, 631, 665, 712
Agn. cast 369, 396, 397, 665, 713
Ail 544, 665, 713
All. c 77, 78, 281, 282, 515, 665, 712
Aloe 18, 29, 30, 119, 260, 462, 494, 497, 515, 552, 577, 614, 711, 712
Alumen 223, 453, 494, 515
Alumina 31, 32, 33, 316, 335, 453, 517, 518, 714, 715
Amm. c 36, 40, 353, 373, 396, 612, 626, 665
Amm. mur 39, 40, 300, 405, 406, 453
Amyl nit 97, 99, 665
Anac 32, 44, 45, 151, 283, 369, 387, 397, 408, 452, 475, 482, 494, 604, 665, 711
Angust 88, 665
Ant. c 30, 35, 48, 49, 100, 169, 187, 218, 339, 340, 377, 382, 411, 451, 481, 567, 582, 614, 643, 663, 665, 714, 715
Ant. tar 54, 55, 99, 116, 117, 217, 339, 340, 341, 342, 381, 641, 665
Anthrac 75, 203, 257, 300, 378, 665
Apis 18, 53, 59, 61, 66, 67, 74, 111, 112, 122, 159, 170, 180, 205, 218, 223, 260, 282, 312, 353, 354, 454, 473, 475, 507, 508, 533, 544, 573, 616, 636, 665, 711, 713
Apocy 61, 205, 665, 711
Apom 340, 665
Aran 53, 273, 461, 665
Arg. m 509, 540, 600, 601, 665, 716
Arg. n 32, 41, 63, 66, 67, 83, 223, 247, 260, 315, 355, 371, 389, 448, 451, 453, 462, 557, 570, 594, 639, 665, 716
Arn 70, 74, 78, 83, 91, 180, 212, 223, 280, 281, 310, 321, 341, 382, 404, 408, 435, 436, 501, 515, 552, 605, 627, 665, 712
Ars 11, 18, 22, 53, 61, 75, 77, 78, 110, 121, 127, 128, 144, 159, 162, 171, 189, 190, 203, 209, 242, 260, 273, 282, 314, 325, 336, 341, 342, 354, 400, 408, 425, 426, 445, 452, 454, 507, 508, 542, 543, 547, 594, 612, 615, 625, 665, 714, 715
Arum. t 665, 711
Asa 88, 210, 408, 665, 713,
Asar 111, 283, 612, 640, 649, 665
Ast. r 245, 247, 248, 665
Aur. m 88, 373, 408, 481, 540, 604, 665

Balsam 251, 666
Bap 61, 70, 295, 330, 408, 501, 543, 551, 666, 712
Baryt. c 36, 49, 91, 95, 96, 115, 116, 274, 311, 315, 316, 397, 489, 543, 587, 590, 666
Bell 11, 18, 99, 100, 112, 121, 122, 136, 147, 190, 215, 231, 247, 269, 284, 289, 295, 299, 300, 311, 316, 322, 323, 330, 336, 341, 371, 407, 408, 415, 416, 451, 452, 515, 518, 533, 544, 562, 579, 596, 598, 616, 626, 657, 666, 713
Bellis 280, 666
Benz. ac 105, 106, 467, 666,
Berb. v 105, 106, 108, 277, 278, 569, 570, 636, 666, 711
Bism 110, 666, 714, 715
Bor 67, 112, 113, 115, 116, 246, 247, 295, 396, 600, 605, 666
Bov 40, 242, 246, 551, 666, 712
Brom 116, 396, 597, 666, 668, 714, 715
Bry 12, 32, 48, 49, 77, 96, 98, 121, 122, 123, 162, 179, 189, 217, 218, 225, 226, 243, 246, 247, 273, 279, 280, 324, 353, 354, 355, 357, 376, 381, 407, 408, 453, 462, 463, 474, 482, 483, 510, 513, 515, 517, 531, 543, 550, 596, 600, 616, 626, 666, 712
Bufo 415, 666
Cact 44
Calad 111, 396, 666
Calc. c 22, 31, 47, 95, 96, 105, 131, 133, 144, 146, 171, 190, 203, 226, 246, 247, 305, 311, 314, 315, 316, 335, 393, 395, 408, 409, 449, 452, 454, 466, 469, 482, 497, 499, 500, 515, 537, 541, 568, 577, 587, 589, 599, 605, 647, 666, 714, 715
Calc. phos 67, 144, 147, 209, 226, 383, 451, 462, 499, 501, 540, 605, 666
Calc. s 589, 666, 714, 715
Calend 605, 666, 712
Camph 148, 262, 313, 408, 474, 574, 612, 652, 653, 666, 712
Cann. sat 155, 205, 582, 636, 642, 666
Canth 158, 159, 161, 179, 205, 236, 251, 277, 278, 388, 408, 418, 497, 544, 616, 636, 666, 713
Caps161, 162,209,210,330 331,342, 388, 408, 409, 418, 581, 616, 666
Carb.a 32, 116, 168, 223, 226, 247, 616, 666
Carb. v 67,77, 78,149, 171, 207, 209, 210, 236, 341, 354, 355, 373, 395, 411, 440, 452, 489, 527, 594, 666, 714, 715
Caul 406, 408, 560, 659, 666, 711
Caust 12, 39, 40, 63, 67, 83, 116, 169, 170, 171, 178, 179, 180, 247, 280, 295, 304, 369, 395, 409, 452, 453, 454, 468, 494, 550, 581, 615, 666, 716
Cedr 78, 127, 666
Cham 11, 48, 55, 99, 112, 141, 187, 189, 217, 218, 231, 232, 233, 241, 242, 329, 363, 364, 377, 397, 403, 404, 408, 480, 481, 515, 518, 531, 567, 604, 606, 616, 659, 666, 712
Chel 27, 203, 247, 407, 425, 453, 462, 494, 509, 521, 596, 600, 666
Cheno 197, 203, 666, 712,
Chim 277, 666, 712
China 61, 67, 70, 147, 169, 171, 206, 207, 209, 210, 236, 260, 284, 285, 305, 314, 327, 341, 355, 370, 387, 395, 396, 403, 408, 451, 453, 462, 499, 501, 515, 522, 527, 537, 595, 596, 666, 710, 711, 713,
Chlorine 561, 715

Cic.v 211, 217, 323, 666, 713
Cimex 39, 40, 454, 713
Cimicif.r 408, 490, 666
Cina 99, 111, 112, 212, 217, 218, 219, 321, 340, 393,537, 557, 712
Cinchona rub 353, 499, 666,
Cinnab 642, 666
Cistus 133, 408, 666, 712,
Clem 63, 221, 247, 540, 667
Cobalt 483, 484, 663, 667
Coc.cact 159, 667
Coca 41, 408, 667
Cocc 32,185, 211, 225, 226, 229, 235, 246, 247, 261, 262, 283, 335, 467, 483, 494, 667, 712, 713
Coff 11, 187, 189, 221, 232, 233, 293, 328, 329, 408, 462, 490, 611, 612, 641, 667, 713
Colch 226, 236, 381, 384, 410, 582, 636, 667, 712
Collin 119, 240, 667, 712
Coloc 189, 242, 243, 260, 267, 397, 408, 409, 543, 600, 604, 667, 712
Como 596, 667
Con 97, 116, 246, 247, 248, 364, 449, 562, 640, 647, 667, 713
Cop 251, 667, 712
Coral. r 253, 269, 448, 667, 713
Croc 256, 293, 341, 400, 474, 517, 560, 585, 625, 667
Crot.t 203, 260, 285, 341, 515, 573, 667, 712
Crotal.h 209, 210, 258, 365, 373, 377, 409, 587, 627, 636, 667, 713
Cupr 54, 67, 97, 148, 329, 408, 483, 515, 587, 652, 662, 662, 667, 716
Cycl 40, 247, 560, 667, 712
Dig 128, 264, 340, 364, 377, 596, 658, 667, 713
Diosc 241, 242, 267, 522, 667, 712
Diphth 398, 667
Dolichos 33, 316, 355, 667,
Dros 280, 321, 507, 584, 667, 712
Dulc 12, 121, 245, 274, 315, 540, 667, 713
Eatherial oil 155
Elap 341, 409, 667
Equis 205, 278, 569, 570, 712
Eug. j 569
Eup. perf 123, 180, 209, 280, 331, 342, 408, 454, 552, 667, 712
Eup. purp 667, 712
Euph 28, 282, 612, 667, 713
Ferr 41, 121, 122, 189, 209, 210, 247, 283, 285, 341, 355, 409, 415, 515, 532, 560, 640, 649, 667
Ferr. phos 667
Fluor. ac 88, 310, 579, 663, 667, 715
Gamb 573, 667, 712
Gels 49, 53, 65, 66, 92, 93, 112, 178, 179, 247, 264, 289, 295, 300, 311, 330, 376, 377, 398, 408, 410, 468, 501, 546, 582, 594, 667, 712
Glon 41, 42, 49, 97, 99, 100, 128, 284, 296, 300, 375, 377, 408, 415, 416, 448, 663, 667
Gnaf 243, 668
Graph 49, 67, 115, 116, 133, 137, 140, 192, 303, 304, 305, 313, 315, 353, 364, 409, 451, 468, 494, 525, 527, 568, 587, 590, 605, 615, 643, 668, 714, 715
Grat 247, 260, 668, 713
Grind 35, 264, 373, 377, 668
Guaic 454
Ham 310, 409, 435, 605, 668, 712
Hell. n 312, 397, 636, 668, 712
Helod 408, 668
Helon. d 144, 147, 437, 668
Hep. s 12, 33, 61, 97, 99, 112, 116, 117, 133, 147, 210, 303, 312-316, 318, 328, 329, 355, 360, 396, 408, 454, 466, 494, 522, 527, 537, 543, 587, 589, 597, 598, 614, 625, 626, 648, 668

Hydras 77, 112, 158, 330, 509,582, 668, 712
Hyo 99, 143, 260, 269, 322, 323, 329, 341, 489, 490, 501, 508, 668
Hyper127, 383, 668, 712
Ign 11, 18, 77, 123, 179, 189, 209, 231, 232, 255, 256, 283, 293, 311, 320, 328-331, 342, 373, 440, 453, 473, 474, 480, 481, 493, 499, 500, 501, 509, 517, 518, 552, 582, 603, 641, 649, 668, 712
Iod 128, 180, 365, 409, 449, 452, 453, 475, 508, 561, 569, 570, 647, 668, 715
Ipec 54, 74, 209, 330, 340, 341, 342, 409, 515, 605, 668, 713
Iris v 54, 295, 712
Jal 242, 393, 668, 712
Jatr 260, 668, 712
Kali bich 30, 122, 159, 346, 360, 369, 387, 400, 475, 481, 482, 483, 525, 582, 587, 612,668, 714, 715
Kali c 36, 41, 61, 66, 109, 121, 122, 137, 197, 203, 246, 354, 360, 397, 407, 408, 425, 449, 451, 463, 475, 507, 508, 532, 614, 668,
Kali chlor 289, 668
Kali hydro 210, 360, 397, 515, 564, 612
Kali i 88, 581, 601, 668
Kali m 147, 616, 668
Kali n 560, 668
Kali p 561
Kali s 361, 612, 668
Kalm 364, 382, 531, 539, 587, 596, 668, 712
Kreas 110, 280, 366, 373, 475
Lac can 43, 116, 151, 316, 373, 387, 396, 408, 454, 508, 515, 573, 649, 668
Lac def 295, 296, 330, 668
Lach 15, 35, 41, 92, 96, 128, 168, 210, 247, 255, 264, 296, 300, 316, 324, 330, 341, 365, 375-378, 393, 395, 396, 408, 409, 439, 443, 448, 452, 454, 473, 474, 475, 482, 490, 533, 543, 544, 564, 567, 597, 636, 639, 640, 641, 663, 668, 713
Laur 489, 491
Led 40, 49, 363, 364, 382, 426, 605, 626, 627, 663, 668, 712
Lil. t 40, 43, 66, 99, 100, 109, 128, 255, 337, 356, 388, 389, 408, 437, 567, 579, 582, 585, 668, 712
Lith. c 106, 668, 714, 715
Lithic. a 88
Lobel 23, 264, 340, 404, 669, 711
Lod 223
Lyc 32, 36, 39, 49, 78, 88, 96, 106, 109, 112, 116, 133, 141, 177, 189, 198, 209, 236, 247, 251, 300, 303, 304, 316, 355, 376, 377, 378, 382, 387, 388, 395, 396, 397, 407, 408, 409, 453,454, 474, 482, 494, 508, 525, 532, 568, 570, 594, 612, 669, 712
Lyss 100, 296, 393, 448, 669
Mag. c 40, 144, 316, 404, 405, 406, 537, 538, 625, 626, 669, 714, 715
Mag. m 405, 406, 453, 590, 669, 714, 715
Mag. phos 97, 407, 408, 515, 659, 669
Mag. s 415, 669
Mang 40, 321, 529, 669, 715
Medo 49, 409, 411, 412, 493, 512, 567, 569, 570, 594, 614, 616, 641, 669
Meli 97-99, 300, 408, 415, 416, 451, 669, 712
Merc. c 67, 77, 78, 83, 88, 93, 99, 111, 112, 156, 313, 315, 316, 366, 376, 382, 388, 404, 408, 417, 426, 452, 482, 515, 612, 636, 669, 714, 715
Merc. i. fl 409, 669
Merc. proto 396, 421, 550, 669, 716

Merc. s 256, 406, 416, 426, 451, 467, 475, 526, 550, 669, 714, 715, 716
Merc. v 122, 203, 316, 355, 669, 714, 715, 716
Mez 303, 424, 515, 525, 669, 713
Mill 436, 489, 669, 712
Mur. ac 77, 78, 171, 440, 452, 465, 552, 625, 669
Mur. p 99, 387, 437, 567, 579, 582, 669
Myrtus com 203
Naja 87, 88, 443, 598, 669, 713
Nat. ars 451, 669, 716
Nat. c 49, 123, 168, 253, 296, 375, 377, 448, 450, 482, 493, 539, 540, 550, 669, 714, 715, 716
Nat. m 32, 40, 78, 96, 122, 129, 137, 144, 162, 179, 192, 209, 210, 247, 278, 284, 285, 311, 342, 364, 369, 375, 377, 405, 406, 409, 424, 426, 445, 450-454, 456, 474, 481, 482, 501, 508, 551, 552, 567, 568, 569, 600, 647, 669, 714, 715
Nat. phos 669, 714, 715
Nat. s 12, 121, 123, 203, 273, 274, 280, 315, 462, 463, 550, 669, 714, 715, 716
Nit 466, 590
Nit. ac 33, 43, 105, 141, 210, 226, 316, 331, 341, 355, 409, 452, 453, 454, 466, 467, 483, 625, 642, 669, 714, 715
Nuph 462
Nux. m 12, 53, 54, 223, 255, 256, 329, 474, 475,480-483, 518, 531, 540, 543, 579, 639
Nux. v 12, 23, 36, 44, 78, 87, 88, 119, 122, 141, 179, 180, 189, 190, 209, 211, 224, 231, 232, 246, 247, 261, 262, 313, 315, 323, 328-331, 342, 376, 382, 388, 395, 410, 411, 418, 424, 439, 443, 451, 467, 475, 481, 482, 483, 484, 486, 493, 519, 541, 544, 604, 605, 612
Olean 30, 550, 669, 711
Op 11, 32, 54, 119, 231, 321, 323, 329, 373, 397, 453, 475, 490, 501, 521, 567, 669, 712
Oxal. ac 144, 147, 669
Petr 247, 305, 315, 453, 494, 509, 587, 669
Petrosel 157, 366, 669, 713
Phallan 515
Phos 39, 61, 67, 77, 83,97, 121, 122, 136, 141, 169, 171, 1 7 9 , 207,209,210,226,241,242, 243, 246, 247, 251, 300, 321, 341, 350, 353, 365, 366, 373, 383, 393, 397, 408, 409, 493, 500, 507, 508, 509, 510, 515, 521, 525, 532, 540, 549, 550, 573, 596, 598, 600, 615, 669, 714, 715
Phos. ac 77, 136, 171, 179, 207, 353, 373, 408, 440, 451, 501, 543, 561, 579, 594, 604, 605, 616, 670, 714, 715
Phyt 33, 40, 70, 96, 122, 243, 396, 513, 514, 515, 670, 712
Pic. ac 157, 295, 397, 408, 521, 670
Pix liquida 203, 251
Plat 45, 119, 141, 324, 342, 363, 364, 408, 437, 474, 518, 599, 600, 670
Plumb 141, 210, 242, 307, 316, 385, 522, 594, 670, 712, 714, 715
Plumb. ac 670, 714, 715
Podo 18, 30, 197, 260, 342, 407, 425, 513, 550, 552, 670, 711
Potash Nitrate 155
Psor 96, 147, 169, 171, 190, 304, 305, 313, 353, 360, 393, 409, 424, 426, 461, 493, 494, 507, 527, 539, 557, 568, 569, 587, 590, 614, 615, 648, 670

Ptelea 406, 670
Puls 27, 32, 49, 66, 77, 209, 221, 246, 247, 285, 303, 305, 310, 327, 339, 340, 342, 355, 361, 364, 369, 388, 393, 400, 406, 408, 409, 426, 449, 451, 452, 454, 462, 475, 482, 483, 499, 509, 515, 517, 540, 544, 560, 562, 570, 579,582, 587, 589, 590, 612, 640, 642, 643, 648, 649, 663, 670, 712
Pyr 70, 91, 92, 280, 408, 547, 551, 636, 670
Ran. b 23, 280, 547, 626, 670, 712
Ratan 404, 466, 522, 670, 712
Rhe 403, 404, 625, 626, 670, 712
Rho 462, 540, 670, 712
Rhus t 11, 12, 49, 61, 67, 70, 78, 259, 273, 274, 282, 315, 322, 323, 324, 342, 364, 366, 370, 408, 525, 454, 483
Rob 626, 670, 712
Rum. c 269, 462, 550, 670, 712
Rut 70, 331, 383, 408, 440, 451, 552, 555, 627, 631, 670, 713
Saba 100, 376, 448, 670
Sabin 560, 642, 670, 712
Samb 36, 396, 612, 670, 711
Sang 19, 295, 360, 407, 509, 564, 567, 569, 590, 596, 598, 670, 712
Sanic 112, 396, 400, 452, 537, 569, 570, 577, 578, 579, 589, 590, 616, 643, 670
Sarsa 112, 277, 278, 305, 396, 409, 454, 570, 578, 670, 713
Sec 78, 148, 255, 313, 341, 342, 381, 408, 409, 560, 575, 670, 712
Sel 83, 168, 396, 568, 578, 582, 670, 714, 715
Seneg 670
Sep 32, 77, 99, 100, 156, 178, 192, 247, 280, 295, 311, 320, 330, 331, 356, 360, 366, 367, 371, 373, 376, 387, 388, 577, 581, 582, 590, 600, 601, 612, 670, 713
Sil 31, 32, 49, 96, 97, 100, 113, 141, 144, 203, 246, 247, 248, 311, 315, 316, 330, 382, 397, 515, 531, 539, 540, 557, 567, 571, 577, 587, 589, 590, 592, 594, 596, 640, 641, 643, 670, 714, 715
Spig 217, 246, 364, 451, 455, 549, 557, 564, 587, 590, 596, 626, 670
Spon 63, 180, 315, 444, 509, 540, 550, 598, 670, 713
Squil 122, 162, 408, 670
Stan 63, 77, 99, 171, 177, 242, 251, 360, 501, 507, 518, 532, 577, 582, 595, 601, 670, 714, 715
Staph 67, 70, 189, 191, 217, 218, 241, 242, 305, 467, 481, 484, 517, 537, 604, 605, 642, 670, 712
Stict 36, 590, 612, 649, 650, 670, 712
Stram 11, 43, 44, 99, 111, 112, 247, 322, 323, 324, 381, 415, 425, 653, 670, 713
Stron 551, 670
Strych 323, 481, 671
Sul 27, 30, 31, 35, 41, 49, 55, 61, 67, 77, 78, 99, 112, 121, 122, 131, 133, 134, 136, 141, 156, 162, 171, 179, 180, 190, 203, 246, 247, 251, 260, 280, 289, 304, 305, 313, 314, 336, 342, 366, 373, 375, 387, 388, 393, 395, 397, 408, 409, 437, 462, 474, 481, 483, 490, 494, 501, 505, 507, 509, 515, 525, 526, 532, 550, 564, 567, 575, 577, 581, 582, 589, 598, 613, 615, 616, 627, 671, 714, 715
Sul. ac 112, 209, 210, 330, 341, 382, 605, 626, 627, 671, 714, 715
Symp 144, 382, 383, 551, 605, 671, 711

Syph 15, 32, 409, 411, 412, 671
Tab 595, 596, 605, 640, 651, 653, 671, 713
Tarax 452, 640, 671,713
Tarent. cub 283, 378, 671, 713
Tereb 53, 625, 636, 641, 671
Ther 203, 246, 247, 671, 713
Thlaspi 627, 671
Thuj 49, 103, 195, 233, 260, 277, 278, 317, 400, 409, 467, 470, 562, 567, 568, 569, 570, 585, 587, 589, 594, 639, 640, 643, 671, 712
Tilia 426
Tuberc 131, 311, 315, 373, 374, 408, 452, 561, 617, 648, 671
Valer 40, 489, 612, 671, 713
Verat 11, 32, 74, 110, 148, 189, 226, 242, 259, 262, 295, 316, 329, 330, 387, 388, 408, 411, 424, 426, 453, 531, 652, 653, 671,
Verat. v 329, 671, 712
Verb 269, 671, 713
Vib. op 559, 560,671, 711
Vipera 317
Xanth 223, 671
Yebra Santa 251
Zinc 36, 256, 262, 329, 340, 350, 366, 454, 484, 505, 521, 661, 662, 663, 671, 714, 715

Index of Diseases and Symptoms

Abdomen 13, 14, 25, 29, 30, 57, 60, 61, 77, 80, 85, 89, 96, 99, 100, 102, 125,131, 135, 137, 139, 141, 145, 149, 160, 164, 170, 171, 172, 188, 190, 191, 192, 193, 200, 208, 209, 213, 217, 220, 224, 226, 227, 228, 236, 237, 241, 242, 243, 244, 256, 267, 306, 317, 324, 327, 328, 332, 333, 343, 355, 356, 357, 374, 387, 388, 389, 393, 394, 395, 398, 399, 400, 408, 409, 410, 413, 462, 469, 475, 487, 488, 501, 503, 509, 510, 518, 519, 521, 522, 523, 534, 540, 564, 581, 582, 584, 585, 591, 600, 604, 607, 619, 623, 624, 637, 643, 654, 655, 660, 684, 687, 696, 703, 707

- distended *(See distension)* 190, 193, 217, 226, 267, 317, 327, 394, 399, 475, 587, 641,
- plethora of 29, 697
- vomiting after operations of 72

Abortion 15, 72, 74, 91, 175, 215, 255, 309, 356, 394, 438, 473, 476, 542, 549, 559, 560, 641, 659, 692

- after effects of 559
- tendency to 15, 215
- threatened..175, 255, 309, 513, 574

Abscess 59, 69, 75, 98, 161, 182, 208, 291, 397,313, 317, 373, 411, 413, 424, 500, 506, 522, 542, 587, 588, 603, 639, 673, 684, 689, 695, 698, 699, 700

Acetonaemia 673

Achromegaly 673

Acidemia 673

Acidity *(see heartburn)* 65, 84, 86, 127, 131, 169, 171, 188, 410, 459, 625, 673, 685

- infants 459

Acne 23, 25, 98, 167, 169, 177, 181, 205, 251, 267, 303, 349, 365, 480, 525, 530, 587, 614, 647, 673

- rosacea 23, 75, 167, 177, 181, 480, 542, 673

Actinomycosis 181, 480, 542, 673

Addison's disease 359, 465, 673

Adenitis 65, 134, 493, 673

Adenoids 525, 595, 603, 614, 673

Adhesions 673

Adipsia 534, 607

After pain 193, 233

Agalactia 177, 673

Ague 75, 548, 614, 673, 676

Albuminous 113, 228, 523, 635

Albuminuria 294, 311, 363, 374, 394, 447, 493, 513, 521, 574, 635, 636, 637, 647, 707

Alcohol-effects of 87, 131, 580

Alcoholism 43, 53, 75, 119, 208, 291, 319, 374, 391, 480, 563, 577, 625, 661

Alimentary canal 61, 76, 89, 161, 171, 241, 261, 346, 439, 479, 625

Alopecia 291, 391, 673

- areata 505

Amaurosis...9, 98, 161, 177, 248, 263, 293, 313, 321, 480, 505, 521, 530, 629, 657, 673

Amblyopia 208, 257, 269, 374, 480, 499, 505, 552, 635, 661, 673

- potatorum 635

Amenorrhoea 75, 87, 119, 175, 303, 311, 353, 365, 391, 567, 580, 586, 614, 651, 657, 673

Amorous 159, 323, 609, 652, 653

Anaemia 32, 65, 69, 131, 143, 145, 208, 217, 283, 284, 286, 287, 339, 348, 353, 354, 355, 357, 438, 449, 450, 493, 505, 506, 507, 521, 524, 530, 587, 599, 614, 629, 651, 661, 673, 686, 699, 710,

Anaesthesia 42, 349, 521, 524, 674

Anasarca 60, 638, 651, 674, 680

Aneurism 95, 127, 167, 359, 374, 394, 521, 597, 674

Anger 9, 89, 119, 188, 189, 190, 191, 193, 194, 213, 224, 226, 229, 241, 242, 255, 283, 327, 331, 350, 397, 439, 450, 455, 456, 480, 481, 483, 484, 491, 604,

- effects of 119, 224, 327, 480
- fits of 603

Angina *(see heart)* 15, 36, 41, 71, 87, 109, 127, 147, 169, 215, 261, 263, 267, 273, 299, 313, 321, 363, 387, 391, 394, 443, 674

- faucium 273
- pectoris 15, 36, 41, 71, 87, 109, 127, 147, 169, 215, 261, 263, 267, 299, 313, 321, 363, 387, 391, 394, 443, 493, 513, 561, 595, 597, 611, 629, 631, 634, 639, 641, 651,

Anidrosis 359, 447, 521, 674

Ankle 59, 131, 143, 167, 168, 270, 309, 382, 384, 385, 411, 429, 447, 448, 454, 546, 554, 609, 622, 704

- itching eruption about 577
- swelling of 59
- weak 131, 143, 309, 447, 454, 587,

Anorexia 286, 674

Anosmia 39, 674

Anterior crural neuralgia 293, 567

Anthrax of Sheep 639, 674

Antrum of Highmore 197, 362, 403, 417, 674

- disease of 362, 403, 417, 505
- inflammation of 197

Anus *(see rectum)* 14, 17, 27, 29, 31, 33, 44, 47, 48, 61, 62, 117, 121, 125, 128, 155, 164, 172, 178, 193, 194, 206, 217, 237, 251, 279, 289, 303, 304, 305, 306, 307, 310, 327, 333, 345, 346, 376, 377, 379, 396, 400, 405, 406, 413, 428, 439, 441, 450, 451, 453, 456, 465, 466, 469, 470, 487, 491, 494, 507, 509, 517, 518, 523, 525, 552, 573, 582, 585, 589, 591, 608, 615, 620, 641, 643, 644, 685, 698

- eczema around 304, 305
- fissure of 345, 465, 493, 505, 513, 542, 643

Anus-fistula of 587, 641

- herpes of 279
- incontinence of 574
- irritation of 47, 217
- itching of 251, 603
- pain in 611
- pressure of 580
- prolapse 289, 439, 552, 614, 629

Anxiety *(see apprehension)* 10, 12, 21, 22, 55, 56, 78, 79, 80, 81, 111, 123, 134, 149, 171, 173, 181, 182, 188, 191, 212, 219, 226, 229, 248, 261, 318, 327, 341, 344, 349, 350, 379, 436, 455, 467, 481, 484, 507, 508, 511, 512, 535, 542, 565, 579, 584, 586, 594, 598, 617, 621, 633, 634, 655, 684, 697

Aortitis 169, 674

Aphasia 169, 177, 203, 273, 283, 293, 299, 349, 394, 489, 549, 563, 577, 674,

Aphonia 110, 115, 180, 187,

192, 321, 357, 366, 373, 442
from fright 489
Aphthae 53, 75, 111, 113, 119, 208, 311, 417, 424, 427, 439, 449, 625, 626, 674
Aphthous 111, 112, 469, 441, 626
Apoplexy 9, 43, 59, 69, 72, 91, 95, 98, 115, 119, 127, 177, 203, 208, 231, 233, 257, 291, 299, 311, 349, 374, 377, 473, 480, 489, 490, 492, 580, 629, 651, 657, 674
Appendicitis 91, 235, 236, 257, 374, 417, 424, 521, 542, 647, 674
Appetite *(see hunger)* 15, 36, 55, 96, 125, 132, 134, 136, 152, 167, 192, 198, 199, 208, 215, 218, 223, 227, 284, 285, 286, 313, 327, 335, 343, 398, 399, 523, 530, 584, 593, 619, 674, 676, 690, 701
- depraved 131, 530, 580, 587
- disordered 15, 167, 208, 215, 313, 327, 335
- lost 542
- want of 138, 192
Apprehension *(see fear)* 12, 66, 80, 447, 542, 544, 545
Arachnitis 674
Ardor Urinae 160, 537, 674
Arms *(see hand)* 19, 57, 113, 117, 139, 153, 155, 170, 183, 194, 212, 213, 220, 228, 237, 248, 270, 280, 336, 369, 456, 503, 526, 528, 545, 609, 615, 621, 623, 624, 631
- varicosis of 369
Arterial circulation 9
Arteries 35, 101, 127, 263, 301, 332, 634, 701, 706
- disease of 505
Arthralgia 63, 524
Arthritis 40, 106, 136, 177, 178, 185, 195, 337, 674, 687, 700
- deformans 40, 674
Articular 674, 675, 696
Ascarides 137, 217, 356, 403, 580, 595, 675
Ascites 13, 27, 155, 381, 399, 413, 638, 675, 680
Asphyxia *(see choking)* 53, 56, 149, 675
- neonatorium 53
Asthenic 384, 583
Asthenopia 169, 217, 255, 374, 387, 451, 539, 552, 553, 574, 675
Asthma *(see breathing)* 9, 35, 55, 59, 73, 75, 80, 85, 86, 87, 105, 117, 119, 127, 155, 169, 188, 194200, 203, 208, 217, 231, 235, 246, 253, 261, 263, 269, 274, 283, 313, 315, 319, 339, 344, 349, 353, 354, 356, 362, 374, 381, 391, 394, 410, 411, 435, 443, 446, 461, 462, 463, 473, 476, 480, 499, 505, 513, 521, 525, 549, 557, 561, 563, 567, 569, 597, 599, 611, 614, 623, 629, 635, 641, 643, 647, 649, 651, 657, 661, 675, 685
- from anger 188
- humidum 274
- hysteric 473
- Milleri 253, 261, 391, 562
Atelectasis 614, 675
Atheroma 127, 374, 675
Atony 314, 440, 493, 675, 706
Atrophy 137, 205, 291, 335, 396, 449, 506, 521, 522, 524, 674, 675, 700
Aural neuralgia 231
Axilla 313, 353, 394, 465, 675
- abscess in 313
- perspiration of 353
Back 15, 17, 18, 19, 24, 32, 37, 39, 51, 63, 67, 69, 70, 80, 100, 107, 108, 112, 137, 143, 152, 156, 164, 165, 181, 183, 190, 194, 219, 200, 203, 208, 213, 215, 216, 219, 220, 224, 225, 228, 240, 243, 244, 260,

270, 274, 275, 279, 280, 295, 296, 327, 333, 336, 343, 353, 354, 356, 357, 360, 366, 369, 382, 385, 389, 394, 396, 397, 399, 400, 410, 413, 425, 429, 454, 459, 504, 508, 514, 515, 516, 526, 527, 543, 545, 546, 547, 554, 559, 560, 568, 578, 580, 585, 586, 588, 589, 590, 591, 616, 618, 620, 621, 622, 624, 637, 644, 648, 652, 655, 659, 660, 687, 693, 696, 700, 701, 704
- stiffness of 625
- weakness of 143, 208, 327, 587
- ache *(see lumbago)* 16, 17, 18, 19, 57, 108, 180, 340, 344, 354, 355, 356, 357, 400, 514, 525, 545,
Balanitis 424, 641, 675
Balanorrhoea 675
Baldness 69, 95, 580, 673
Barber's itch 513, 516, 675
Barrenness 175
Bashfulness 603
Bazin's disease 675
Beard *(see chin)* 567, 675, 703
- eruptions of 313
- sycosis of 131
Bearing-down pains 175, 620
Bed-sores 69, 147, 374, 493, 614, 649
Bee-stings 60, 567
Belching *(see eructation)* 51, 55, 66, 67, 68, 72, 172, 409, 632
Beri Beri 675
Bile 107, 237, 258, 280, 342, 345, 537, 584, 565, 675, 683, 688
Biliary colic 107
Bilious 17, 53, 91, 97, 107, 119, 198, 199, 201, 208, 257, 258, 267, 279, 293, 328, 345, 479, 480, 534
- attack 107, 119, 208, 345, 480
- fever 257, 279, 293,
Bite 25, 100, 148, 289, 332, 374, 382, 466, 473, 493, 513, 514, 515, 623
Black-eye 69, 309, 381, 627
Bladder 59, 72, 91, 98, 105, 107, 108, 127, 128, 133, 137, 156, 157, 158, 159, 160, 162, 164, 170, 171, 177, 178, 179, 184, 205, 211, 246, 251, 268, 273, 277, 289, 309, 310, 316, 317, 321, 370, 373, 389, 400, 418, 424, 441, 465, 480, 488, 490, 491, 492, 493, 530, 551, 569, 570, 581, 585, 608, 635, 637, 645, 660, 680, 683, 684, 695, 698, 705
- inflammation of 246
- irritable 251, 580, 635
- paralysis of 127, 211, 289, 321,490, 574
- paresis of 405
- weakness 98
Bleeding 18, 49, 83, 113, 128, 164, 169, 170, 172, 181, 182, 185, 210, 239, 240, 255, 256, 258, 275, 310, 341, 344, 366, 367, 374, 376, 377, 413, 418, 425, 427, 429, 436, 441, 451, 452, 453, 469, 470, 495, 503, 509, 510, 560, 614, 618, 620, 643, 644, 645, 682, 685, 691, 702
Blenorrhagia 251, 675
Blenorrhoea pulmonum 51
Blepharites 188, 427, 605, 606
Blepharophathalmia 50, 273
Blepharospasm 188, 255, 530, 676
Blindness 9, 311, 322, 363, 456, 480, 497, 525, 618, 630, 673, 693
- sudden 9
Blisters 157, 158, 159, 160, 163, 185, 306, 398, 412, 452, 455, 548, 673, 676, 688, 696
Blood 5, 14, 17, 30, 32, 33, 35,

39, 40, 54, 56, 66, 68, 69, 72, 73, 75, 90, 91, 97, 98, 99, 100, 101, 102, 108, 132, 156, 158, 159, 160, 164, 169, 170, 183, 190, 193, 207, 208, 209, 219, 248, 255, 256, 257, 258, 248, 283, 284, 286, 287, 289, 299, 301, 302, 309, 310, 340, 341, 343, 344, 375, 376, 378, 379, 383, 384, 390, 393, 398, 390, 403, 413, 415, 416, 418, 425, 429, 433, 436, 439, 443, 449, 461, 465, 466, 467, 468, 469, 470, 475, 476, 486, 487, 505, 508, 509, 512, 520, 533, 534, 535, 551, 614, 615, 616, 617, 620, 621, 623, 625, 626, 645, 636, 637, 660, 661, 662, 673, 674, 675, 679, 680, 681, 682, 683, 685, 686, 689, 690, 691, 695, 697, 699, 700, 704, 705, 706, 709, 710,

Blushing 41, 42, 415

Boils 33, 69, 70, 98, 143, 257, 313, 349, 373, 374, 499, 513, 525, 528, 559, 573, 574, 588, 592, 593, 614, 616, 624, 677

- blind 567

Bone 19, 24, 63, 67, 70, 85, 88, 89, 90, 103, 120, 131, 132, 133, 140, 143, 144, 145, 163, 213, 220, 224, 228, 238, 270, 279, 280, 291, 315, 331, 342, 355, 360, 408, 412, 417, 423, 424, 427, 431, 432, 480, 505, 511, 513, 519, 521, 553, 564, 569, 583, 589, 592, 606, 639, 641, 655, 662, 674, 676, 677, 678, 682, 683, 685, 686, 692, 694, 696, 698, 701, 702, 704, 706, 709

- bruised 552

Bone-disease 85, 131, 423, 424, 425, 505, 513, 603

- exostoses on 521
- lesions and fracture 555
- nodes on 480
- pains 279, 331, 342, 360, 408, 412, 432, 542
- caries of 647
- inflamed 433
- necrosis of 588

Bone-set 280

Borborygmi 217, 394, 549, 567, 676

Bowels *(see stool)* 32, 33, 37, 49, 65, 92, 134, 148, 169, 170, 171, 200, 227, 237, 243, 244, 400, 440, 462, 503, 513, 548, 559, 616, 619, 620, 622, 625,

- looseness of *(see diarrhoea)* 625

Brachial 131, 676

- neuralgia 131, 635

Brachialgia 676

Brain 13, 17, 21, 35, 43, 53, 61, 63, 69, 71, 74, 83, 91, 95, 98, 101, 119, 123, 127,143, 152, 161, 163, 185, 191, 212, 215, 216, 217, 231, 232, 243, 245, 255, 263, 291, 293, 295, 296, 299, 300, 301, 311, 312, 317, 332, 335, 342, 397, 415, 424, 426, 449, 461, 473, 479, 480, 485, 490, 502, 505, 606, 617, 618, 648, 657, 658, 661, 662, 663, 633, 674, 677, 679, 680, 682, 683, 686, 690, 709,

- anaemia of 629
- atrophy of 291, 335
- concussion of 588, 625
- congestion of 127, 215, 255, 299, 614
- infantile affections of 505
- inflammation of 424
- injuries of 461
- irritation of 161, 255
- paralysis of 661
- softening of 23, 91, 521

- fag 21, 43, 63, 91, 143, 449, 499, 506, 588, 629, 661
Breast *(see mammae) 15, 60,* 115, 119, 122, 131, 203, 205, 215, 245, 246, 248, 249, 305, 313, 336, 370, 515, 516, 564, 587, 588, 591, 661, 683, 687, 690 *(see also mastitis)*
Breasts-abscess of 506
- atrophy of 205
- cancer of 115, 167
- inflamed 119
- pain 203, 515
- scirrhus of 569
- sore/hot/hard 122, 138, 245, 246, 370
- tumour of 115, 563, 564
- distended 138
- erysipelas of 169
- indurated 303
Breath 14, 34, 35, 55, 56, 60, 69, 73, 77, 80, 209, 219, 227, 228, 249, 264, 269, 270, 271, 315, 316, 318, 330, 335, 336, 338, 344, 360, 377, 379, 396, 398, 424, 425, 433, 440, 450, 465, 470, 471, 480, 495, 564, 621, 626, 653, 655
- cold 171
- foetid/offensive/sour 69, 87, 424, 465, 480, 493, 516, 523, 537, 625
Breathing *(see respiration)* 34, 55, 56, 73, 80, 90, 93, 199, 200, 219, 228, 253, 262, 286, 340, 341, 344, 356, 357, 371, 373, 377, 399, 400, 429, 470, 489, 490, 492, 508, 509, 579, 585, 675, 681, 691
- difficult, laboured 56
Bright's disease 263, 289, 299, 350, 359, 363, 394, 521, 569, 614, 676
Bronchi *(see lungs)* 10, 27, 116, 279, 320, 337, 344, 373, 391, 613
Bronchial 56, 98, 131, 136, 251, 344, 600
- catarrh 136, 251, 637
- glands-disease of 98, 131
Bronchitis 9, 10, 29, 35, 39, 53, 56, 57, 69, 75, 120, 127, 136, 169, 171, 177, 217, 246, 251, 269, 289, 313, 314, 321, 353, 424, 465, 506, 512, 530, 549, 563, 564, 599, 611, 614, 635, 647, 651, 676
Bronchitis-capillary 499
- membranous 506
Broncho-pneumonia 56
Bronchorrhoea 676
Brow ague 75, 676
Bruises *(see injuries)* 246, 249, 309, 381, 552, 555
Bubo 31, 167, 168, 313, 359, 374, 428, 465, 676
Bulimia/Bulimy 676
Bunions 676
Burning 13, 14, 18, 24, 28, 33, 39, 51, 59, 60, 61, 62, 75, 76, 77, 78, 79, 80, 81, 85, 100, 101, 102, 103, 110, 116, 125, 135, 137, 138, 140, 149, 152, 157, 158, 159, 160, 161, 162, 163, 164, 171, 172, 173, 178, 179, 180, 181, 182, 188, 190, 194, 195, 201, 205, 213, 214, 219, 229, 236, 237, 243, 248, 278, 280, 300, 306, 307, 334, 337, 341, 345, 346, 367, 368, 373, 375, 384, 389, 393, 399, 400, 408, 413, 418, 424, 427, 428, 429, 432, 433, 440, 451, 454, 469, 470, 482, 487, 488, 491, 564, 565, 567, 568, 570, 574, 575, 581, 582, 584, 585, 588, 591, 598, 604, 605, 606, 607, 608, 609, 614, 615, 616, 618, 620, 621, 622, 623, 624, 633, 634, 636, 637, 654, 662, 663, 677, 685
Burns 28, 98, 158, 159, 160,

169, 173, 177, 182, 309, 313, 447, 793, 677
Bursa 676, 686
Bursitis 552, 676
Cachetic 342, 449, 573, 574, 580
Cachexia 278, 676
Caecum 75, 374, 676, 696, 705
- inflammation of 374, 542, 657
Calculi 6, 107, 131, 396, 400, 480, 569
Callosities 47, 48, 49, 631, 676, 700
Cancer 59, 64, 75, 91, 109, 115, 120, 167, 197, 205, 211, 221, 246, 253, 257, 258, 281, 303, 304, 307, 309, 319, 335, 337, 354, 359, 365, 394, 407, 435, 490, 508, 510, 513, 514, 525, 563, 574, 580, 588, 595, 625, 630, 631, 641, 676, 689, 690, 701
- of bone 506
Cancrum oris 75, 417, 424, 625, 676
Canthi 50, 66, 306, 343, 398, 553, 607
Carbuncles 59, 60, 69, 75, 98, 169, 257, 313, 365, 374, 574, 588, 676
Carcinoma 677
Cardiac *(see heart)* 152, 173, 239, 240, 311, 348, 387, 443, 677
Cardialgia 261, 391, 405, 607, 677,
Carphology 323
Carriage-sickness 480
Cartilage 64, 551, 553, 608, 677, 682, 688, 696, 709
Caruncle 677
Catalepsy 9, 151, 211, 283, 327, 374, 473, 490, 597, 630, 641, 677
Catamenia 113, 134, 137, 339, 344, 429, 530, 653
Catarrh 27, 31, 47, 50, 51, 53, 88, 102, 107, 136, 169, 177, 187, 188, 201, 235, 251, 253, 261, 269, 273, 281, 303, 315, 319, 337, 339, 353, 362, 375, 398, 403, 424, 446, 447, 448, 449, 459, 465, 468, 480, 485, 508, 514, 530, 537, 549, 561, 563, 582, 588, 595, 611, 612, 614, 618, 637, 642, 645, 652, 654, 677, 685, 696
- intestinal, nasal 530
Catarrhal 27, 53, 55, 57, 109, 205, 208, 253, 273, 274, 275, 281, 318, 319, 335, 359, 365, 403, 446, 447, 461, 479, 516, 529, 561, 563, 582, 599, 611, 698, 702
- aphonia 549
- irritation 563, 565
- pneumonia 647
Catheter 677
- fever 497
Catheterism 407
Cauliflower excrescences 603, 644
Cellulitis 411, 588, 677, 695
Cerebral 36, 41, 43, 93, 101, 203, 299, 321, 439, 541, 618, 658, 661, 674, 677, 686
- deafness 203, 439
Cerebrospinal 9, 15, 147, 211, 214, 224, 231, 235, 255, 257, 293, 321, 373, 391, 443, 557, 651
- meningitis 293
- system 9, 147, 255, 321, 373, 391, 443, 573, 599, 631, 639, 649, 657, 659, 661,
Cervix 438, 706
Cervix uteri 438, 677
Chafing 172, 625, 626, 677
Chagres fever 614
Chalazae 604, 605, 606, 643
Chalazion 603, 677
Chancre 5, 59, 65, 253, 257, 369, 374, 417, 424, 465, 499, 614, 677, 703
Chancroid 319, 677

Change of life *(see menopause)* 15, 215, 327, 353, 365, 374, 580, 649, 691
Chaps 140, 163, 303, 317, 530, 677
Cheeks 13, 14, 25, 50, 79, 385, 412, 468, 563, 565, 584, 607, 623
Cheloid 465, 588, 614
Chest 9, 11, 14, 15, 17, 19, 25, 39, 51, 53, 55, 57, 69, 73, 74, 77, 80, 86, 90, 102, 113, 117, 121, 123, 125, 128, 134, 137, 138, 139, 140, 145, 149, 160, 164, 165, 171, 172, 178, 181, 182, 183, 191, 193, 194, 197, 200, 203, 215, 219, 228, 237, 249, 256, 269, 270, 275, 280, 286, 300, 307, 324, 339, 341, 343, 344, 354, 356, 357, 360, 374, 375, 383, 389, 391, 397, 398, 399, 400, 429, 462, 463, 476, 486, 500, 501, 503, 507, 508, 510, 511, 528, 530, 552, 554, 564, 565, 586, 596, 598, 599, 600, 601, 608, 616, 621, 623, 624, 634, 640, 647, 655, 658,
- burning 171
- oppression of 561
- pains in 15, 215, 530, 552, 563, 614
Chicken-pox 9, 53, 424, 686, 706
Chilblains 23, 24, 25, 61, 131, 169, 309, 313, 335, 353, 374, 439, 465, 473, 490, 493, 494, 495, 499, 506, 530, 542, 574, 599, 614, 625, 647, 657, 661, 677
Chill 14, 15, 16, 50, 51, 73, 78, 120, 139, 149, 162, 190, 209, 229, 270, 274, 275, 280, 284, 285, 294, 295, 318, 325, 328, 331, 334, 340, 342, 395, 401, 426, 456, 457,482, 487, 516, 531, 543, 544, 548, 562, 593, 655, 656, 673
Chin *(see beard)* 275, 618, 624, 644
- affections of 597
- eruption on 588, 661
Chloasma 175, 580, 584, 614, 677
Chlorosis 39, 64, 120, 138, 140, 145, 261, 283, 286, 303, 313, 435, 493, 506, 517, 661, 677, 709
Choking easy *(see asphyxia)* 465
Cholera 9, 21, 22, 53, 75, 109, 110, 136, 143, 144, 145, 147, 148, 149, 169, 172, 175, 235, 259, 261, 262, 273, 311, 339, 340, 346, 349, 365, 366, 413, 453, 467, 475, 492, 499, 513, 574, 630, 655, 661, 678
- Asiatica 147, 172, 620, 651, 652, 654
- Infantum 9, 21, 22, 54, 110, 136, 143, 144, 145, 340, 346, 349, 365, 366, 413, 453, 475, 492, 525, 527, 531,574, 582, 630,
- Morbus.53, 54, 175, 262, 654
Cholerine 473, 651, 678
Chordee 147, 151, 158, 164, 349, 635, 678
Chorea 23, 24, 25, 41, 47, 69, 85, 131, 134, 136, 143, 177, 179, 184, 197, 215, 216, 217, 224, 246, 255, 261, 267, 283, 321, 327, 329, 362, 407, 410, 439, 449, 506, 539, 574, 580, 622, 631, 635, 641, 657, 661, 678
Choroiditis 293, 542, 678
Chyluria 335, 678
Cicatrix 2191, 513, 588, 678
Cilia 678
Ciliary 241, 257, 374, 678
- Neuralgia 15, 16, 241, 257, 374, 513, 539, 506, 595, 596, 635
Circulation 9, 10, 23, 149, 207,

377, 379, 455, 616, 657
- feeble 542, 588
Cirrhosis 678
Clairaudience 473, 678
Clairvoyance 151, 473, 649, 678
Clavus 327, 353, 480, 530, 573, 641, 678
Clergyman's sore throat 32, 83, 611, 678
Climacteric *(see menses)* 16, 41, 128, 203, 245, 255, 263, 303, 365, 373, 375, 377, 438, 465, 493, 563, 580, 586, 621, 625, 626, 627, 645, 678
- flushes and vertigo 499, 563
- sufferings 438
Climaxis 563, 569, 639, 645
- sufferings of 614, 625
Clonic 25, 211, 261, 323, 411, 481
- spasms 25, 261, 411
Clots 32, 72, 73, 193, 232, 284, 341, 342, 416, 660
Clumsiness 597
Coccygodynia.53, 167, 177, 211, 291, 365, 431, 499, 506, 588, 631, 678
Coccyx 183, 520, 591, 622, 678
-soreness of 567
Coffee-effects of 188
Coitus 534, 608
Cold *(see chill)* 9, 10, 12, 14, 18, 25, 27, 28, 35, 39, 41, 47, 48, 49, 51, 53, 60, 61, 69, 70, 73, 75, 76, 78, 80, 81, 96, 97, 99, 100, 110, 117, 119, 120, 122, 124, 129, 131, 132, 133, 134, 136, 138, 139, 140, 141, 144, 145, 147, 148, 149, 152, 160, 163, 164, 169, 170, 171, 172, 173, 178, 180, 181, 182, 183, 185, 188, 189, 190, 193, 194, 198, 200, 209, 218, 219, 221, 225, 227, 228, 229, 232, 233, 236, 238, 242, 259, 267, 270, 271, 273, 274, 275, 281, 282, 289, 291, 301, 306, 309, 312, 313, 314, 315, 317, 318, 330, 334, 336, 346, 348, 356, 357, 360, 382, 383, 385, 393, 395, 400, 407, 409, 410, 411, 413, 424, 425, 426, 427, 429, 432, 449, 462, 463, 465, 474, 476, 477, 481, 482, 487, 491, 494, 495, 503, 507, 509, 512, 516, 525, 526, 527, 530, 531, 532, 533, 535, 539, 540, 543, 544, 548, 549, 550, 552, 563, 565, 573, 575, 581, 586, 589, 590, 591, 592, 593, 596, 598, 607, 614, 615, 617, 619, 622, 623, 629, 630, 633, 642, 647, 648, 651, 652, 653, 654, 655, 656, 674, 690, 694, 701, 711,
Coldness 14, 16, 23, 39, 54, 75, 80, 110, 132, 133, 135, 136, 145, 147, 148, 149, 165, 170, 195, 209, 236, 294, 295, 307, 408, 519, 520, 555, 574, 575, 586, 588, 599, 620, 629, 651, 652, 653, 654, 655,
Colic 22, 29, 33, 55, 68, 98, 107, 188, 190, 193, 195, 208, 213, 217, 224, 226, 227, 231, 232, 235, 240, 241, 242, 243, 244, 261, 267, 268, 274, 275, 289, 303, 339, 340, 343, 349, 383, 394, 399, 400, 403, 404, 407, 408, 409, 410, 411, 425, 469, 474, 480, 487, 490, 491, 494, 521, 522, 523, 534, 538, 569, 599, 600, 604, 605, 607, 619, 620, 635, 651, 654, 655, 658, 660, 678, 681, 683, 700
Collapse 56, 115, 147, 148, 149, 170, 172, 173, 262, 341, 411, 574, 575, 651, 652, 653, 675
Coma 54, 57, 208, 321, 477, 491, 656, 678, 699

Coma vigil 321, 679
Comedo 577, 679
Commissures 75, 305, 307, 679
Complexion pale 395, 678
Concussion 71, 72, 74, 211, 212, 311, 588, 625, 679
Condylomata 281, 359, 424, 461, 465, 466, 470, 499, 559, 567, 580, 603, 605, 641, 642, 643, 644, 679
Congenital 365, 530, 679
- syphilis 365
Congestion 9, 10, 17, 29, 35, 41, 65, 97, 100, 127, 135, 149, 161, 187, 191, 197, 198, 215, 239, 255, 284, 286, 295, 296, 299, 300, 301, 302, 311, 339, 341, 387, 389, 413, 415, 426, 435, 446, 468, 474, 505, 525, 559, 581, 614, 616, 618, 619, 620, 621, 623, 624, 635, 637, 657, 658, 677, 682
Conjunctiva 27, 57, 152, 541, 677, 679, 696
Conjunctivitis 57, 281, 382, 459, 495, 514, 567, 679, 684, 685
- phlyctenular 588
- granular 684
Constipation 17, 29, 30, 31, 32, 34, 39, 40, 43, 47, 48, 50, 98, 119, 120, 125, 131, 155, 167, 169, 178, 179, 193, 197, 200, 208, 239, 240, 267, 293, 303, 305, 320, 335, 345, 356, 365, 389, 393, 394, 395, 403, 405, 406, 431, 449, 450, 453, 456, 465, 470, 479, 480, 481, 483, 488, 489, 490, 491, 492, 493, 506, 507, 509, 513, 517, 518, 519, 521, 522, 523, 525, 537, 552, 567, 568, 569, 577, 578, 582, 588, 589, 595, 597, 614, 619, 623, 625, 630, 641, 643, 651, 652, 654, 661, 679, 711
- during pregnancy 585
- of children 567
- of suckling 31, 34, 59
Constriction 32, 41, 44, 92, 100, 117, 127, 128, 155, 162, 192, 199, 200, 211, 294, 307, 344, 374, 375, 376, 377, 383, 388, 408, 417, 446, 487, 488, 519, 522, 523, 537, 557, 614, 630, 652, 655, 674
Consumption *(see tuberculosis)* 9, 120, 134, 138, 143, 269, 283, 309, 313, 335, 339, 353, 359, 360, 365, 394, 412, 435, 506, 512, 598, 599, 614, 679
Contraction 148, 178, 184, 185, 211, 228, 256, 263, 269, 293, 333, 395, 396, 427, 456, 469, 479, 488, 503, 551, 573, 619, 651, 660, 678, 679, 680, 702
Convulsion 9, 21, 22, 23, 36, 65, 67, 73, 98, 100, 103, 139, 147, 177, 188, 203, 209, 211, 212, 213, 217, 220, 223, 224, 228, 231, 235, 245, 257, 261, 262, 293, 299, 300, 302, 312, 321, 322, 324, 327, 328, 329, 339, 373, 435, 479, 480, 488, 492, 506, 517, 521, 524, 530,573, 574, 599, 641, 660, 657, 658
Coprophagia 651, 679
Corn 47, 48, 49, 69, 111, 367, 614, 625, 678
Cornea 85, 95, 136, 248, 259, 282, 313, 403, 447, 567, 618, 675, 679, 688, 695, 696, 703
- opacity of 259, 403, 631, 647
- ulcers of 525
Corpulency *(see obesity)* 506, 679
Coryza 18, 27, 28, 36, 39, 78, 102, 117, 120, 125, 131, 147, 164, 181, 280, 282, 335, 376, 397, 426, 427, 429, 446, 447, 485, 533,

534, 539, 544, 549, 557, 561, 567, 584, 588, 608, 612, 618, 679, 684
Costiveness 481, 609, 679
Cough 10, 14, 17, 21, 23, 24, 27, 29, 35, 36, 39, 40, 43, 47, 49, 53, 55, 57, 64, 69,75, 76, 77, 78, 131, 135, 138, 140, 153, 161, 162, 165, 167, 169, 177, 178, 179, 180, 182, 183, 188, 190, 192, 194, 197, 198, 208, 216, 217, 219, 228, 235, 244, 246, 249, 251, 253, 258, 259, 261, 262, 267, 269, 270, 271, 274, 275, 279, 281, 282, 283, 285, 286, 289, 304, 313, 314, 315, 317, 318, 321, 322, 323, 324, 328, 333, 335, 337, 339, 340, 341, 342, 343, 344, 350, 353, 354, 356, 359, 360, 362, 366, 370, 374, 377, 379, 383, 391, 394, 398, 400, 401, 403, 405, 407, 415, 424, 429, 433, 439, 444, 449, 450, 462, 463, 465, 466, 470, 473 480, 485, 486, 490, 495, 499, 500, 501, 503, 506, 507, 509, 510, 511, 513, 525, 526, 528, 530 534, 543, 544, 545, 548, 549, 550, 561, 563, 564, 565, 569, 580, 586, 588, 592, 597, 598, 600, 601, 603, 611, 612, 614, 619, 635, 639, 642, 645, 652, 655, 662, 679, 690, 696, 707
- of pregnancy 569
Coxalgia 75, 131, 241, 269, 499, 641, 649, 679
Cracks 50, 105, 279, 305, 307, 407, 449, 456, 466, 618, 661, 700
- in skin 449, 493
Cramp 23, 69, 138, 148, 160, 182, 183, 184, 188, 194, 213, 219, 235, 242, 261, 262, 267, 283, 286, 294, 304, 379, 394, 406, 407, 409, 412, 427, 488, 519, 520, 552, 555, 568, 574, 588, 593, 599, 620, 622, 645, 649, 651, 652, 653, 654, 655, 659, 660, 678, 679, 707
Cretinism 143, 679
Croup 9, 10, 12, 53, 75, 98, 115, 116, 117, 132, 188, 261, 289, 313, 314, 315, 318, 327, 335, 336, 337, 369, 391, 506, 509, 563, 597, 598, 679
Crusta lactea *(see breasts)* 132, 136, 273, 275, 345, 431, 525, 679
Crusta serpiginosa 525, 614, 679
Cyanosis 173, 261, 264, 374, 542, 679
Cyst 289, 359, 539, 603, 604, 677, 680, 686
Cystitis 9, 57, 109, 155, 205, 206, 251, 277, 289, 311, 394, 497, 521, 631, 635, 559, 580, 680
Dandruff 75, 353, 362, 456, 506, 567, 580, 641, 643, 680, 702
Deafness 169, 177, 179, 181, 203, 208, 293, 303, 306, 320, 324, 339, 366, 381, 391, 403 405, 424, 439, 447, 468, 493, 508, 517, 537, 618
Debauchery 577
Debility 6, 43, 67, 97, 132, 137, 138, 139, 143, 167, 169, 172, 207, 208, 209, 224, 235, 245, 248, 263, 283, 289, 319, 327, 335, 336, 338, 353, 354, 355, 357, 359, 366, 391, 394, 401, 403, 439, 440, 441, 447, 449, 461, 468, 471, 473, 499, 501, 503, 525, 526, 527, 528, 557, 567, 577, 587, 588, 592, 599, 600, 601, 616, 623, 651, 675
- of drunkards 461

Decubitus 291, 680
Deglutition 93, 102, 178, 179, 330, 370, 452, 700
Delirium 11, 12, 15, 21, 23, 24, 53, 71, 75, 78, 83, 93, 97, 98, 99, 100, 101, 109, 120, 132, 140, 151, 158, 161, 208, 215, 257, 264, 289, 321, 322, 323, 324, 341, 374, 480, 489, 494, 508, 521, 539, 542, 543, 545, 625, 653, 661, 680
- Tremens 15, 23, 24, 53, 71, 75, 98, 109, 132, 151, 161, 215, 257, 264, 289, 321, 374, 489,
Deltoid 333, 473, 680
- rheumatism 473
Delusions 91, 151, 349, 350, 517, 653, 680
Dementia 257, 322, 387, 680
- senilis 322
Dengue fever 9, 293, 542
Dentition *(see teething)* 9, 21, 55, 111, 114, 120, 132, 136, 140, 141, 143, 177, 187, 188, 190, 192, 193, 194, 195, 211, 212, 217, 261, 327, 365, 366, 406, 407, 409, 424, 435, 513, 514, 517, 537, 538, 588, 599, 603, 635, 647, 661,
- abnormal 424
- difficult 513, 537
Depression 53, 75, 87, 88, 98, 115, 179, 207, 224, 245, 246, 311, 323, 327, 340, 348, 375, 388, 389, 394, 397, 438, 449, 451, 455, 479, 489, 501, 579, 587, 632, 644, 661, 684
- of spirits 75, 246, 311, 327, 388, 389, 517, 521, 631
Despondent 87, 89, 207, 304, 305, 374, 431, 432, 525, 526, 530, 599, 600
Diabetes 64, 69, 132, 143, 205, 235, 241, 289, 335, 345, 349, 411, 438, 449, 453, 459, 461, 489, 499, 567, 574, 588, 611, 614, 625, 633, 645, 680
- mellitus 490
Diaphragm 15, 120, 127, 200, 213, 215, 400, 651, 680
- cramp in 574
- pains in 599
- rheumatism of 15, 120, 127, 215, 611
- stitches in 595
Diaphragmitis 313, 657, 680
Diarrhoea *(see stool)* 9, 27, 29, 39, 47, 48, 49, 51, 57, 59, 62, 65, 66, 67, 68, 75, 85, 93, 98, 105, 109, 111, 113, 120, 122, 125, 132, 133, 135, 137, 140, 144, 145, 147, 148, 149, 161, 169, 188, 190, 192, 193, 194, 197, 200, 207, 208, 217, 231, 233, 239, 240, 241, 242, 259, 260, 261, 267, 273, 274, 275, 279, 283, 284, 286, 289, 293, 294, 295, 296, 304, 305, 311, 313, 314, 316, 321, 335, 339, 343, 345, 346, 365, 379, 387, 391, 403, 405, 413, 417, 424, 428, 435, 440, 456, 459, 462, 465, 467, 469, 475, 480, 487, 488, 493, 494, 499, 500, 501, 503, 505, 506, 507, 510, 513, 525, 527, 530, 534, 537, 538, 539, 549, 550, 552, 563, 567, 568, 573, 574, 580, 594, 611, 614, 615, 616, 617, 619, 620, 623, 625, 630, 641, 643, 654, 656, 678, 680
- chronic 542
- nervous; with stupor 661
Diathesis 506, 507, 513, 541, 549, 551, 569, 573, 574, 595, 597, 624, 647, 680, 685
Digestion 48, 50, 170, 239, 348, 393, 399, 453, 479, 489, 529
- slow 567
Diphtheria 59, 60, 61, 75, 83, 91, 115, 116, 117, 118, 158,

161, 257, 258, 393, 394, 396, 293, 327, 335, 369, 374, 376, 421, 439, 441, 444, 446, 452, 456, 468, 513, 516, 525, 542, 545, 557, 563, 625, 680
- after effects of 525
Diplopia 513, 521, 597, 680
Disappointments-effects of 31
Dislocation 35, 334, 383, 551, 552, 608
- pains from 35
Dissection wounds 59
Distension *(See abdomen)* 80, 164, 169, 172, 201, 213, 224, 226, 227, 228, 306, 341, 343, 355, 394, 398, 399, 487, 530, 584, 681, 686, 687, 705
Distortions 574
Dog-bite 374
Dreams 14, 90, 120, 123, 152, 165, 214, 229, 318, 351, 371, 385, 456, 490, 542, 555, 578, 593, 609, 623
Dropsy 9, 59, 60, 105, 120, 127, 132, 203, 205, 208, 235, 238, 239, 240, 264, 265, 273, 277, 291, 303, 311, 312, 336, 353, 359, 363, 374, 387, 394, 449, 506, 521, 568, 635, 674, 675, 680
- cardiac 239
- during pregnancy 567
Drowsiness *(see sleepiness)* 54, 55, 74, 93, 198, 293, 471, 476, 477, 502, 609, 622, 702
Drowsy 21, 22, 24, 92, 93, 152, 294, 473, 477, 492, 500, 504, 637
Duodenum 76, 680, 699
- catarrh of 107, 537
Dupuytren's contraction 680
Dyscrasia 5, 291, 305, 449, 465, 681
Dysentery 9, 29, 31, 70, 72, 91, 98, 158,161, 164, 169, 235, 237, 238, 239, 240, 241, 242, 251, 267, 273, 274, 275, 289, 293, 339, 345, 387, 394, 509, 513, 537, 542, 545, 554, 603, 605, 614, 620, 635, 661, 681
Dysmenia 246, 255, 293, 443, 447, 473, 490, 493, 513, 517, 530, 569, 681
- membranous 246
Dysmenorrhoea 9, 23, 43, 107, 115, 116, 175, 176, 188, 226, 303, 322, 327, 353, 363, 369, 391, 394, 405, 407, 410, 411, 415, 435, 438, 542, 559, 563, 580, 631, 635, 639, 641, 651, 657, 658, 659, 660, 681
Dyspareunia 449, 641, 680
- in newly married women 603
Dyspepsia 15, 21, 31, 43, 44, 53, 65, 72, 76, 85, 120, 132, 143, 163, 169, 188, 197, 208, 215, 236, 239, 257, 267, 289, 316, 319, 345, 353, 356, 362, 374, 391, 394, 403, 405, 424, 447, 449, 459, 461, 465, 473, 480, 563, 569, 580, 599, 625, 681, 687
- of drunkards 461
- of pregnancy 557
Dysphagia 574, 681
Dyspnoea 76, 86, 237, 261, 317, 327, 344, 396, 400, 444, 476, 511, 516, 526, 581, 608, 681
Dysuria 277, 497, 521, 569, 661, 681
Ear 9, 14, 21, 24, 60, 66, 72, 76, 98, 103, 111, 112, 189,191, 199, 208, 209, 219, 248, 257, 258, 259, 264, 275, 284, 289, 303, 304, 306, 307, 313, 315, 317, 319, 332, 334, 341, 353, 359, 365, 367, 370, 374, 378, 381, 383, 394, 398, 409, 423, 427, 431, 432, 466, 467, 469, 493, 513, 527, 528, 542, 553, 588, 591, 607, 614, 618, 619,

659, 675, 694, 695, 704, 709
- discharge from 21, 111, 257
- eczema of 394, 542
- inflammation of 128, 353, 381
- polypi of 374, 563, 641
- wax in 374
- ache 188, 189, 192, 275, 530, 539, 557, 661
Ears-ring holes-ulceration of 599
Ecchymosis 70, 257, 382, 443, 501, 505, 506, 626, 627, 681
Eclampsia 500, 699
Ecthyma 53, 424, 542, 681
Eczema 31, 43, 47, 76, 77, 120, 133, 140, 158, 211, 212, 259, 260, 303, 304, 305, 306, 307, 313, 319, 345, 362, 381, 394, 398, 417, 424, 431, 433, 454, 493, 494, 525, 528, 542, 548, 567, 577, 580, 603, 605, 614, 661, 681, 704
- impetiginoides 319
Effusion 119, 120, 311, 491, 616
Elephantiasis 43, 588, 681
Emaciation 134, 145, 177, 184, 273, 287, 307, 335, 336, 337, 338, 348, 359, 385, 409, 424, 447, 449, 450, 453, 456, 468, 501, 502, 521, 522, 523, 524, 561, 564, 567, 568, 569, 570, 571, 577, 647, 648, 675, 681
Embolism 674, 681
Emissions 137, 143, 158, 208, 261, 286, 304, 345, 350, 405, 480, 503, 608, 609, 611
Emmenagogue 551, 681
Emotions 163, 231, 233, 293, 328, 456, 500, 561
Emphysema 56, 115, 169, 313, 341, 391, 652, 681
Endometritis 76, 681
Enteralgia 268, 409, 459, 681, 684
Enteric fever 23, 76, 91, 309, 322, 335, 339, 374, 417, 439, 499, 506, 542, 635, 681
Enteritis 9, 57, 681
Enterocolitis 340
Entropion 111, 681
Enuresis 35, 64, 105, 143, 177, 217, 277, 283, 365, 407, 410, 435, 461, 499, 525, 552, 567, 569, 573, 577, 581, 588, 614, 641, 661, 681
- diurna 283, 681
- nocturna 65, 681
Ephelis 394, 439, 506, 681
Epidemic 6, 280, 516
Epididymitis 659, 682
Epigastric 125, 355, 519, 534
Epigastrium 74, 200, 227, 320, 237, 356, 399, 483, 486
Epiglottis 102, 682
Epilepsy 21, 23, 65, 67, 98, 132, 139, 143, 147, 151, 177, 203, 211, 213, 215, 257, 261, 293, 299, 311, 322, 324, 325, 327, 349, 374, 377, 411, 415, 435, 449, 461, 466, 480, 490, 506, 521, 530, 574, 588, 599, 614, 630, 631, 635, 641, 652, 682, 696
- traumatic 461
Epistaxis 12, 36, 71, 72, 122, 163, 269, 285, 299, 300, 317, 322, 394, 412, 415, 427, 428, 461, 530, 539, 549, 552, 557, 574, 580, 583, 599, 631, 682
Epistaxis-menstrual 461
Epithelial tissue-affections of 64
Epithelioma 76, 211, 362, 365, 394, 682
Epithelium 637
Epulis 132, 369, 521, 641, 682
Erethism 10, 87, 293, 499, 505, 517, 661, 682
Ergot poisoning 573
Erotomania 143, 158, 322, 480, 506, 517, 631, 682
Eructation *(see belching)* 13, 48, 50, 65, 68, 70, 71, 72, 121, 125, 132, 167, 169, 182, 188, 193, 208, 227, 237, 243, 284, 285, 286, 337,

343, 365, 395, 399, 456, 459, 469, 486, 528, 626, 682
Eruption 6, 9, 35, 48, 50, 51, 54, 57, 59, 60, 76, 77, 81,120, 139, 140, 147, 167, 168, 172, 177, 178, 180, 185, 188, 194, 211, 214, 253, 257, 261, 270, 273, 274, 275, 303, 304, 305, 306, 307, 313, 319, 345, 349, 356, 365, 381, 394, 431, 432, 441, 449, 450, 456, 494, 516, 525, 526, 527, 528, 541, 542, 544, 548, 563, 569, 571, 577, 579, 588, 605, 613, 614, 615, 616, 617, 618, 622, 623, 634, 645, 661, 662, 673, 680, 684, 686, 691, 698
- moist; itching 525
- suppressed 661
Erysipelas 35, 36, 60, 61, 65, 76, 87, 98, 111, 147, 158, 159, 169, 188, 208, 246, 257, 261, 289, 304, 313, 374, 449, 459, 542, 547, 548, 551, 555, 647, 657, 682
- bullosa 635
Erythema 9, 60, 319, 349, 359, 381, 431, 635, 647, 674, 682
- nodosum 9, 60, 319, 349, 359, 381, 513, 542, 625
Eustachian catarrh 362
Eustachian tubes 495, 513, 682
Examination funk 43
Exanthema 548
Exanthemata 60, 77
Excitement 9, 42, 98, 134, 137, 188, 224, 228, 231, 233, 245, 285, 294, 295, 296, 299, 321, 348, 350, 401, 438, 490, 534, 592, 594, 597, 598, 631, 632, 633
Excoriation 21, 33, 70, 93, 188, 394, 400, 424, 432, 585, 620, 621, 682
Excrescences 51, 466, 588, 603, 605, 641, 642, 644, 682
Exhaustion 70, 75, 80, 149, 187, 207, 229, 238, 261, 262, 307, 357, 375, 377, 379, 456, 499, 501, 503, 504, 512, 577, 586, 587, 599, 661
Exophthalmos 41, 597, 682
Exostosis 64, 273, 431, 506, 542, 552, 682
Exposure 10, 25, 96, 97, 120, 181, 273, 274, 299, 309, 314, 315, 508, 516, 544, 598, 648, 698
Extravasation 682
Exudation 433, 516, 605, 682
Eye 9, 10, 13, 15, 21, 22, 27, 28, 31, 33, 50, 55, 65, 67, 69, 71, 72, 76, 79, 85, 87, 89, 92, 97, 98, 99, 101, 102, 105, 107, 109, 111, 115, 123, 124, 132, 134, 135, 136, 138, 139, 141, 145, 152, 155, 158, 159, 161, 163, 171, 172, 177, 179, 181, 185, 188, 191, 195, 199, 217, 221, 235, 246, 247, 257, 259, 265, 280, 281, 282, 285, 291, 293, 295, 296, 301, 303, 306, 309, 313, 319, 322, 323, 324, 330, 335, 337, 340, 343, 346, 349, 353, 355, 359, 364, 369, 371, 373, 374, 378, 381, 382, 383, 387, 391, 394, 397, 398, 403, 409, 411, 412, 427, 431, 446, 449, 451, 466, 417, 424, 426, 432, 439, 440, 441, 447, 449, 455, 465, 468, 470, 476, 477, 480, 483, 485, 490, 491, 502, 505, 506, 508, 522, 529, 539, 544, 552, 553, 564, 565, 567, 569, 580, 583, 588, 595, 596, 603, 604, 607, 613, 614, 627, 629, 630, 632, 634, 639, 640, 641, 644, 647, 655, 661, 677, 678, 680, 682, 687, 688, 692, 694, 695, 699, 700
Eye-corneal opacity 155

- dry 102
- inflamed 33, 39, 53, 158, 211, 403, 411, 521
- pains in 595
- polypi of canthus 394
- strain 451, 449, 500, 552
- swollen 191
- tumours of 105, 603, 641

Eyeball 25, 124, 191, 216, 243, 279, 427, 502, 678, 679, 684, 688, 693, 694, 700, 702, 703

Eyelashes 112, 468, 506, 675, 705

Eyelids 24, 25, 33, 49, 50, 60, 62, 79, 178, 179, 184, 195, 242, 243, 263, 264, 281, 282, 294, 295, 295, 304, 305, 353, 354, 355, 367, 398, 468, 580, 582, 603, 604, 605, 606, 615, 643, 675, 676, 678, 679

Eye-teeth-pains in 639

Face 10, 12, 13, 14, 22, 25, 35, 36, 41, 54, 55, 56, 57, 60, 61, 69, 70, 79, 92, 93, 97, 98, 99, 100, 101, 102, 103, 110, 113, 115, 116, 189, 190, 191, 192, 193, 195, 198, 199, 209, 211, 213, 214, 217, 218, 219, 221, 227, 241, 244, 257, 263, 264, 271, 275, 285, 286, 294, 296, 300, 302, 303, 304, 306, 307, 322, 324, 328, 331, 332, 334, 336, 340, 341, 342, 343, 344, 349, 353, 355, 364, 367, 370, 371, 375, 377, 381, 385, 394, 395, 398, 409, 412, 415, 416, 418, 423, 426, 433, 447, 449, 451, 456, 469, 480, 482, 484, 485, 490, 491, 492, 493, 507, 508, 515, 516, 520, 522, 530, 533, 537, 544, 547, 548, 563, 569, 577, 578, 579, 580, 582, 583, 584, 586, 587,589, 593, 596, 617, 618, 621, 623, 624, 634, 643, 652, 653, 654, 655, 656, 658, 662, 673, 675, 686, 691, 704, 705
- blotches on 353
- boils on 143
- complexion unhealthy 449
- erethema of 303
- eruption on 76, 167, 211, 257, 394
- flushing of 10
- pale 209, 219, 149, 322, 336, 340, 343, 491, 573, 629, 634, 655
- pimples on 221, 381
- rough 493
- yellow 580

Facial bones 694

Facial muscles 212, 398, 491

Facial neuralgia 208, 432

Facial paralysis27, 177, 493, 698
- from cold 552

Fag 449, 499, 506, 588, 629, 661, 676, 683,

Fainting 75, 76, 128, 172, 188, 190, 247, 255, 261, 314, 327, 374, 377, 473, 506, 531, 597, 622, 632, 639, 652
- fits 188
- with flooding 645

Faintness 15, 81, 120, 121, 208, 209, 215, 223, 224, 225, 235, 236, 258, 264, 265, 319, 337, 341, 391, 424, 425, 476, 488, 524, 569, 579, 581, 586, 614, 616, 619, 623,

Fatty degeneration 73, 357, 505, 506

Fatty tumours 642

Fauces 18, 57, 68, 93, 102, 117, 125, 270, 271, 351, 370, 428, 433, 486, 557

Favus 411, 683

Fear *(see anxiety)* 10, 11, 12, 16, 70, 71, 76, 78, 79, 80, 98, 99, 111, 112, 127, 128, 134, 152, 189, 216, 219, 224, 232, 233, 293, 294, 370, 371, 389, 415, 467, 489,

490, 491, 517, 527, 530, 579, 632, 680, 686
- of death 10, 11, 127, 128, 134, 216, 232, 233, 370, 467, 653
Fear-of falling 112, 294, 370
Feet 14, 27, 39, 47, 49, 60, 70, 80, 96, 97, 115, 132, 133, 134, 138, 139, 140, 160, 169, 170, 171, 172, 175, 184, 188, 194, 200, 224, 225, 228, 229, 235, 237, 295, 303, 317, 350, 356, 381, 382, 384, 394, 429, 439, 441, 466, 471, 494, 505, 509, 530, 532, 545, 546, 547, 554, 567, 571, 574, 575, 577, 581, 586, 588, 590, 592, 593, 594, 614, 615, 616, 617, 620, 621, 622, 623, 624, 652, 656, 662, 676, 702
- burning 60, 588, 614
- cold 169, 614, 617
- cramps in 574
- foetid 642
- pain in 39, 115, 235, 381, 542
- perspiring 394, 466, 588
- soles painful 439, 493
- sore 70, 499
- tender 549
Fester 313, 588, 683
- tendency to 313, 493
Fever 9, 10, 23, 24, 27, 32, 35, 47, 51, 53, 60, 69, 70, 72, 73, 76, 78, 79, 81, 83, 87, 91, 92, 93, 97, 98, 99, 103, 107, 112, 116, 119, 120, 127, 128, 132, 139, 140, 149, 160, 162, 163, 170, 173, 178, 188, 195, 205, 207, 208, 209, 217, 218, 224, 229, 232, 235, 257, 258, 261, 264, 270, 273, 275, 258, 261, 264, 270, 273, 275, 279, 283, 289, 293, 295, 299, 302, 309, 311, 316, 318, 322, 328, 331, 335, 339, 340, 342, 344, 348, 354, 362, 373, 374, 375, 376, 394, 401, 409,417, 421, 424, 426, 434, 439, 441, 443, 449, 454, 456, 459, 468, 474, 480, 482, 497, 500, 506, 512, 515, 516, 520, 525, 528, 539, 541, 542, 545, 548, 552, 593, 597, 598, 599, 611, 614, 615, 618, 624, 562, 564, 635, 637, 652, 656, 657, 658, 662, 673, 676, 680, 681, 682, 684, 685, 686, 688, 689, 690, 691, 692, 694, 699, 700, 701, 702, 703, 705, 707
-hectic 139, 208, 499, 511, 599
- intermittent 112, 120, 127, 132, 139, 178, 208, 217, 224, 235, 279, 283, 289, 328, 331, 339, 342, 374, 449, 473, 480, 493, 497, 522, 530,
- remittent 120, 217, 257, 279, 293, 339
Fibroma 359, 387, 394, 574, 588, 631, 635, 683
Fibroma-haemorrhage from 645
Finger joints-ulcers on 111
Fingers 14, 24, 37, 48, 49, 51, 111, 155, 184, 200, 213, 218, 244, 262, 275, 295, 305, 307, 336, 470, 495, 511, 526, 546, 571, 592, 609, 622, 632, 680, 683, 700
Finger-nails 48, 49
Fissure 27, 31, 193, 303, 305, 345, 398, 441, 465, 466, 470, 493, 505, 513, 542, 580, 587, 641, 676
Fistula 23, 31, 107, 115, 127, 132, 138, 143, 145, 178, 197, 251, 291, 319, 345, 356, 374, 435, 466, 493, 495, 506, 587, 588, 591, 641, 683
- dentalis 178, 291, 603, 614,
- lachrymalis 23, 115, 197, 291, 374, 435, 466, 588, 599

Flatulence *(see flatus)* 65, 85, 134, 137, 144, 145, 170, 171, 172, 188, 208, 209, 224, 227, 240, 267, 268, 285, 286, 327, 354, 355, 374, 394, 395, 399, 453, 462, 469, 473, 476, 499, 506, 534, 607, 683
Flatulent colic 13, 164, 188, 224, 226, 227, 343, 409, 410, 534, 654, 683
Flatus *(see gas)* 13, 30, 67, 68, 71, 72, 85, 89, 117, 172, 193, 208, 209, 226, 227, 243, 306, 393, 399, 400, 456, 462, 534, 591, 607, 608, 619, 637, 654, 676
- incarcerated 539, 642
Flushing 10, 41, 284, 365, 617, 623, 625
Foetid 14, 69, 85, 89, 93, 192, 242, 258, 304, 305, 316, 360, 366, 419, 427, 429, 441, 469, 470, 516, 523, 525, 526, 527, 574, 581, 621, 642
Foetus 490, 643, 683, 705, 706
- excessive movements of 490
Fontanelles 132, 133, 135, 140, 141, 143, 144, 587, 589
Forehead 13, 14, 36, 53, 55, 85, 89, 101, 123, 124, 135, 148, 153, 163, 172, 181, 199, 212, 227, 243, 275, 301, 302, 304, 305, 312, 332, 346, 385, 412, 455, 502, 515, 519, 535, 565, 569, 583, 590, 592, 606, 611, 612, 617, 626, 629, 651-655, 683, 702,
Foreign bodies 589
- expulsion of 588
Foreskin 695, 696, 698
Forgetful 43, 71, 151, 322, 324, 369, 494, 577, 578
Formication 332, 503, 519, 574, 575, 624, 634
Fracture 69, 71, 74, 143, 145, 279, 551, 552, 555, 588, 605, 683
Freckles 353, 373, 473, 466, 580, 614, 630, 681
Frontal sinuses-catarrh of 642
Frost-bite 25, 289, 466, 473, 493, 683
Frowning 537
Fungus 374, 573, 673, 683, 697, 701
- haematoides 374, 506
Furuncle 618, 683
Galactorrhoea 138, 246, 683
Gall stone 107, 132, 197, 201, 208, 480
- colic 208, 339, 394, 399
Gall-Bladder 91, 268, 683
Ganglion 499, 521, 552, 588, 614, 642, 683
Ganglionic nervous system 35, 267, 405, 439, 447, 613
Gangrenous 36, 511, 676, 693
- ergotism 573
Gas *(see flatulence)* 92, 169, 236, 354, 355, 409, 447, 448, 475, 514, 682, 683, 697, 705
Gastralgia 109, 110, 172, 190, 193, 268, 303, 331, 353, 363, 391, 459, 473, 549, 599, 603, 625, 661, 683
Gastric 17, 45, 49, 50, 51, 65, 66, 67, 76, 91, 122, 173, 197, 201, 255, 261, 263, 299, 309, 311, 319, 339, 340, 343, 346, 348, 373, 391, 435, 439, 440, 459, 479, 482, 486, 563, 588, 595, 652, 654, 683, 685, 697
- disorders 122, 255, 261, 340, 439, 639
- fever 51, 91, 173
- ulcer 65, 76, 309, 339, 493
Gastritis 57, 109, 115, 158, 251, 289, 506, 574, 576, 683
Gastrodynia 76, 345, 480, 684
Gastro-enteralgia 684
Gastroenteritis 542, 684
Gastromalacia 365, 367, 684
General paralysis 23, 277, 349, 652
Genito-urinary 64, 97, 221, 393, 479, 603, 641

Giddiness 147, 248
Glanders 374, 684
Glands 10, 21, 36, 39, 59, 95, 96, 98, 113, 115, 116, 117, 118, 131, 136, 137, 139, 140, 173, 192, 199, 205, 245, 246, 249, 253, 274, 307, 317, 328, 332, 335, 336, 337, 338, 345, 359, 370, 394, 418, 428, 431, 459, 465, 469, 514, 516, 528, 541, 544, 545, 548, 551, 569, 591, 603, 614, 629, 676, 677, 686, 691, 692, 694, 702, 704
- inflamed 253, 542
- inguinal 635
- scrofulous swelling of 459
- swollen 10, 136, 139, 394, 548, 574, 611
Glaucoma 241, 506, 595, 618, 684
Gleet 132, 143, 156, 205, 277, 291, 303, 362, 411, 431, 466, 497, 506, 514, 525, 563, 580, 581, 614, 635, 642, 684
Globus hystericus 330, 363, 614, 684
Glossitis 10, 365, 514, 625, 684
Glossopharyngeal 443, 449, 684
- paralysis 443, 449
Glottis 684, 686, 693
Goitre 98, 115, 127, 132, 178, 283, 291, 299, 335, 336, 394, 574, 597, 598, 684
- exophthalmic 127, 283, 595, 597
Gonorrhoea 10, 29, 65, 87, 132, 143, 145, 147, 151, 155, 156, 158, 160, 164, 175, 197, 205, 221, 251, 264, 277, 283, 289, 291, 293, 319, 359, 362, 369, 411, 418, 428, 431, 449, 461, 462, 470, 493, 497, 514, 525, 530, 533, 540, 559, 569, 571, 580, 614, 635, 641, 642, 644, 675, 684
- suppressed 411
Gonorrhoeal rheumatism 411
Gout 15, 24, 60, 71, 74, 76, 98, 105, 162, 175, 184, 188, 215, 235, 238, 261, 279, 336, 359, 363, 381, 382, 384, 394, 411, 424, 459, 480, 499, 514, 517, 521, 525, 530, 542, 559, 560, 569, 614, 623, 684, 700
Gravel 107, 240, 277, 303, 394, 497, 499, 569, 580, 684
Gravid 573
Griping 227, 243, 244, 267, 343, 394, 404, 409, 491
Grippe 56, 294
Groin 96, 389, 676, 684, 688, 687, 697
Gumma 359, 684
Gums 35, 50, 170, 171, 172, 182, 192, 366, 367, 412, 417, 418, 424, 425, 427, 452, 466, 469, 503, 513, 514, 522, 523, 605, 607, 626, 645, 702
- itching of 539
- painful, sore 366, 466, 533, 605
- sensitive 35, 605
- spongy 171, 418
- swollen 425, 427
- ulceration of 506
- unhealthy 424
Haematemesis 70, 261, 309, 339, 435, 685
Haematocele 685
Haematuria 70, 72, 257, 277, 309, 394, 431, 435, 436, 466, 574, 635, 636, 637, 647, 685
Haemoglobinuria 506, 685
Haemophilia 685
Haemoptysis 14, 73, 197, 255, 286, 289, 313, 322, 381, 415, 435, 446, 470, 507, 521, 563, 599, 647, 685
Haemorrhage 10, 32, 33, 35, 69, 70, 71-73, 87, 102, 127, 128, 155, 157, 160, 170, 171, 173, 176, 207-210, 239, 255-258, 269, 273, 283, 284,

287, 289, 301, 309, 310, 322, 337, 339, 340, 341, 342, 344, 353, 359, 365, 366, 374, 375, 377, 409, 415, 421, 435, 441, 443, 466, 467, 473, 474, 493, 500, 505, 506, 512, 517, 529, 530, 542, 552, 559, 560, 573, 574, 577, 579, 580, 583, 591, 595, 597, 621, 625, 626, 632, 636, 637, 642, 645, 685
- ante-partum, post-partum 645
Haemorrhagic 35, 257, 258, 284, 287, 309, 365, 366, 574, 636
- diathesis 35, 257, 284, 287, 309, 365, 366, 506, 507, 509, 573, 574, 685
Haemorrhoidal 17, 240, 391, 620
- discharge 391
Haemorrhoids 10, 17, 18, 29, 30, 35, 39, 43, 60, 87, 95,98, 162, 164, 167, 170, 178, 179, 182, 197, 200, 201, 208, 224, 239, 240, 251, 268, 273, 291, 307, 309, 313, 319, 328, 335, 339, 349, 353, 374, 375, 376, 394, 400, 439, 440, 470, 479, 480, 484, 487, 493, 514, 517, 521, 525, 530, 542, 591, 614, 619, 620, 635, 642, 685, 697
- strangulated 10
- swollen 440
Haemorrhophilia 287
Hair 210, 217, 291, 300, 306, 313, 327, 335, 353, 373, 391, 394, 398, 412, 432, 439, 450, 452, 454, 456, 465, 468, 479, 489, 491, 493, 500, 505, 506, 529, 530, 577, 579, 580, 583, 591, 595, 597, 621, 625, 632, 642
- dry; tangling 352, 525, 641, 643
- falling off. 170, 291, 394, 499, 577, 643
- grey 557
Hallucination 685
Hand/Hands 24, 35, 36, 54, 57, 60, 66, 98, 109, 120, 123, 125, 129, 132, 137, 140, 149, 153, 160, 170, 172, 175, 182, 183, 184, 198, 201, 214, 224, 225, 228, 237, 244, 271, 275, 280, 286, 289, 291, 294, 295, 301, 307, 317, 336, 337, 343, 349, 350, 356, 364, 370, 371, 381, 383, 384, 385, 388, 394, 400, 409, 419, 429, 447, 450, 477, 488, 493, 494, 495, 503, 507, 509, 530, 547, 548, 555, 571, 577, 578, 581, 586, 592, 621, 622, 623, 624, 634, 655
- chapped 394, 447, 493, 569
- cold 477
- pains in 381, 542, 552
- perspiring 291
- swollen 60, 65, 120, 289
- tremble 137, 225
Hang-nails 685
Hay-asthma 76, 557, 685
Hay-fever 27, 273, 293, 359, 374, 376, 443, 525, 611, 685
Head 12, 13, 14, 15, 21, 45, 51, 54, 66, 68, 71, 73, 76, 79, 85, 96-103, 113, 114, 123, 124, 125,132, 133, 134, 135, 138, 139, 140, 141, 144, 148, 152, 155, 162, 163, 167, 172, 181, 183, 188, 189, 191, 195, 197, 198, 212, 213, 216, 224, 225, 226, 227, 228, 229, 232, 233, 238, 241, 242, 246, 248, 259, 264, 269, 275, 284, 294, 296, 299, 300, 301, 302, 303, 304, 305, 306, 309, 312, 319, 322, 328, 330, 332, 340, 341, 342, 356, 364, 383, 389, 395, 397, 406, 407, 416, 418, 424, 426, 427,

431, 432, 467, 468, 469, 473, 485, 495, 502, 504, 507, 514, 515, 517, 519, 525, 530, 533, 549, 553, 564, 565, 567, 579, 582, 583, 588, 589, 590, 592, 593, 595, 596, 598, 605, 606, 607, 617, 618, 619, 623, 629, 632, 633, 640, 651, 655, 661, 662, 679, 680, 691, 693, 694, 699, 704, 705,
- congestion of 525
- convulsive movement of 473
- lice 557
- rush of blood to 614
- ache 10, 11, 13-17, 19, 21, 23, 24, 25, 31, 41, 45, 47, 49, 51, 57, 62, 65, 71, 75, 76, 83, 85, 91, 97, 98, 100, 101, 103, 105, 109, 119, 120, 121, 122, 123, 124, 127, 132, 134, 135, 139, 143, 144, 151, 155, 162, 163, 165, 167, 170, 172, 173, 178, 188, 191, 197, 203, 208, 209, 212, 215, 219, 221, 223, 224, 225, 226, 227, 231, 232, 233, 241, 248, 255, 257, 264, 268, 269, 273, 285, 291, 293, 294, 295, 296, 299, 300, 301, 302, 303, 311, 313, 316, 328, 329, 330, 332, 335, 340, 342, 343, 344, 345, 346, 353, 363, 368, 369, 373, 374, 375, 376, 389, 391, 396, 397, 405, 406, 407, 409, 411, 412, 415, 426, 432, 443, 447, 448, 449, 450, 451, 454, 455, 456, 457, 461, 468, 473, 475, 476, 480, 483, 485, 489, 493, 494, 499, 500, 501, 502, 506, 514, 516, 519, 521, 522, 525, 527, 531, 533, 537, 557, 561, 563, 564, 565, 567, 569, 571, 577, 579, 581, 582, 583, 586, 588, 589, 590, 591, 595, 596, 597, 599, 606, 611, 612, 614, 618, 619, 629, 630, 631, 632, 633, 637, 639, 641, 642, 643, 647, 649, 653, 659, 660, 711

Headache-bilious, sick 91, 651
- catarrhal 561
- nervous 589, 657, 661, 662
- neuralgic 411
- occipital 493
- of school children 499

Heart *(see angina)* 10, 11, 12, 14, 15, 17, 35, 41, 42, 43, 53, 60, 64, 65, 70, 73, 76, 80, 85, 90, 95, 98, 115, 116, 120, 127, 128, 129, 139, 147, 149, 155, 156, 170, 173, 178, 213, 215, 231, 235, 237, 239, 255, 257, 258, 263, 264, 283, 289, 293, 294, 296, 299, 302, 328, 335, 336, 337, 340, 348, 353, 354, 355, 357, 363, 364, 371, 373, 374, 377, 378, 382, 387, 388, 390, 391, 394, 405, 406, 424, 443, 444, 449, 451, 455, 456, 470, 475, 480, 505, 511, 514, 521, 530, 549, 595, 596, 597, 598, 616, 621, 630, 633, 634, 647, 655, 657, 674, 677, 686, 689, 696, 700
- degeneration of 506
- disease 115, 170, 293, 363 394, 543
- hyperaesthesia of 231

Heart-hypertrophy of 335, 597
- inflammation of 120
- palpitation of 289, 574, 649
- burn *(see scidity)* 162, 163, 495, 530, 625

Heat-effects of 293

Heat-spots 60

Heel-blistered 178, 447
- pain in 649, 661

Hemicrania 66, 192, 685, 704
- of women 582

Hemiplegia 203, 374, 599, 685

Hepatic 199, 203, 279, 345, 346, 393, 399, 479, 553, 579
Hepatisation 685
Hepatitis *(see jaundice)* 199, 201, 319, 685
Hernia 27, 31, 120, 132, 143, 162, 188, 193, 224, 227, 231, 311, 374, 393, 396, 400, 403, 431, 449, 480, 487, 490, 521, 525, 542, 567, 588, 597, 630, 642, 652, 685
- incarcerated 490
- inguinal 595, 625, 661
- strangulated 521, 635
Herpes 21, 107, 111, 132, 135, 158, 178, 183, 303, 313, 346, 363, 365, 374, 424, 431, 447, 449, 450, 456, 466, 470, 493, 495, 499, 542, 569, 614, 635, 642, 685, 686, 707
- circinatus 135, 516, 580
- facialis 374
- preputialis 313, 466, 493, 569
- zoster 76, 158, 178, 346, 363, 431, 542, 543
- neuralgia after 363
Herpetic Dyscrasia 305
Hiccough 21, 120, 211, 213, 279, 322, 324, 328, 332, 335, 428, 449, 473, 534, 569, 574, 607, 625, 630, 631, 657, 661, 686
Hip-joint disease 64, 208, 313, 353, 499, 588, 603, 614,
Hives 624, 686, 706
Hoarseness 14, 64, 67, 83, 103, 117, 134, 138, 165, 171, 180, 183, 194, 241, 270, 279, 280, 313, 374, 473, 476, 495, 503, 509, 561, 577, 578, 598, 632, 679
Hodgkin's disease 10, 76, 686
Homesickness 311, 405, 499, 502, 588
Hopelessness 71, 89
Housemaid's knee 60, 359, 542, 588, 611, 686
Hunger *(see appetite)* 36, 125, 136, 152, 170, 207, 218, 219, 227, 284, 285, 336, 337, 394, 395, 398, 453, 511, 512, 528, 584, 604, 654
Hydraemia 461, 686
Hydroa 449, 686
Hydrocele 87, 120, 143, 264, 291, 303, 311, 480, 506, 525, 530, 539, 542, 561, 588, 614, 686,
Hydrocephaloid 217, 652
Hydrocephalus 59, 60, 74, 98, 120, 132, 135, 136, 264, 283, 311, 335, 506, 614, 661, 686
Hydrogenoid 461, 462, 642
- constitution 53, 461, 641
Hydronephrosis 686
Hydropericardium 394, 686
Hydrophobia *(see rabies)* 98, 158, 257, 322, 374, 424, 635, 686, 700
Hydro-salpingitis 293, 686
Hydrothorax 60, 76, 237, 354, 614, 686
Hygroma 73, 143, 686
Hyperaemia 55, 134, 299, 652, 686, 710
Hyperaesthesia 97, 231, 521, 522, 524, 687
Hyperpyrexia 10, 15, 23, 147, 215, 657, 662, 687
Hypersensitiveness 85
Hypertrophy 62, 96, 115, 116, 127, 167, 248, 274, 316, 335, 336, 338, 396, 443, 514, 597, 687, 698
Hypochondriac 198, 337, 399, 432, 451, 485,
Hypochondriasis 15, 44, 45, 76, 132, 215, 246, 248, 249, 394, 435, 447, 449, 480, 599, 603, 614, 617, 635, 649, 662, 687
Hypochondrium 117, 137, 199, 343, 687
Hypogastrium 89, 102, 164, 216, 389, 503, 607, 637
Hypopion 259, 521, 588, 687

Hysteria 15, 29, 35, 41, 44, 85, 86, 92, 132, 155, 211, 215, 216, 231, 248, 249, 253, 255, 261, 294, 328, 329, 339, 354, 374, 387, 391, 394, 405, 435, 447, 473, 477, 506, 517, 530, 574, 580, 611, 631, 632, 639, 649, 652, 659, 662, 687, 684
Hysterical 64, 85, 180, 188, 232, 255, 256, 293, 321, 328, 329, 330, 331, 365, 405, 406, 473, 474, 476, 477, 501, 517, 612, 649, 660, 662
- joint 63, 188, 328, 687
- vomiting 365
Hystero-epilepsy 490, 631
Ichthyosis 76, 208, 369, 447, 521, 642, 687
Idiocy 21, 630, 687
Ileum 687
Ileus 235, 490, 561, 687
Illiciuma 251
Imaginary diseases 557
Impetigo 53, 65, 211, 345, 431, 687
Impotence 70, 132, 137, 178, 208, 264, 349, 394, 396, 412, 439, 480, 499, 506, 514, 526, 574, 577, 603, 614, 625,
Incontinence 274, 277, 284, 321, 350, 366, 530, 574, 580, 588, 687
Indigestion 76, 122, 127, 167, 169, 239, 279, 289, 349, 350, 405, 531, 549, 567, 619, 681, 687,
Induration 405, 468, 517, 526, 580, 621, 687
Infantile 32, 96, 136, 155, 320, 473, 627
- leucorrhoea 155
- paralysis 21

Infammation 9, 10,13, 18, 25, 27, 35, 50, 53, 56, 57, 59, 60, 71, 74, 83, 97, 98, 99, 100, 103, 109, 115, 117, 119, 120, 121, 127, 136, 138, 140, 155, 156, 157, 158, 159, 161, 167, 177, 197, 198, 205, 215, 217, 221, 235, 241, 246, 247, 248, 251, 258, 261, 284, 289, 291, 299, 306, 310, 311, 316, 324, 335, 353, 356, 359, 362, 373, 374, 381, 387, 394, 403, 417, 424, 431, 446, 447, 449, 450, 465, 480 494, 495, 497, 504, 505, 513, 526, 530, 541, 542, 544, 548, 559, 577, 588, 589, 591, 597, 599, 607, 614, 618, 642, 657, 673-700, 702, 703, 705, 706, 707
Influenza 3, 10, 27, 92, 147, 149, 170, 178, 180, 197, 207, 273, 279, 280, 281, 294, 303, 359, 360, 394, 461, 514, 525, 542, 557, 563, 567, 611, 614, 647, 652, 657, 687, 690,
Inframammary pain 175, 687
Inguinal 595, 608, 625, 635, 661, 687
- glands-swelling of 635
Injuries 60, 69, 70, 71, 72, 73, 74, 273, 289, 314, 318, 344, 374, 461, 462, 525, 551, 555, 626, 685
Insanity 44, 415, 443, 632, 635, 691
Insomnia 687
Intercostal 407, 662, 688
- neuralgia 407
Inter-menstrual flow 559, 688
Intermittent pulse 129, 263, 264, 629, 658
Interscapular pain 446, 688
Intertrigo 170, 177, 178, 394, 459, 688,
Intestines 14, 23, 29, 31, 45, 91, 111, 120, 158, 159, 160, 170, 177, 178, 237, 244, 311, 317, 343, 394, 417, 459, 469, 488, 490, 507, 635, 637, 654, 676, 681,

684, 688
- obstruction of 490, 521
- ulcerated 417, 635
Intoxication 163, 248, 294, 381, 485, 533, 680
Intra-menstrual haemorrhage 359
Intussusception 417, 506, 521, 642, 652, 688
Iris 54, 71, 295, 345, 447, 626, 712, 688
- circinatus 447
Iritis 74, 85, 281, 335, 417, 421, 466, 595, 635, 688
- syphilitic 466, 603
Irritable 64, 80, 119, 120, 147, 149, 180, 188, 191, 197, 217, 241, 251, 273, 283, 311, 321, 325, 373, 394, 395, 397, 403, 439, 449, 466, 479, 484, 537, 567, 580, 583, 587, 604, 622, 632, 635, 660
Irritation 15, 21, 23, 31, 47, 60, 65, 76, 107, 109, 115, 125, 155, 156, 157, 159, 161, 170, 194, 215, 216, 217, 219, 224, 239, 241, 249, 251, 255, 261, 268, 273, 277, 303, 314, 328, 333, 339 353, 354, 365, 369, 387, 388, 394, 403, 410, 431, 443, 493, 497, 514, 541, 545, 549, 563, 565, 574, 579, 580, 588, 597, 614, 615, 618, 625, 631, 635, 639, 641, 649, 660, 687, 696, 697
Ischuria 72
Itch 6, 18, 23, 24, 25, 30, 31, 51, 56, 57, 61, 81, 159, 259, 362, 513, 514, 516, 525, 528, 567, 613, 614, 675, 701,
- suppressed 368
Jarring-effects of 299
Jaundice 10, 17, 23, 76, 87, 107, 120, 197, 201, 205, 207, 208, 246, 257, 258, 264, 265, 279, 294, 313, 319, 335, 342, 374, 417, 424, 469, 522, 537, 550, 580, 614, 635, 688, 707
- malignant 506
- of anaemia, of pregnancy 506
Jaw 33, 83, 89, 117, 124, 136, 179, 181, 213, 274, 291, 296, 383, 394, 397, 412, 427, 431, 439, 440, 441, 466, 468, 490, 519, 634, 705
- carries of 588
- cracking in 542
- disease of 506
- easily dislocated 493, 603
- growth on 642
- tumour of 522
- joint painful 83, 595, 597
Jealousy-effect of 60
Joints 10, 14, 39, 51, 57, 60, 64, 83, 103, 105, 108, 111, 120, 121, 129, 140, 145, 175, 184, 194, 228, 235, 236, 238, 270, 271, 325, 334, 337, 344, 362, 381, 382, 384, 411, 424, 454, 456, 494, 499, 530, 541, 546, 547, 551, 552, 554, 587, 609, 622, 647, 674, 684, 689, 696, 700, 709
- cracking in 381, 642, 662
- pain in 120
Joints-scrofulous 499
Joy-ill effects of 231
Keratitis 257, 259, 363, 506, 563, 618, 688
Kerato-iritis 421, 688
Kidney 59, 60, 76, 98, 107, 108, 158, 159, 160, 161, 183, 205, 237, 263, 283, 289, 311, 313, 348, 354, 394, 396, 400, 413, 499, 505, 513, 523, 537, 568, 635, 636, 637, 638, 645, 676, 686, 693, 699, 700, 703
- Bright's disease of 60, 289
- congestion of 311, 635
- inflammation of 417
Kleptomania 631, 688
Knees 49, 90, 134, 137, 139,

153, 162, 170, 172, 173, 184, 225, 228, 334, 356, 383, 384, 476, 512, 546, 582, 593, 609, 622, 623, 624, 686,
- cracking in 184
- pain in 105, 107, 268
- weakness of 224
- white swelling of 354
Labia 113, 137, 367, 688
Labour 10, 29, 41, 56, 70, 73, 138, 175, 176, 188, 190, 193, 208, 216, 231, 233, 239, 294, 296, 321, 324, 356, 357, 374, 394, 409, 417, 448, 482, 490, 508, 559, 560, 574, 579, 580, 581, 587
- constipation after 652
- disorders of 188
- false pains of 659
- pains 138, 176, 190, 193, 231, 356, 394, 482, 490, 574, 660
- pains afer 374
Lachrymal duct 303, 688
- inflamed 303
Lachrymal gland 591, 688
Lachrymal sac 495, 530, 688
- suppuration of 599
Lachrymation 13, 28, 33, 124, 136, 255, 281, 282, 427, 455, 553, 583, 618, 685, 688
Lactation *(see milk)* 10, 85, 120, 132, 138, 139, 167, 175, 205, 208, 336, 499, 506, 514, 530, 579, 580, 588, 688
- abnormal, defective 132, 499, 514
- disordered 85, 120, 205, 336, 506
Lameness 19, 25, 108, 138, 237, 270, 274, 541, 542, 544, 551, 552, 555, 565
Landry's 246
Laryngismus 115, 197, 349, 374, 514, 561, 597, 688
Laryngitis 10, 27, 53, 57, 60, 64, 170, 178, 269, 314, 336, 350, 359, 374, 506, 597, 611, 614, 688
- scrofulous, tubercular 577
Larynx 10, 14, 83, 103, 115, 116, 117, 172, 177, 178, 183, 194, 199, 219, 228, 249, 261, 270, 314, 324, 333, 336, 343, 344, 351, 354, 373, 378, 379, 391, 400, 470, 486, 507, 509, 510, 577, 597, 598, 655, 679, 684, 688,
- catarrh of 354
- spasm of 261
Lascivious 322, 323, 632, 652, 653
Lassitude 66, 91, 98, 524, 565, 619
Laughter 100, 152, 232, 255, 322, 323, 476, 529, 567, 623, 633
Lead colic 490, 521
Lead poisoning 178, 517, 519
Legs 103, 133, 139, 141, 156, 160, 162, 167, 184, 192, 194, 212, 294, 355, 410, 429, 441, 454, 494, 503, 520, 535, 546, 547, 548, 554, 570, 577, 580, 593, 623, 631, 632, 650, 655, 660, 675, 681, 695
Leprosy 374, 647, 689
Lesion 526, 674, 682, 690, 693, 707
Leucophlegmatic 131
Leucorrhoea 17, 18, 19, 31, 32, 56, 76, 87, 107, 112, 113, 132, 137, 138, 143, 155, 167, 175, 178, 193, 203, 208, 223, 217, 245, 255, 303, 307, 309, 314, 319, 320, 337, 354, 365, 366, 367, 369, 405, 415, 424, 426, 429, 431, 435, 438, 441, 449, 459, 514, 526, 530, 559, 567, 573, 580, 585, 600, 614, 647, 660, 689
- in chldren, little girls 424, 435
- in place of Menses 223
Leukemia 461, 689

Leukocythemia 132, 449, 689
Leukocytosis 459, 689
Levitation 499, 506, 611, 631, 642, 649, 689
Lichen 60, 76, 273, 514, 549, 611, 614, 689, 712
Lienteria 188, 208, 283, 500, 506, 526, 539
Ligaments 14, 64, 178, 703, 709
Lips 22, 50, 76, 77, 83, 93, 102, 120, 121, 136, 149, 185, 218, 263, 281, 283, 303, 306, 313, 332, 340, 412, 428, 449, 450, 451, 452, 454, 469, 474, 475, 615, 616, 617, 618, 619, 658, 662, 686
- chapped 136
- cracked 303, 652
- eruption on 76, 449
- stiffness of 281
- swollen 314
Lisping 447, 480, 689
Liver 10,17, 29, 39, 53, 74, 88, 107, 119, 120, 187, 197, 198, 200, 201, 205, 207, 208, 210, 246, 257, 258, 268, 279, 291, 294, 303, 306, 313, 314, 319, 336, 337, 345, 354, 359, 374, 393, 394, 395, 396, 399, 405, 406, 411, 413, 424, 447, 449, 452, 453, 461, 469, 480, 505, 506, 514, 521, 522, 526, 537, 563, 577, 614, 625, 639, 675, 678, 685, 689
- abscess of 411, 542
- cough 563
- enlarged 461, 246, 574
- hyperaemia of 652
- indurated 291, 303
- soreness of 279, 567
- spots 394, 580
- torpid 580
Location-sense of-lost 299
Lochia 322, 366, 368, 435, 637, 689
- foetid 574
- suppressed 322, 662
- too profuse 435
Lockjaw 213, 491, 522, 652, 689, 704, 705
Locomotor ataxy 31, 65, 76, 87, 178, 179, 291, 294, 328, 349, 359, 363, 374, 377, 394, 407, 474, 480, 500, 506, 522, 588, 631, 689
Loose teeth 469
Loss of memory 43, 44, 45, 95, 349, 350, 474, 475, 522
Love-disappointed 500
Lumbago *(see backache)* 17, 23, 29, 53, 70, 107, 120, 143, 167, 215, 235, 268, 273, 319, 354, 359, 363, 424, 474, 476, 480, 514, 539, 542, 544, 567, 574, 614, 635, 659, 689
Lumbar abscess 603, 689
Lumbrici 595, 600, 689
Lump 44, 50, 66, 247, 357, 330, 370, 413, 528, 591, 653, 655, 684
Lungs 10, 35, 53, 54, 55, 86, 119, 123, 127, 128, 145, 165, 170, 171, 172, 198, 200, 219, 309, 310, 335, 337, 344, 357, 359, 360, 374, 435, 450, 470, 505, 509, 510, 511, 598, 620, 637, 645, 651, 657, 658, 673, 688, 689, 697
- congested 170
- haemorrhage from 127
- hepatisation of 359
- oedema of 35, 450, 647, 652
Lupus 76, 132, 314, 319, 365, 367, 514, 614, 647, 689
Lymph nodes 697, 696, 702
Lymphatic 91, 96, 133, 140, 141, 221, 313, 335, 336, 359, 365, 449, 541, 549, 613, 675, 676, 686, 706
- swellings 336
Malar bones 662, 690
Malaria 73, 209, 461, 550, 673, 676, 690, 716
Malignant pustule 76, 374, 690
Malnutrition 65, 690

Mammae *(see breasts)* 121, 138, 194, 513, 516, 533, 690
Mania 10, 15, 98, 148, 151, 158, 215, 216, 255, 261, 294, 299, 322, 323, 375, 424, 491, 530, 557, 588, 603, 614, 631, 633, 647, 652, 653, 658, 690
Marasmus 136, 144, 314, 440, 474, 490, 506, 568, 569, 570, 690
Mastitis 60, 74, 122, 188, 257, 260, 369, 370, 515, 690
Mastoid 88, 163, 219, 519, 553
Masturbation 480, 483, 484, 500, 517, 662, 690, 694, 702
- effects of 569, 603, 630
Measles 10, 35, 51, 60, 76, 98, 120, 123, 148, 149, 162, 169, 170, 194, 251, 253, 257, 261, 269, 273, 279, 281, 289, 294, 374, 417, 424, 439, 490, 530, 533, 542, 611, 614, 652, 657, 684, 690, 694
- cough of 611
Medulla oblongata 299, 629, 661
Melaena 690
Melancholia 15, 39, 76, 132, 215, 245, 311, 328, 336, 349, 350, 415, 424, 490, 517, 522, 557, 569, 617, 647, 652, 690
- religious 526
Melancholy 87, 89, 128, 179, 180, 311, 397, 447, 450, 455, 525, 567, 690
Melanoma 690
Melanosis 87, 690
Membranous dysmenorrhoea 116, 193, 407, 410, 660
Memory 12, 43, 44, 45, 71, 87, 95, 148, 181, 224, 236, 245, 248, 264, 318, 349, 350, 375, 394, 412, 418, 426, 447, 467, 474, 475, 522, 603, 606
- defective 95
- lost 44, 148, 264
- weak 224, 245, 418, 426, 539, 614, 662
Mendacity 652, 690
Meniere's disease 178, 208, 374, 381, 537, 630, 631, 639, 690
Meningeal headaches 391, 690
Meningitis 23, 60, 70, 71, 98, 120, 211, 215, 224, 257, 261, 262, 264, 273, 293, 294, 299, 311, 312, 322, 407, 424, 490, 588, 614, 618, 652, 658, 662, 690
Menopause *(see Climacteric)* 41, 355, 375, 474, 678, 691
Menorrhagia16, 151, 314, 319, 354, 403, 438, 474, 482, 506, 517, 542, 560, 625, 645, 691
Menses 32, 40, 51, 102, 121, 122, 123, 128, 131, 134, 137, 138, 168, 203, 216, 223, 239, 241, 245, 246, 247, 284, 285, 286, 299, 300, 301, 305, 311, 335, 350, 354, 356, 367, 368, 370, 398, 404, 406, 449, 450, 451, 474, 476, 481, 482, 488, 509, 510, 517, 518, 520, 532, 560, 563, 569, 580, 585, 586, 589, 593, 607, 648, 660, 661, 662, 663, 673, 688, 691
- profuse 481, 645
- scanty 20
- suppressed 203, 239, 299, 474, 517, 658
- too early 131, 137, 168, 356, 481, 586, 647
- vicarious 510
Menstrual colic 190, 193, 224, 241, 410, 658
Menstrual headache 224, 255
Mentagra 303, 691
Mental alienation 70, 691
Mental excitement- effects of 224
Menyanthes 375
Mephitis 561
Mercurial poisoning 87, 691, 698
- syphilis 500
- ulceration 439
Mercury 64, 85, 87, 88, 185, 172, 208, 313, 359, 360,

374, 417, 421, 423, 433, 466, 467, 468, 469, 470, 513, 540, 642, 711
- abuse of 569
- effects of 85, 208, 374, 431, 514
Meteorism 410, 500, 637
Metritis 424, 637
Metrorrhagia 137, 176, 190, 231, 255, 294, 319, 354, 394, 403, 438, 466, 474, 522, 542, 560, 574, 586, 588, 625, 645, 691
Micturition 249, 523, 531, 585, 621, 633
Migraine 115, 345, 461, 590, 611, 631, 685, 691, 702, 704
Milia 691
Miliaria 10, 120, 128, 691
Miliary eruption 35, 76, 188, 691
Milk *(see lactation)* 21, 22, 98, 123, 125, 132, 133, 137, 138, 145, 188, 193, 257, 273, 307, 369, 370, 405, 406, 435, 456, 503, 515, 553, 568, 580, 582, 585, 591, 620, 673, 679, 683, 688, 691, 716
- abnormal, defective 537, 599, 662
- absent, suppressed 574
- fever 98, 120, 132, 188,
- scanty, thin 138, 567, 611
Milk-leg 257, 691
Mind 7, 21, 44, 88, 92, 93, 96, 103, 134, 151, 181, 189, 212, 225, 226, 232, 233, 236, 261, 262, 268, 296, 322, 323, 371, 374, 375, 388, 394, 401, 432, 467, 474, 475, 479, 481, 483, 487, 491, 499, 501, 518, 527, 580, 599, 604, 606, 617, 620, 632, 637,
- weakness of 21, 44, 499, 662
Miner's asthma 691
Miscarriage *(see abortion)* 10, 70, 132, 176, 188, 417, 559, 574, 588, 614, 659, 660, 692
Moaning 160, 187, 191, 192, 212, 439, 440, 441
Mole 447, 692
- promotes expulsion of 559
Mollities ossium 336, 424, 506, 692
Molluscum 132, 614, 692
- contagiosum 132, 588
- fibrosum 588
Morbus 523, 654, 678
- Basedowii 285
Morbus Brightii 523
Morning sickness 345, 391, 692
- of drunkards 391
- of pregnancy 584
Morphia habit 391
Morphinomania 459, 692
Morphoea 76, 506, 588, 692
Morvan's disease 574, 588, 642
Mouth 13, 18, 22, 36, 45, 47, 48, 50, 51, 57, 61, 65, 71, 72, 77, 79, 81, 83, 91, 97, 98, 102, 111, 112, 113, 120, 124, 136, 149, 152, 158, 162, 163, 181, 189, 192, 193, 199, 217, 218, 219, 221, 226, 232, 233, 258, 279, 284, 304, 307, 314, 319, 324, 332, 341, 344, 345, 346, 355, 367, 373, 374, 377, 383, 396, 398, 399, 412, 417, 419, 425, 427, 428, 431, 433, 439, 440, 441, 450, 451, 452, 455, 456, 459, 465, 466, 468, 469, 473, 474, 475, 476, 495, 507, 515, 516, 530, 531, 534, 549, 561, 591, 607, 619, 626, 643, 654, 658, 676, 687, 694, 700, 703, 707
- cracks of 279
- dry 475, 476
- inflammation of 450
- mucous in 537
- sore 83, 314, 319, 374, 466, 567
- ulcerated 92, 162, 427, 428, 468, 514, 549

Mucous 18, 19, 24, 27, 30, 31, 32, 33, 35, 39, 40, 47, 48, 51, 53, 54, 55, 59, 64, 65, 66, 68, 91, 97, 98, 107, 108, 111, 113, 115, 116, 120, 121, 125, 147, 155, 157, 158, 159, 161, 162, 163, 164, 169, 170, 171, 177, 178, 180, 182, 183, 187, 193, 194, 199, 205, 206, 219, 228, 236, 237, 240, 248, 251, 253, 259, 273, 274, 275, 277, 278, 279, 281, 282, 283, 284, 286, 291, 304, 305, 306, 307, 313, 314, 319, 320, 324, 335, 339, 341, 343, 344, 345, 346, 348, 349, 353, 359, 362, 365, 366, 367, 370, 378, 381, 393, 396, 403, 405, 411, 412, 417, 418, 423, 424, 425, 428, 431, 433, 435, 446, 447, 448, 449, 450, 465, 466, 469, 470, 485, 486, 487, 489, 493, 497, 505, 509, 510, 511, 513, 516, 529, 530, 532, 537, 538, 541, 544, 549, 557, 561, 563, 584, 587, 591, 595, 611, 613, 625, 629, 635, 641, 643, 644, 645, 654, 675, 676, 677, 679, 681, 682, 683, 684, 685, 688, 692, 693, 694, 696, 697, 700, 702, 703, 709

- patches 424, 466, 642

Mumps 10, 92, 98, 170, 188, 289, 374, 417, 424, 514, 530, 533, 692, 694

Muscles 15, 23, 24, 25, 39, 40, 64, 93, 102, 131, 140, 160, 175, 177, 178, 179, 180, 181, 183, 212, 213, 216, 219, 220, 224, 225, 226, 228, 244, 248, 256, 271, 279, 295, 313, 317, 322, 324, 341, 355, 356, 357, 383, 398, 406, 432, 452, 489, 491, 522, 541, 544, 546, 548, 609, 651, 660, 662, 676, 677, 688, 693, 694, 695, 697, 698, 700, 702, 705

Muscoe volitantes 208, 466, 480, 506, 642, 692

Myalgia 10, 15, 53, 74, 98, 178, 215, 235, 274, 294, 658, 692

Mycosis 569, 692

Myelitis 10, 76, 211, 273, 480, 522, 692

- diffusa 574

Myopia 23, 466, 493, 597, 625, 642, 692

Myosotis 251

Myrtus com 203

Naevus 132, 291, 289, 394, 506, 642, 692

Nails 31, 47, 48, 49, 76, 178, 184, 200, 264, 303, 304, 305, 307, 319, 385, 362, 450, 454, 466, 477, 506, 592, 593, 599, 655

- blue 170, 200
- brittle, cracked 454, 643
- crippled 49, 178
- diseased 303, 362, 588
- pains under 580
- ulceration of 506, 563

Nasal catarrh 253, 281, 319, 337, 446, 447, 448, 459, 468, 508, 532, 595, 611, 612, 642,

Naso-pharynx 693

Naso-pharyngeal catarrh 87

Nausea 13, 21, 48, 49, 50, 51, 54, 55, 79, 102, 120, 121, 122, 134, 135, 181, 198, 199, 216, 223, 224, 225, 226, 227, 235, 237, 265, 269, 275, 285, 286, 295, 317, 339, 340, 342, 343, 344, 346, 368, 389, 391, 403, 405, 428, 456, 457, 468, 469, 485, 486, 487, 488, 493, 494, 495, 500, 503, 523, 555, 564, 565, 583, 584, 603, 629, 637, 639, 640, 652, 654, 658, 660, 690, 691, 693

Navel 45, 89, 243, 244, 333, 343, 607
Neck 10, 14, 15, 16, 44, 53, 72, 95, 96, 101, 102, 120, 123, 139, 140, 143, 145, 160, 164, 183, 198, 200, 213, 216, 235, 251, 274, 300, 307, 349, 368, 375, 376, 379, 409, 450, 453, 456, 476, 488, 502, 514, 516, 539, 545, 551, 567, 570, 589, 590, 591, 593, 604, 623, 624, 634, 662, 663, 673, 677, 693, 701
- cracking in 642
Necrosis 88, 505, 588, 639, 640, 693
Nephritic scarlatina 461
Nephritis 10, 72, 73, 120, 155, 197, 205, 235, 522, 559, 647, 676, 693
- rheumatic and gouty 235
Nervous 6,9, 15, 16, 22, 31, 35, 41, 43, 44, 65, 69, 75, 85, 92, 97, 103, 110, 111, 119, 120, 132, 141, 147, 149, 151, 161, 165, 167, 169, 179, 187, 188, 189, 207, 208, 215, 223, 224, 229, 231, 232, 235, 241, 245, 255, 267, 293, 294, 295, 299, 317, 318, 320, 329, 330, 349, 354, 363, 369, 401, 403, 405, 406, 407, 409, 410, 415, 439, 447, 456, 465, 466, 467, 468, 473, 475, 479, 481, 489, 491, 499, 500, 506, 516, 517, 518, 521, 525, 539, 557, 573, 583, 587, 588, 589, 613, 614, 624, 631, 633, 643, 649, 651, 652, 657, 660, 661, 662, 663, 683, 700
- fever 132,
- headache 406, 468, 595
Nervousness 92, 249, 285, 350, 403, 612
Nettlerash 47, 60, 76, 273, 362, 450, 614
Neuralgia 10, 15, 16, 23, 39, 65, 76, 85, 98, 107, 127, 128, 131, 132, 158, 162, 175, 178, 180, 184, 188, 197, 199, 201, 208, 215, 216, 217, 231, 241, 243, 257, 259, 261, 268, 273, 283, 289, 293, 294, 299, 322, 345, 359, 363, 365, 369, 374, 376, 403, 407, 408, 409, 410, 411, 412, 417, 431, 432, 433, 415, 446, 506, 513, 514, 517, 530, 539, 542, 557, 563, 565, 567, 574, 580, 588, 595, 596, 599, 603, 611, 614, 631, 635, 639, 642, 649, 661, 662, 674, 693, 694
- intercostal, subcostal 662
- palpebralis 652
- supraorbital 417, 635
Neurasthenia 374, 403, 500, 504, 517, 567, 599, 662, 693
Neuritis 60, 76, 630, 693
Night-blindness 311, 322, 480, 497, 693
Nightmare 349, 480, 506, 539, 623, 625,
Night sweats 132, 133, 145, 289, 357, 360, 471, 502, 565, 586
Night-terrors 88, 90, 567, 647
Nipple 73, 111, 125, 183, 203, 259, 260, 309, 314, 319, 435, 516, 550, 591
- cracked 183, 516
- painful 259, 537
- retracted 569
- sore 111, 183, 309, 314, 319, 435, 506, 514, 614, 662,
Nisus 579, 693
Nocturnal emissions 345, 405
Nodes 88, 359, 471, 480, 588, 696, 697, 700
Nodosities 382, 384, 516, 604, 605, 606
Noises in ears 359
- in head 264, 303, 309, 319, 424

Noma pudendi 76, 693
Nose 24, 28, 33, 35, 36, 60, 70, 72, 73, 77, 79, 83, 89, 98, 101, 103, 111, 112, 116, 120, 121, 128, 133, 135, 136, 138, 148, 155, 162, 164, 167, 170, 171, 178, 181, 182, 198, 199, 217, 218, 219, 243, 251, 253, 255, 256, 258, 281, 289, 291, 303, 306, 309, 310, 315, 316, 319, 324, 332, 334, 335, 341, 343, 344, 349, 355, 367, 370, 371, 373, 374, 375, 378, 394, 396, 416, 426, 427, 432, 435, 436, 446, 447, 452, 465, 466, 468, 480, 484, 485, 495, 502, 507, 508, 509, 510, 533, 544, 561, 580, 582, 584, 588, 593, 608, 611, 612, 614, 617, 618, 623, 624, 642, 643, 645, 653, 656, 679, 682, 683, 690
- bleed 35, 36, 120, 121, 124, 155, 170, 198, 251, 255, 258, 289, 303, 309, 341, 344, 374, 416, 435, 436, 427, 468, 506, 510,
- block 396
- cancer of 281
- catarrh 253, 639
- crusts in 178, 567
- eruption on 349
- inflamed 580
- pain in 537
- redness of 60, 526, 662
- sore 136, 493
- swollen 355, 447, 510,
Nosode 411, 525, 647, 693, 716
Nostrils 47, 48, 50, 79, 89, 306, 468, 485, 584, 615,
Nucha 443, 693
Numbness 10, 11, 23, 25, 32, 33, 76, 85, 108, 129, 145, 188, 189, 211, 224, 228, 246, 296, 307, 328, 363, 364, 408, 452, 459, 506, 517, 518, 519, 520, 522, 523, 537, 548, 574, 620, 624, 575
Nurselings 537, 693
Nursing painful 514
Nursing women-sore mouth of 319
Nyctalopia 98, 618, 652, 693
Nymphomania 98, 143, 158, 291, 322, 374, 394, 438, 480, 500, 506, 517, 518, 530, 559, 603, 631, 634, 662, 693, 701
Nystagmus 23, 294, 359, 693
Obesity *(see corpulency)* 85, 133, 162, 164, 303, 304, 305, 307, 349, 353, 356, 679
Occipital 181, 216, 247, 482, 493, 494, 500, 502, 590
Occiput 16, 71, 93, 101, 123, 124, 135, 172, 183, 184, 199, 216, 219, 223, 296, 306, 389, 407, 476, 485, 502, 553, 564, 565, 583, 590, 592, 606, 633, 693
Odour of body-abnormal 359
- changed 506
- foetid, offensive 526
Oedema 35, 56, 59, 60, 61, 62, 129, 159, 237, 353, 359, 374, 450, 506, 507, 508, 647, 652, 680, 693
- glottidis 359, 563, 647
- of lungs 56, 374
Oesophagitis 170, 574, 625, 693
Oesophagus 10, 57, 85, 92, 93, 95, 162, 192, 199, 211, 213, 227, 294, 328, 332, 346, 356, 417, 443, 446, 522, 565, 685, 693, 694
- constriction of 92, 162, 211, 294, 417, 446, 522, 537, 557, 614, 630, 652
- inflammation of 10
- pain in 506
- spasm of 95, 658, 662
- spasmodic stricture of 443
Onanism 29, 64, 137, 139, 172, 503, 603, 604, 608, 631, 634, 642, 694
Operation-effects of 60, 255

Ophthalmia 107, 136, 188, 255, 259, 273, 279, 328, 455, 461, 468, 530, 563, 644, 694
- acute, rheumatic 614
- neonatorum 65, 468, 644
- scrofulous 526
- tarsi 567
Opisthotonos 213, 413, 599, 694
Opium habit 339
Optic 694
- neuritis 60, 630
Orbital neuralgia 199, 694
Orchitis 74, 170, 221, 310, 514, 658, 682, 694
Orthopnoea 56
Os uteri-dilated 567
Ossification 567, 694
Osteoma 431, 694
Osteo-myletis 500, 694
Otitis 618, 690, 694
Ovaries 15, 60, 64, 158, 215, 241, 243, 246, 257, 303, 309, 314, 335, 336, 349, 365, 369, 374, 375, 387, 394, 411, 424, 443, 473, 517, 530, 559, 603, 694, 660
- enlargement of 631
- pain in 60, 411, 530, 635, 659
Ovaritis 128, 694
Over-sensitiveness 191, 194, 195, 231, 480, 618, 640, 650
Overstrain-bodily or mental 224
Oxaluria 107, 694
Ozaena 31, 85, 88, 257, 319, 336, 362, 405, 447, 466, 468, 506, 514, 526, 567, 580, 584, 611, 639, 642, 694
Pain 10, 11, 12, 13, 14, 15, 16, 17, 18, 21, 22, 23, 24, 25, 29, 33, 35, 37, 39, 40, 41, 44, 45, 48, 49, 50, 51, 56, 59, 60, 61, 62, 64, 68, 69, 71, 73, 74, 75, 76, 77, 78, 80, 81, 83, 85, 86, 88, 89, 90, 91, 92, 93, 107, 108, 110, 112, 113, 115, 116, 117, 119, 120, 121, 122, 123, 124, 125, 128, 135, 136, 137, 138, 145, 147, 152, 153, 156, 157, 158, 159, 160, 162, 163, 164, 165, 167, 172, 173, 175, 178, 179, 180, 181, 182, 183, 184, 187, 188, 189, 190, 191, 192, 193, 194, 195, 197-201, 203, 208, 215, 216, 219, 224, 225, 227, 228, 213-216, 219, 220, 231, 232, 233, 235, 237, 238, 240, 241, 242, 243, 244, 247, 249, 259, 260, 267, 268, 270, 271, 275, 277, 278, 279, 280, 283, 285, 286, 287, 289, 294, 296, 299, 300, 301, 304- 306, 314, 316, 317, 318, 320, 328, 329, 330, 331, 332, 333, 343, 344, 346, 354, 355, 356, 360, 363, 364, 369, 370, 376, 377, 378, 379, 382, 383, 384, 387, 389, 396, 397, 398, 399, 435, 438, 446, 466-471, 476, 482, 484-489, 491, 494, 495, 502, 503, 506, 511, 514-517, 520-524, 529-532, 534, 535, 537-550, 553, 554, 560, 564, 565, 568, 569, 570, 571, 580, 583, 584, 585, 586, 590, 591, 592, 593, 595, 596, 599, 600, 606, 607, 608, 609, 611, 612, 615, 616, 618, 620, 621, 622, 625, 629, 633, 634, 635, 637, 639, 640, 642, 647, 648, 649, 650, 652, 653, 654, 655, 657, 658, 659, 660, 661, 662, 673, 674,
Palm 564, 622, 623, 655, 699
Palpitation 12, 14, 44, 73, 80, 86, 89, 127, 128, 134, 139, 140, 155, 213, 224, 227, 237, 239, 249, 257, 262, 283, 285, 289, 296, 299, 302, 337, 379, 387, 391, 405, 406, 444, 451, 470, 511, 530, 535, 574, 596, 620, 621, 623, 647, 649, 655, 695

Palsy 695
Panaris 95
Panaritium 27, 37, 60, 394, 461, 588, 592
Pancreas 167, 345, 506, 695
- indurated 167
Pancreatitis 359, 424, 695
Pannus 60, 695
Panophthalmitis 514, 625
Paralysis 10, 21, 23, 25, 27, 31, 44, 53, 54, 56, 65, 70, 71, 73, 88, 91, 93, 95, 98, 127, 132, 151, 153, 162, 172, 173, 177-182, 184, 185, 203, 211, 223, 224, 246, 261, 263, 274, 277, 283, 289, 293, 294, 295, 297, 299, 303, 311, 321, 322, 324, 328, 329, 348, 349, 353, 359, 370, 374, 377, 394, 397, 417, 444, 449, 450, 452, 456, 466, 480, 489, 490, 491, 492, 493, 505, 506, 516, 522, 524, 539, 542, 544, 547, 548, 552, 629, 630, 642, 647, 652, 655, 657, 661, 695
- left side 377, 466
- agitans 53, 294, 322, 349, 394, 631
- diphtheritic 514, 522
- lead 625
- of viscera 283
- pseudo-hypertrophic 506
- spastic 480
Parametritis 314, 588, 695
Paraphimosis 241, 264, 374, 417, 480, 542, 695
Paraplegia 294, 363, 695
Paresis 177, 695
Paronychia 268, 470, 695
Parotid glands 115, 345, 545, 695
- induration of 115
Parotitis 35, 95, 132, 172, 188, 224, 268, 281, 303, 322, 424, 514, 695
Paroxysms 42, 117, 190, 192, 228, 244, 249, 269, 271, 317, 344, 523, 560, 609, 618, 632, 695
Pediculosis 381, 431, 449, 526, 603, 695
Pelvic cellulitis 411, 695
Pelvic haematocele 309, 614, 695
Pelvis 30, 356, 389, 408, 435, 474, 567, 579, 581, 585, 634, 658, 686, 695, 699, 701
- congestion of 474
Pemphigus 44, 178, 274, 417, 542, 642, 696
Penis 72, 153, 159, 621, 675, 677, 678, 686, 696, 698
- cartilaginous swelling on 559
Pericarditis 235, 696
Pericardium 237, 400
Perichondritis 98, 188, 522, 552, 696
Perimetritis 98, 417, 696
Periosteum 24, 70, 359, 383, 384, 426, 431, 433, 511, 513, 551, 553, 555, 587, 696
- pains in 542
Periostitis 163, 506, 511, 551, 552, 555, 696
Peritoneum 417, 696
Peritonitis 10, 60, 76, 98, 120, 132, 158, 188, 208, 241, 246, 257, 291, 324, 394, 417, 424, 545, 614, 637, 652, 696
- tubercular 526
Perityphlitis 76, 257, 374, 696
Pernicious fevers 652
Perspiration *(see sweat)* 14, 29, 110, 132, 167, 208, 229, 275, 289, 291, 353, 373, 374, 394, 395, 411, 424, 426, 429, 465, 466, 471, 474, 490, 492, 493, 500, 512, 561, 567, 580, 581, 586, 588, 592, 593, 594, 603, 621, 622, 625, 632, 651, 654, 655
- abnormal 506
- absent, altered 167
Perspiration-bloody, hysterical 374, 474
- offensive 493, 588, 603
- profuse 208, 500, 567, 625

Pertussis 51, 696
Petit mal 506, 696
Pharyngitis 563, 690, 696
Pharynx 79, 192, 399, 433, 469, 565, 684, 693
Phimosis 155, 309, 424, 466, 549, 560, 580, 588, 614, 696
Phlebitis 60, 257, 421, 696
Phlegm 275, 344
Phlegmasia alba dolens 10, 309, 374, 461, 614, 696
Phlyctenulae 281
Phlyctenular 328, 696
-ophthalmia 328
Phobia 618, 697
Phosphaturia 143, 500, 697, 706
Photophobia 13, 135, 136, 181, 247, 461, 510, 583, 639, 697
Photopsia 662, 697
Phthiriasis 224, 697
Phthisis 23, 29, 51, 64, 88, 132, 145, 245, 269, 289, 344, 354, 459, 461, 511, 549, 561, 611, 625, 647, 648, 697
- florida 563, 639
- haemorrhagica 289
- mucosa 51
- pituitosa 599
Phymosis 72
Physomet 631
Physometra 394, 500, 563, 697
Piles 18, 47, 51, 178, 239, 240, 328, 333, 377, 413, 441, 470, 487, 697
Pimples 181, 201, 221, 281, 307, 371, 381, 469, 500, 617, 621, 673
Pining boys 87, 88
Pityriasis 76, 175, 291, 303, 431, 446, 516, 635, 697
- rubra 446
- versicolor 580
Placenta 158, 160, 319, 530, 674, 697, 698
- adherent 319
- retained 158, 560, 574
Plague 92, 374, 443, 506, 697
Plethora 29, 76, 132, 137, 167, 200, 201, 286, 658, 697, 709
Plethoric 9, 17, 41, 69, 97, 127, 131, 141, 161, 299, 301, 350, 614, 657
Pleurisy 10, 60, 73, 76, 98, 111, 120, 155, 158, 167, 208, 289, 314, 354, 359, 391, 542, 580, 585, 614, 621, 647, 697
Pleurodynia 10, 15, 70, 76, 120, 198, 215, 237, 354, 542, 697
Pleuro-pneumonia 56, 162, 697
Plica polonica 53, 111, 394, 526, 569, 652, 697
Pneumogastric 98, 373, 391, 443, 629, 657, 697
- paralysis 98
Pneumonia 10, 27, 39, 53, 54, 55, 56, 76, 98, 120, 128, 155, 162, 172, 198, 200, 261, 289, 314, 322, 341, 360, 374, 393, 394, 396, 415, 506, 509, 510, 511, 512, 545, 564, 614, 625, 637, 647, 652, 658, 697
- acute 563, 647
- typhoid 542
Polypi 107, 132, 133, 136, 137, 138, 143, 145, 167, 313, 349, 362, 374, 394, 411, 466, 506, 563, 565, 641, 642, 643, 697
- of ear, eye, nose 394
- rectal 349
Pollutions 64
Post-nasal catarrh..253, 319, 446, 447, 459, 595, 611, 642
Post-partum 155, 645, 698
- haemorrhage 155, 341, 574
Pot-bellied children 567, 604
Pott's disease 611, 698
Pregnancy 10, 15, 31, 44, 98, 120, 132, 138, 158, 162, 170, 175, 178, 188, 192, 199, 215, 223, 239, 246, 255, 268, 283, 286, 294, 314, 340, 345, 354, 363, 365, 367, 368, 391, 403, 405, 424, 438, 473, 474, 476, 480, 493, 500, 506, 530, 557, 564, 567, 579,

580, 582, 584, 585, 586, 614, 629, 630, 659, 660, 662, 692
- nausea of 403, 405, 603
- painful breasts during 246
- albuminuria of 294, 363
Pregnancy-constipation of 31
- diarrhoea of 500
- false pains of, spurious 574
- imaginary 255, 642, 652
- morning cough of 120
- morning sickness of 345
- pyrosis of 268
- sickness of 120, 314, 493, 568, 625, 639
- vomiting of 365, 506
Prepuce 155, 534, 675, 686, 698
- eruption on 588
- warts on 500
Presbyopia 447, 494, 698
Priapism 148, 155, 157, 160, 303, 381, 411, 447, 497, 530, 577, 698
Prickly heat 381, 698
Proctalgia 328, 354, 394, 506, 522, 631, 658, 698
Proctitis 29, 205, 239, 466, 506, 698
Progressive muscular atrophy 506, 522
Prolapsus 18, 29, 47, 72, 88, 281, 328, 331, 333, 431, 438, 454, 518, 533, 585, 600, 698
- ani 72, 281, 431, 522
- uteri 29
Prosopoplagia 132, 179, 181, 208, 232, 417, 600, 698
Prostate 17, 29, 65, 95, 105, 128, 248, 264, 281, 336, 359, 365, 424, 466, 514, 530, 603, 644, 698
- disease of 424, 642
- enlarged 65, 95, 264, 336
- irritation of 365
- suppuration of 466
Prostatitis 60, 151, 178, 205, 235, 246, 251, 394, 494, 577, 698
Prostatorrhoea 31, 530, 577, 595, 615, 630, 662, 698
Prostrate 512, 545, 570
Prostration 21, 22, 29, 35, 41, 43, 56, 65, 75, 76, 77, 81, 91, 92, 93, 109, 110, 147, 148, 168, 207, 224, 225, 258, 280, 285, 293, 294, 295, 373, 377, 391, 401, 408, 421, 444, 510, 516, 524, 543, 565, 579, 586, 593, 599, 608, 626, 637, 651, 653, 654, 655
Protoplasm 613
Prurigo 549, 698
Pruritus 138, 239, 251, 303, 314, 387, 580, 630, 698
- vulvae 239, 387, 517
Psoas abscess 500, 588, 603, 698
Psora 5, 6, 525, 613, 616
Psoriasis 53, 76, 111, 132, 208, 211, 253, 257, 261, 303, 345, 349, 362, 391, 439, 494, 506, 516, 580, 699
- palmaris 132, 257, 411, 577
Psoric 95, 177, 178, 304, 311, 314, 342, 357, 365, 395, 409, 494, 525, 526, 615, 616, 618, 642
Psychosis 699
Psychotic 411
Pterygium 205, 595, 699
Ptosis 178, 246, 281, 294, 303, 363, 411, 470, 474, 542, 580, 599, 642, 652, 662, 699
Ptyalism 264, 368, 699
Puerperal 15, 98, 120, 211, 215, 216, 258, 294, 311, 322, 324, 354, 374, 530, 699
- convulsion 211, 294, 311, 435, 474, 490, 506, 530, 658
- eclampsia 500
- fever 10, 120, 258, 354, 374, 417, 435, 530
- mania 15, 98, 215, 216, 322, 530, 658
- spasms 324
Pulse 9, 14, 53, 54, 55, 56, 73, 74, 80, 86, 97, 101, 103,

129, 140, 148, 149, 153, 171, 183, 237, 263, 264, 265, 294, 296, 300, 301, 348, 363, 364, 381, 441, 455, 492, 516, 629, 637, 657, 658,
- hard, rapid 56, 658
- intermittent 129, 170
Punctured wounds 60, 382, 383, 385
Pupils 13, 98, 101, 102, 136, 141, 212, 215, 216, 245, 294, 295, 312, 322, 324, 343, 383, 491, 492, 510, 606, 655, 658
Pupils-dilated 491
Purpura 10, 70, 76, 170, 253, 257, 424, 438, 500, 506, 574, 625, 699
- haemorrhagica 508, 626, 635, 636, 637
Pus 67, 71, 72, 74, 135, 248, 315, 413, 424, 427, 432, 433, 470, 527, 589, 617, 618, 643, 673
Pustules 57, 74, 103, 136, 201, 304, 365, 433, 528, 583, 592, 699
Pyaemia 70, 76, 257, 373, 374, 424, 510, 542, 652, 699, 710
Pyelitis 76, 699
Pylorus 208, 314, 394, 480, 699
- induration of 580
- suppuration of 588
- thickening of 506
Pyrexia 340
Pyrosis 171, 268, 564, 630, 699
Pyuria 699
Qualmishness 343, 487, 495
Quarrelsome 329, 331, 479, 484, 493, 633, 658
Quinsy 10, 95, 96, 274, 425, 526, 564, 580, 631, 700
Rabies 374, 686, 700
Rage 158, 322, 323
Ranula 132, 369, 424, 450, 466, 603, 642, 643, 700
Rat bites 382, 385
Rawness 18, 62, 64, 68, 117, 172, 178, 179, 180, 182, 183, 194, 280, 378, 469, 485, 486, 510, 549, 598
Raynaud's disease 289, 574, 700
Reaction defective 662
Rectum 14, 17, 18, 29, 30, 32, 33, 44, 45, 128, 145, 158, 162, 164, 172, 178, 179, 193, 228, 235, 237, 239, 240, 283, 303, 307, 319, 328, 331, 333, 345, 356, 376, 389, 400, 407, 418, 424, 428, 440, 453, 456, 465, 466, 469, 476, 482, 487, 491, 510, 551-555, 581, 585, 591, 613, 615, 620
- burning in 345
- cancer of 514, 580, 595
- cramp in 568
Rectum-fissure of 580
- paralysis of, stricture of 630
- prolapse of 235, 283, 328, 407,
Red-gum 47, 60, 188, 542
Regurgitation 285, 286, 701, 707
Relapsing fever 92, 120, 279, 542, 700
Renal calculi 480, 700
Renal colic 107, 132, 268, 394, 400, 411, 474, 569, 700
Respiration *(see breath)* 14, 23, 41, 54, 56, 77, 115, 149, 264, 293, 337, 341, 344, 383, 441, 443, 491, 492, 511, 593, 597, 598, 608, 655, 689, 696
- abnormal, irregular 264, 514
- anxious 511
- very difficult 510
Restlessness 9, 10, 11, 12, 14, 56, 75, 76, 78, 79, 81, 109, 134, 149, 189, 191, 229, 233, 271, 323, 341, 363, 385, 441, 507, 508, 532, 542, 543, 545, 547, 548, 552, 554, 592, 631, 632, 644, 660
Retina 294, 700
Retinitis 363, 506, 700
- albuminurica 363
Retrocession 616

Reveries 577, 700
Rhagades 31, 132, 140, 307, 314, 394, 466, 569, 622, 700
Rheumatic 14, 15, 16, 55, 64, 76, 105, 119, 120, 144, 145, 162, 175, 180, 181, 183, 188, 189, 194, 195, 215, 216, 235, 238, 273, 328, 336, 362, 363, 381, 382, 384, 385, 409, 426, 461, 513, 516, 529, 539, 540, 544, 548, 551, 570, 595, 614, 652, 700
- diathesis 105, 119, 195, 513, 541, 595
- fever 328, 597, 615
- gout 15, 76, 162, 176, 215, 336, 382, 384, 560
- pains 14, 63, 145, 181, 183, 188, 189, 194, 216, 238, 362, 363, 381, 384, 539, 564, 565, 622, 655
Rheumatic-tendency 120
- troubles 144, 570
Rheumatism 10, 15, 23, 44, 53, 60, 64, 70, 74, 76, 98, 105, 107, 108, 120, 121, 127, 128, 129, 132, 143, 145, 148, 162, 175, 178, 180, 181, 188, 198, 201, 208, 215, 221, 224, 235, 237, 239, 241, 257, 259, 268, 274, 279, 284, 289, 294, 299, 310, 314, 316, 336, 345, 359, 360, 362, 363, 364, 365, 369, 381, 382, 384, 394, 411, 424, 431, 447, 459, 462, 473, 474, 494, 500, 515, 517, 530, 531, 537, 539, 542, 543, 548, 549, 552, 557, 564, 595, 597, 603, 611, 612, 625, 652, 662, 700
- acute 615
- chronic 588
- gonorrhoeal 570, 642
- paralytic 506
- syphilitic 514
Rheumatoid 185, 541
Rhinitis 700
Rhus poisoning 198, 259, 304, 315, 362, 564
Ribs 200, 334, 399, 608, 688, 697, 703
Rickets 35, 76, 131, 132, 143, 359, 424, 466, 504, 506, 568, 588, 639, 642, 701
Riding in carriage-effects of 224
Rigg's disease 417, 424
Rigid os 391
Ring-worm 53, 76, 701
Rodent ulcer 435, 514, 701
Roseola 10, 98, 701
Rubella 684
Rumination 363, 701
Rupia 359, 701
Sacrum 14, 17, 19, 107, 188, 194, 219, 333, 391, 476, 559, 584, 701
- pain in 17, 23 29, 107, 580
Saliva 124, 152, 192, 199, 227, 337, 343, 346, 376, 383, 392, 425, 468, 619, 652, 654, 699, 707
- profuse 469
Salivation 113, 188, 336, 337, 339, 345, 419, 424, 466, 514, 537, 545, 652
- nocturnal 188
Satyriasis 151, 153, 158, 160, 291, 693, 701
Scabies 170, 178, 185, 577, 613, 635, 701
Scabs 135, 140, 303, 306, 432, 433, 493, 495, 593, 605, 618, 643
Scald-head 76, 198
Scalp 178, 306, 426, 432, 456, 468, 494, 527, 528, 533, 537, 567, 617, 704
- dry 525
- eczema of 577
Scapula 197, 200, 203, 213, 244, 259, 310, 400, 508, 511, 621, 688, 701
- pain in 203
- rheumatism of 310
Scars 336, 700
Scarlatina 10, 35, 36, 37, 60, 65, 76, 83, 98 103, 120,

123, 158, 217, 257, 262, 274, 311, 312, 314, 323, 374, 439, 441, 461, 542, 545, 595, 635, 636, 637, 638, 652, 701
Scarlet fever 441, 468, 528, 694, 701
School-headache 407, 447
Sciatica 15, 39, 40, 73, 76, 132, 162, 188, 215, 231, 241, 242, 243, 268, 269, 299, 320, 328, 345, 354, 369, 359, 374, 394, 407, 411, 461, 500, 514, 515, 522, 526, 542, 543, 552, 580, 603, 615, 636, 642, 649, 650, 701
Scirrhus 249, 368, 569, 701
Scleroderma 363, 702
Sclerosis 522, 524, 631, 702
Sclerotitis 363, 702
Scorbutic 367, 449, 452
Screaming 53, 111, 114, 120, 160, 188, 211, 213, 349, 350, 506, 525, 537, 653, 662
- of children 537
Scrofula 31, 88, 115, 131, 132, 140, 162, 167, 178, 205, 246, 274, 281, 304, 314, 359, 432, 447, 459, 702
Scrofulosis 639
Scrofulous 76, 85, 95, 96, 115, 118, 136, 137, 143, 144, 173, 185, 245, 246, 249, 273, 314, 335, 336, 338, 365, 459, 461, 468, 499, 504, 526, 551, 555, 561, 577, 589, 595, 614, 616, 618, 623, 624,
Scrotum 60, 228, 260, 307, 318, 494, 495, 620, 621, 624, 704
Scurf 306, 561, 702
Scurvy 39, 170, 310, 374, 424, 439, 500, 506, 526, 568, 603, 625, 702
Sea-bathing-effects of 76
Sea-sickness 41, 76, 111, 162, 165,224, 227, 480, 494, 568, 604, 630, 639,
Seaside-effects of 115
Sebaceous cysts, tumours 23, 350
Sebaceous glands 528, 702, 703
Seborrhoea 320, 336, 350, 391, 450, 570, 586, 604, 702
Self-abuse 44, 60, 143, 208, 350, 450, 500, 604, 615, 702
Semen/seminal fluid 620, 698, 702, 703
Seminal emissions 286, 304, 350, 429, 608, 609, 611, 662, 702
- nocturnal 429, 642
Sensibility-loss of 350
Sensitiveness 14, 51, 85, 96, 98, 102, 112, 157, 187, 188, 191, 194, 195, 199, 207, 208, 210, 231, 233, 316, 317, 318, 328, 355, 391, 448, 480, 481, 484, 519, 525, 543, 591, 592, 618, 637, 640, 650, 687
Sepsis/septic 173, 631, 702
Septicaemia 69, 71, 74,
Serous 59, 119, 120, 121, 122, 303, 311, 354, 381, 391, 417, 423, 433, 513, 686, 696, 702, 709
Sewer-gas poisoning 92, 514
Sexual excess-effects of 23, 294
- mania, perversion 148, 480, 517
Shivering 10, 25, 76, 92, 148, 164, 165, 170, 192, 195, 343, 410, 486, 506, 593, 609, 623, 655
Shock 72, 74, 149, 152, 213, 231, 232, 301, 502, 579, 581, 582, 655, 679
Shoulder 110, 139, 153, 162, 342, 564, 565, 600, 608, 621, 622, 640, 680, 701
- pains in 283, 381, 383, 384, 391, 411
- rheumatism of 564, 568
Shyness 415
Sick headache 199, 225, 226, 248, 345, 346, 563-565, 611, 629, 702
Side pain 15, 107, 215, 268

Sighing 54, 145, 216, 328, 342, 459, 490, 492, 500,
Sight-affections of 217
Sigmoid flexure 702
- cancer of 595
Sinciput 219, 243, 301, 389
Sinking 15, 42, 73, 75, 76, 81, 149, 178, 184, 215, 216, 264, 265, 328, 438, 507, 579, 584, 586, 600, 605, 615, 651, 653, 654, 655
- sensation 216
Sinuses 588, 642, 683, 702
Skin 5, 6, 11, 14, 24, 44, 47, 57, 59, 60, 61, 74, 77, 80, 97, 98, 100, 103, 112, 115, 132, 133, 139, 141, 149, 157, 158, 159, 163, 168, 177, 178, 184, 185, 198, 201, 221, 243, 258, 259, 262, 264, 273, 303, 304, 307, 313, 314, 315, 318, 327, 345, 349, 353, 357, 362, 365, 371, 376, 378, 381, 393, 394, 411, 412, 418, 423, 431, 433, 439, 441, 449, 450, 454, 461, 465, 466, 473, 477, 490, 491, 493, 494, 495, 499, 505, 513, 516, 522, 524, 525, 526, 527, 528, 533, 541, 544, 547, 548, 549, 550, 561, 569, 570, 571, 573, 575, 579, 582, 586, 587, 589, 592, 603, 605, 609, 613, 614, 615, 616, 618, 620, 623, 624, 625, 626, 627, 641, 652, 653, 655, 656, 673, 676, 677, 679, 680, 681, 682, 685, 686, 687, 688, 689, 690, 691, 692, 696, 697, 698, 699, 700, 701, 702, 704, 706, 709
- blue 653
- cracked 495, 677
- dry 77, 139, 526
- eruptions on 178, 381, 494, 544, 680, 684, 686
- hot 97, 103, 441, 490, 573
- unhealthy 577
Skull 71, 140, 163, 165, 199, 301, 342, 432, 468, 486, 686, 694
Sleep 11, 14, 24, 25, 57, 60, 61, 72, 73, 81, 92, 98, 99, 100, 103, 112, 114, 120, 123, 132, 135, 136, 139, 153, 157, 160, 161, 165, 170, 172, 185, 191, 194, 195, 201, 208, 209, 214, 217, 218, 219, 223, 224, 225, 228, 229, 232, 233, 246-248, 249, 261, 262, 264, 275, 294, 312, 315, 316, 318, 322, 325, 328, 334, 340, 343, 344, 350, 351, 356, 357, 366, 370, 373, 375, 376, 377, 379, 384, 393, 394, 395, 398, 400, 427, 430, 441, 467, 471, 474, 475, 476, 481, 492, 500, 501, 504, 506, 508, 535, 542, 547, 562, 565, 578, 580, 581, 585, 586, 593, 598, 606, 608, 611, 617, 622, 633, 661, 662, 687, 702, 711
- abnormal 394, 480, 490
Sleep-affections from loss of 224
- anxious dreams in 120
- disordered 98, 132, 170, 208, 294, 322, 328, 506, 615
- disturbed, restless 229, 542, 617
- dreamful 658
- overpowering 474
- whining in 652
Sleepiness *(see drowsiness)* 21, 51, 53, 54, 57, 62, 153, 185, 340, 342, 473, 475, 476, 477, 512, 662, 702
Sleeplessness 10, 15, 16, 21, 132, 148, 161, 185, 189, 216, 231, 232, 233, 257, 261, 321, 325, 350, 354, 385, 489, 490, 524, 535, 599, 606, 611, 612, 644, 649
Small-pox 53, 65, 178, 258, 310, 359, 374, 424, 542, 574, 702, 706

Smell 10, 35, 36, 44, 71, 72, 85, 86, 88, 92, 98, 102, 103, 105, 132, 133, 136, 137, 192, 227, 231, 235, 236, 268, 304, 306, 404, 405, 468, 469, 476, 484, 525, 527, 530, 537, 564, 573, 582, 583, 584, 618, 626, 637
- disordered 10, 88, 98, 132, 268, 304, 405
- illusions of 44, 530, 564, 615
- sense of-too acute 580
Snake-bites 148
Sneezing 28, 34, 179, 182, 376, 423, 429, 456, 485, 534, 544, 557, 608, 618, 629, 685
Snoring 334, 490, 491, 492, 537
Snow-headache 299
Snuffles 561, 702
Sobbing-spasmodic 407
Soles 48, 49, 51, 96, 138, 184, 188, 194, 225, 228, 382, 384, 411, 439, 471, 493, 503, 564, 567, 592, 620, 622, 702
Somnambulism 350, 363, 450, 506, 588, 662, 702
Somnolence 37, 224, 702
Soreness 50, 64, 68, 70, 72, 73, 74, 75, 83, 89, 92, 108, 117, 121, 125, 137, 163, 178, 179, 180, 183, 184, 200, 216, 279, 280, 304, 306, 307, 310, 318, 328, 337, 356, 367, 370, 379, 408, 453, 463, 469, 471, 486, 495, 528, 543, 547, 550, 551, 567, 568, 582, 585, 598, 620, 621, 624, 658
Spasm 10, 15, 23, 25, 37, 72, 86, 95, 97-99, 127, 134, 139, 148, 149, 175, 179, 180, 182, 188, 190, 193, 211, 213, 214, 215, 219, 220, 227, 237, 261, 262, 286, 310, 328, 350, 391, 406, 480, 481, 491, 517, 519, 522, 523, 553, 555, 588, 590, 649, 657, 658, 660, 661, 662, 678, 688, 695, 700, 702, 705, 706,
Spastic 480, 574, 702
Speech 102, 179, 182, 188, 275, 314, 324, 350, 394, 419, 450, 456, 471, 474, 480, 555, 689
- disordered 394, 474, 480
- embarrassed 450, 630
Speechlessness 182
Spermatic cords 604, 702, 706
- neuralgia of 107
- swelling of 570
Spermatorrhoea 143, 158, 208, 246, 264, 268, 450, 480, 500, 570, 577, 580, 588, 603, 604, 636, 662, 703,
Spina bifida 120, 143, 520, 703
Spine 14, 15, 19, 23, 132, 133, 140, 153, 165, 219, 223, 297, 325, 359, 454, 466, 495, 504, 507, 521, 522, 523, 530, 554, 555, 592, 622, 658, 663, 698, 701
- congestion of 658
- curvature of 506, 615
- diseases of 522, 542
- injury to 466
- Pott's curvature of 359,
Spleen 23, 39, 74, 85, 107, 207, 208, 268, 337, 359, 449, 461, 522, 526, 552, 625, 703
- congested 658
- enlarged 337, 405, 450, 506,
- neuralgia of 662
- pain in.39, 268, 403, 514, 539
- swollen 652
Splenalgia 70, 291, 703
Spotted fever 35, 279
Sprain 35, 39, 70, 74, 289, 334, 368, 494, 506, 539, 542, 548, 551, 552, 703
Squint 703
Stammering 151, 155, 178, 279, 322, 394, 419, 447, 474, 506, 552, 574, 577, 595
Staphyloma 281, 703
Starting 23, 81, 149, 170, 184,

192, 195, 324, 490, 561, 590, 615,
Steatoma 604, 703
Sterility 111, 246, 336, 506, 625
Sternum 35, 90, 125, 153, 183, 194, 219, 337, 360, 503, 511, 545, 552, 564, 565, 592, 608, 652, 703
Stiff-neck 10, 15, 44, 53, 120, 143, 198, 216, 235, 274, 514, 539, 604
Stiffness 102, 108,145, 175, 179, 180, 183, 200, 201, 216, 228, 274, 281, 364, 541, 542, 544, 545, 546, 547, 586, 591, 622, 625,
Stings 60, 70, 74, 258, 374, 381, 382, 385, 567
Stitch in side 23
Stomacace 172, 619
Stomach 13, 21, 37, 44, 47, 48, 50, 53, 57, 65, 71, 76, 77, 79, 80, 85, 87, 93, 109, 110, 120, 121, 122, 125, 127, 128, 133, 136, 137, 139, 140, 147, 148, 155, 158, 160, 163, 164, 165, 169, 170, 171, 172, 182, 190, 192, 193, 198, 199, 200, 213, 219, 224, 225, 226, 227, 236, 242, 246, 256, 260, 264, 265, 284, 285, 286, 304, 306, 311, 316, 320, 324, 328, 330, 332, 336, 339, 340, 341, 343, 345, 346, 348, 354, 355, 366, 367, 369, 379, 397, 398, 399, 400, 407, 408, 409, 412, 413, 452, 470, 475, 476, 481, 483, 486, 494, 503, 507, 510, 513, 530, 537, 553, 565, 580, 582, 583, 584, 586, 599, 600, 604, 617, 619, 621, 626, 630, 633, 640, 657, 658, 660, 677, 682, 683, 684, 685, 694, 697, 699, 703, 709
- ache 452
- cancer of 109, 407, 574
- cramp in 304
- disordered 170, 450, 537
- hanging down 605
- neurosis of 564
Stomatitis 92, 109, 162, 170, 419, 424, 450, 466, 615, 676, 703
Stone-cutter's phthisis 132
Stool *(see bowels)* 14, 18, 22, 29, 30, 32, 33, 34, 40, 44, 45, 48, 50, 51, 54, 55, 62, 66, 67, 70, 72, 76, 80, 85, 89, 92, 93, 109, 110, 112, 113, 117, 120, 121, 125, 135, 137,144, 148, 158, 159, 164, 178, 179, 182, 188, 190, 198, 237, 249, 259, 260, 274, 285, 295, 304, 305, 306, 316, 317, 321, 323, 324, 330, 331, 333, 346, 366, 376, 388, 389, 393, 396, 399, 400, 403, 404, 405, 406, 413, 418, 424, 428, 430, 440, 453, 456, 462, 466, 467, 469, 470, 475, 476, 481, 482, 487, 488, 491, 497, 501, 509, 510, 518, 519, 522, 528, 531, 534, 537, 538, 552, 553, 567, 568, 577, 578, 582, 585, 588, 589, 591, 600, 607, 608, 619, 620, 621, 626, 635, 642, 643, 645, 652, 553, 654, 655, 704,
- green, slimy 403, 425
- involuntary, white 440, 491, 503
- knotty 304, 305, 406
Strabismus 31, 132, 167, 211, 212, 217, 574, 595, 630, 662, 703
Strains 76, 132, 394, 584, 588
Strangury 98, 148, 157, 158, 159, 161, 164, 374, 474, 559, 560, 570, 588, 635, 636, 637, 703
Stricture 148, 205, 221, 391, 411, 443, 494, 497, 506, 508, 522, 542, 588, 630,

636, 703
- spasmodic 574
Stumps-neuralgia in 39
Stupor 11, 36, 54, 60, 61, 70, 71, 91, 92, 93, 322, 474, 475, 489, 490, 492, 500, 508, 542, 637, 638, 661, 705, 711
Stuttering 182, 211, 703
Styes 289, 314, 398, 580, 599, 603-606, 643, 703
Subcostal 534, 662, 703
Subinvolution 703
Sub-maxillary glands 370, 469, 544, 545
Subsultus tendinum 322, 324
Suffocation 116, 117, 129, 164, 208, 213, 341, 511, 512, 598, 655
- fits of 208
Sun-effects of 128, 577
Sun-headache 294, 299,363, 375,
Sunstroke 41, 47, 128, 148, 258, 294, 299, 300, 394, 447, 450, 490, 658
- chronic effects of 447
Suppressed eruptions-effects of 60, 120
Suppressions 662
Suppuration 70, 74, 76, 96, 116, 118, 168, 182, 291, 313, 314, 315, 396, 424, 425, 428, 466, 495, 513, 516, 527, 574, 588, 589, 591, 592, 597, 699, 703
Surgical fever 424, 703
Swallowing 68, 102, 163, 178, 179, 182, 199, 213, 218, 315, 317, 324, 328, 330, 332, 344, 356, 370, 376, 378, 398, 428, 469, 503, 516, 543, 598, 619, 681, 684
- constant while talking 604
Sweat(see persipiration) 11, 14, 25, 30, 41, 49, 51, 53, 55, 56, 57, 76, 81, 93, 95, 96, 98, 109, 110, 129, 131, 132, 133, 135, 137, 138, 139, 140, 141, 144, 145, 148, 149, 153, 160, 170, 171, 172, 188, 189, 191, 192, 193, 195, 201, 207, 209, 233, 237, 242, 248, 249, 258, 274, 289, 295, 312, 316, 318, 334, 340, 342, 354, 355, 356, 357, 384, 385, 395, 405, 429, 450, 469, 477, 490, 512, 528, 532, 535, 537, 562, 567, 586, 587, 588, 589, 593, 600, 601, 615, 620, 629, 630, 633, 634, 642, 652, 653, 654, 655, 656, 661, 682,
- glands 454
Swelling 15, 19, 25, 39, 59, 61, 62, 74, 76, 79, 83, 85, 95, 96, 98, 102, 113, 116, 117, 118, 121, 132, 135, 136, 139, 140, 162, 163, 167, 168, 172, 173, 182, 184, 192, 206, 213, 229, 236, 246, 247, 249, 274, 316, 317, 337, 343, 353, 354, 355, 360, 366, 367, 368, 370, 376, 378, 382, 384, 396, 398, 409, 412, 413, 418, 424, 425, 427, 428, 429, 432, 455, 459, 466, 468, 469, 470, 495, 516, 524, 539, 544, 547, 551, 552, 591, 597, 615, 616, 618, 619, 624, 635, 677, 681, 685, 686, 687, 692, 693, 694, 695, 696, 702, 703, 705, 706, 709,
Sycosis 5, 53, 60, 105, 131, 132, 281, 435, 461, 466, 560, 641, 642, 691, 703
- Hahnemanni 435, 500
- menti 132
Sycotic 304, 409, 465, 641, 642, 643, 644
- diathesis 304, 569
Syncope 655
Synovial 119, 235, 529, 696, 703, 709
Synovitis 53, 530, 588, 703
Syphilis 5, 60, 65, 85, 87, 88,

167, 178, 205, 253, 258, 284, 291, 314, 320, 336, 350, 359, 365, 374, 417, 423, 424, 432, 466, 468, 494, 500, 506, 514, 526, 564, 570, 577, 611, 642, 684, 691, 703

Syphilitic 88, 89, 105, 111, 173, 279, 409, 412, 423, 424, 431, 465, 466, 468, 471, 504, 513, 514, 540, 603, 642, 643, 644
- deafness 366
- eruptions 514, 571
- pains 279
- sore-throat 111, 363
- ulcers 89, 677

Syringo-myelia 506, 703

Tabes mesenterica 92, 132, 336, 417, 494, 522,

Tape-worm.132, 137, 517, 557, 599

Tarsal cysts, tumours 283, 606, 643, 662

Taste bad, foul 163, 537
- disordered 17, 31, 53, 66, 70, 98, 111, 132, 148, 198, 208, 320, 417, 424
- illusions of 615
- lost 450

Tea-effects of 208, 268, 391, 480, 642

Teeth 50, 71, 93, 100, 124, 132, 136, 169, 170, 171, 172, 177, 181, 182, 190, 192, 197, 198, 199, 211, 217, 233, 242, 243, 291, 295, 301, 322, 324, 325, 342, 351, 354, 366, 367, 374, 376, 398, 403, 406, 409, 418, 424, 425, 427, 428, 432, 457, 469, 503, 513, 514, 515, 548, 605, 607, 634, 639, 643,
- black 418
- carious 132, 366, 588, 604, 642
- decay 242, 366, 604
- defective 291
- grating of 322

Teeth-loose 418

Teething *(see dentition)* 97, 132, 137, 138, 145, 192, 211, 294, 350, 409

Temple 71, 102, 124, 163, 275, 367, 389, 398, 412, 502, 519, 583, 606, 633

Tendo Achilles 439

Tendons 47, 105, 178, 180, 184, 322, 384, 432, 541, 546, 548, 592, 709
- contracted 178, 432
- inflamed 47

Tenesmus 29, 72, 98, 157, 158, 159, 160, 164, 237, 240, 286, 314, 328, 388, 389, 404, 417, 418, 424, 425, 428, 480, 482, 491, 509, 538, 588, 615
- of bladder, of rectum 418, 423, 570, 637

Testicles *(see scrotum)* 10, 64, 88, 98, 115, 183, 221, 245, 246, 310, 335, 533, 539, 540, 597, 604, 620
- hard and swollen 143, 540
- induration of 115
- inflamed 221, 310, 597
- neuralgia of 446
- undeveloped 88

Tetanic 327, 344, 479

Tetanus 10, 148, 155, 211, 212, 258, 311, 322, 339, 350, 382, 435, 514, 630, 636, 639

Tetany 10

Tetters 31, 246, 454, 456, 500
- moist and itching 31

Thirst 10, 13, 22, 48, 50, 51, 54, 55, 61, 62, 70, 75, 76, 77, 79, 81, 98, 109, 120, 121, 122, 124, 152, 158, 159, 164, 182, 188, 192, 193, 195, 207, 208, 209, 219, 227, 233, 236, 258, 271, 274, 279, 289, 328, 331, 340, 341, 342, 344, 385, 395, 398, 503, 509, 512, 516, 530, 531, 545, 586, 592, 593, 609, 615, 637, 654, 655, 656

Thirstlessness 59, 60, 61
Thorax 311
Threadworms 286, 459
Throat 10, 13, 17, 18, 31, 32, 33, 36, 55, 60, 61, 65, 66, 67, 68, 70, 76, 77, 83, 85, 86, 89, 91, 95, 96, 97, 98, 99, 100, 102, 105, 111, 115, 117, 136, 143, 145, 152, 158, 159, 162, 163, 172, 178, 179, 182, 183, 188, 190, 192, 194, 199, 213, 218, 220, 249, 253, 269, 274, 314, 315, 317, 320, 328, 330, 332, 333, 336, 337, 343, 344, 345, 346, 349, 354, 355, 357, 363, 369, 370, 373, 374, 375, 376, 378, 379, 383, 394, 398, 417, 418, 421, 424, 426, 428, 443, 447, 448, 469, 474, 476, 485, 486, 495, 503, 511, 513, 514, 523, 528, 534, 545, 549, 557, 565, 578, 585, 595, 607, 608, 611, 619, 633, 643, 650, 652, 654,
- deafness 320, 424
- mucus in 60, 76, 95, 98, 105, 111, 115, 117, 143, 158, 162, 314, 320, 328, 332, 354, 369, 370, 374, 383, 394, 421, 424, 443, 447, 506, 514, 516, 526, 549, 557, 568, 615, 618, 662,
Throbbing 13, 18, 41, 85, 98-101, 148, 152, 163, 164, 165, 181, 191, 209, 213, 243, 255, 299-302, 316, 332, 341, 346, 376, 379, 397, 408, 413, 415, 450, 451, 476, 554, 565, 581, 653
- pain 165, 316
Thrombosis 574
Thyroid 118, 285, 335, 337, 597, 716
Tibia 86, 274, 433, 452, 511, 609
- burning in 662
- pains in 274, 604
Tic convulsif 23
Tic douloureux 294, 359, 407
Tinea 92, 135, 181
- capitis 92, 181, 432, 526, 527
- ciliaris 405
- favosa 135
- versicolor 432
Tinnitus 15, 203, 208, 216, 359, 363, 381, 403, 540, 564, 595
- aurium 15, 216
Tobacco 76, 122, 125, 143, 148, 158, 208, 244, 294, 296, 330, 331, 332, 344, 363, 391, 480, 486, 534, 629
- effect of 294, 363, 604
Tobacco-habit 76, 143, 148, 208, 480, 506, 522, 595
Toenail-ingrowing 466, 604
Toes 24, 25, 32, 51, 62, 96, 138, 184, 220, 262, 305, 307, 336, 384, 471, 454, 571, 574, 592, 593, 594, 623, 656
Tongue 10, 13, 17, 24, 47, 48, 50, 54, 55, 60,66, 68, 71, 76, 77, 79, 83, 88, 92, 93, 98, 99, 102, 105, 113, 120, 124, 136, 148, 158, 162, 167, 170, 172, 178, 179, 182, 184, 185, 192, 197-199, 235, 238, 258, 263, 264, 274, 275, 291, 294-296, 306, 316, 320, 324, 332, 339, 340, 342, 345, 346, 355, 359, 374, 376, 394, 398, 406, 409, 412, 417, 418, 419, 424, 425, 427, 428, 432, 439, 440, 441, 452, 454, 455, 459, 468, 469, 474, 475, 476, 480, 491, 516, 528, 530, 531, 533, 542, 543, 545, 548, 555, 591, 617, 635-637, 642, 643, 655, 658,
- biting of 574
- blistered, heavy 450, 456
- burning, ringworm of 568
- coated 47, 50, 54, 120, 182, 394, 421, 530, 615

- cramp in 552
- inflammation of 158, 258
- mapped 450, 452
- neuralgia of 359
- nodules on 88
- numbness of 537
- oedema of 60
- paralysis of 162, 522
- protruded 258
- sore 105
- swollen 316
- ulcerated 66, 93, 291, 466

Tonsils 39, 93, 96, 97, 99, 316, 370, 396, 428, 468, 469, 514, 619
- concretions in 526
- swollen 469, 514, 516
- inflamed 97, 370

Tonsilitis 163, 274, 376, 557, 604, 615

Torpid 53, 133, 295, 313, 580

Trachea 55, 60, 76, 86, 115-117, 120, 132, 156, 162, 167, 170, 177, 178, .183, 374, 480, 510, 549, 588, 597, 599
- dryness of 170
- irritation in 60, 115, 615
- mucus in 155
- pain in 120
- tickling in 162, 506

Trachiitis 57

Trauma 27, 70, 299

Traumatic fever 10, 69, 70, 73, 76, 128, 208, 374,

Trembling 24, 54, 56, 57, 66, 67, 68, 134, 139, 148, 173, 176, 178, 184, 208, 213, 220, 228, 294, 295, 297, 373, 375, 377, 383, 419, 429, 471, 490, 491, 523, 535, 545, 546, 557, 622, 626, 634, 662, 663

Tremors 15, 23, 54, 216, 294, 328, 424, 661

Trichiasis 111, 304

Trifacial-nerve paralysis 450

Trismus 21, 31, 212, 213, 246

Tuberculosis *(see consumption)* 98,115, 131, 132, 139, 269, 381, 446, 506, 510, 528, 597, 647, 648

Tumours 23, 60, 70, 88, 95, 105, 107, 132, 198, 241, 246, 249, 255, 274, 291, 303, 304, 336, 359, 374, 403, 513, 514, 515, 564, 588, 603, 606, 631, 634, 641, 642, 643, 662
- erectile/polypoid/cancerous 506
- tarsal 604

Turgescence 170

Turpentine-effects of 474

Twitching 15, 24, 25, 33, 56, 98, 124, 148, 179, 217, 219, 220, 256, 262, 322, 323, 327, 328, 333, 340, 341, 398, 480, 481, 548, 557, 609, 658, 662

Tympanites 85, 170, 208, 490, 636, 637

Tympany 224

Typhlitis 235, 522

Typhoid 3, 23, 32, 73, 74, 78, 83, 92, 93, 121, 132, 140, 169, 170, 173, 235, 274, 295, 311, 323, 354, 373, 376, 378, 394, 440, 441, 490, 501, 527, 542, 543, 545, 548, 574, 636, 652, 656, 658, 662
- haemorrhage in 474

Typhus 23, 31, 60, 72, 73, 76, 81, 92, 170, 320, 424, 439, 441, 500, 506, 512, 542, 637

Ulcer 5, 39, 40, 65, 76, 77, 81, 85, 88, 89, 92, 93, 98, 105, 111, 112, 115, 161, 167, 170, 173, 178, 181, 185, 188, 201, 205, 246, 248, 253, 258, 261, 291, 304, 309, 310, 311, 317, 320, 339, 359, 366, 369, 374, 432, 435, 450, 466, 493, 500, 506, 514, 554, 570, 574, 588, 593, 615, 625, 642, 662, 677, 701, 705
- malignant 205

Ulceration 60, 65, 85, 93, 111, 112, 136, 167, 173, 255, 313, 319, 357, 398, 439, 447, 465, 468, 506, 513, 563, 567, 599, 624, 637, 647, 695, 705,
Umbilicus 200, 242, 243, 267, 268, 343, 637, 655, 705
- abscess of, hernia of 522
Unconsciousness 74, 323, 350, 373, 439, 456, 678
Uraemia 35, 151, 490, 636, 705
Urea 39, 348
Urethra 10, 65, 80, 108, 148, 156, 157, 159, 160, 178, 179, 183, 221, 251, 277, 351, 389, 391, 424, 429, 465, 470, 480, 497, 507, 553, 570, 581, 604, 605, 608, 613, 615, 620, 635, 637, 644, 698, 705, 706
- spasm of 480
- spasmodic stricture of 10, 148
- stricture of 221, 391, 494, 506, 588
Urethral caruncle 155
Urethral fever 10
Urethritis 60, 178, 251, 642, 678, 684, 706
Uric acid 105, 238, 348, 393, 684, 706
Uric acid diathesis 105, 238, 393
Uric-acidaemia 522
Urinary disorders 151, 178, 205, 264, 304
Urination 113, 149, 152, 157, 160, 178, 180, 205, 277, 278, 286, 294, 296, 297, 325, 328, 370, 387, 389, 396, 400, 429, 482, 491, 533, 552, 570, 578, 637, 642, 681
- difficult 164, 537
Urine 10, 14, 30, 33, 34, 59, 60 70, 72, 73, 86, 92, 93, 102, 105, 107, 108, 112, 113, 125, 143, 148, 152, 155, 156, 158, 159, 160, 162, 164, 179, 182, 183, 198, 200, 205, 206, 207, 217, 218, 221, 228, 237, 242, 245, 246, 247, 249, 251, 258, 265, 274, 277, 278, 284, 289, 295, 296, 300, 311, 312, 314, 316, 317, 321, 322, 328, 330, 333, 343, 345, 348, 350, 354, 366, 370, 378, 388, 394, 396, 400, 405, 406, 418, 429, 440, 441, 454, 456, 465, 466, 500, 501, 503, 530, 551, 568, 569, 570, 573, 581, 585, 608, 620, 635, 636, 638, 652, 655, 662, 673, 678, 681, 684, 685, 686, 687, 694, 697, 699, 703, 705, 706
- abnormal 60, 158, 328, 394
- albuminous 523
- black 637
- brown 72
- clear but irritating 569
- cloudy, milky 217, 343,637
- dark yellow 200
- disorders of 105, 107, 162
- dribbles 152, 534, 578
- difficulty in passing 274
- frequent passing of 354, 388, 480
- incontinence of 284, 289, 350, 366, 580, 588
- involuntary 577
- like ink 237
- pale, straining to pass 405, 406
- phosphatic 500
- red 537, 636
- sandy reddish 581
- scalds 159
- scanty 413, 637
- strong smelling 111
- suppression of 10, 148, 490, 636
- thick, very acid 72
Urticaria 59, 60, 132, 136, 251, 258, 314, 354, 411, 454, 459, 542, 543, 548, 549, 615, 684, 686, 693, 706

Uterine 15, 16, 98, 132, 145, 175, 216, 226, 245, 246, 255, 294, 296, 301, 310, 320, 336, 337, 353, 366, 369, 376, 387, 388, 389, 394, 404, 405, 406, 514, 522, 600, 660, 691, 697,
- atony, spasm 175, 706
- trouble 376, 388, 406, 522, 582
Uterus 10, 17, 18, 40, 61, 64, 88, 90, 102, 111, 115, 128, 133, 143, 145, 167, 168, 188, 193, 241, 256, 304, 309, 310, 320, 331, 337, 340, 343, 354, 368, 387, 388, 389, 405, 411, 438, 473, 474, 480, 530, 551, 559, 560, 573, 584, 585, 637, 645, 659, 660, 677, 681, 694, 695, 696, 706,
- air in 115
- bearing down in 580
- bleeding from 560
- cancer of 63, 167, 304, 354, 631
- congestion of 658
- cramps in 659
- diseases of 188
- induration of 88, 517
- inertia of 490, 574
- pain in 241, 405
- prolapse of 10, 17,144, 438, 474, 480, 500, 599, 615, 625
- soreness of, tumour of 568, 631
Uvula 68, 516, 706
- elongated 417, 557
Vaccination 10, 60, 258, 304, 424, 431, 432, 587, 588, 589, 615, 642, 643, 644, 706
- effects of 10, 258, 304
Vaccinia 506, 706
Vaccinosis 369, 642, 706
Vagina 31, 111, 115, 117, 128, 138, 241, 310, 328, 367, 368, 376, 387, 388, 389, 391, 393, 465, 580, 581, 585, 587, 621, 686, 688, 698, 706
- air in 115
- cysts in 540
- pains in 241
- prolapse of 480, 599, 625
- serous discharge from 391
- spasm of 310, 328, 522, 588
Vaginismus 107, 128, 407, 450, 517, 522, 523, 642, 706
Valvular 598
Varicella 381, 706
Varices 117, 132, 137, 356, 435, 439, 450, 469, 494, 500, 706
Varicocele 258, 310, 552, 615, 630, 706
Varicose 60, 140, 178, 185, 208, 289, 309, 310, 369, 374, 529, 530, 552, 580, 706
Varicosis 258, 291, 309, 369, 394, 421, 597, 615, 625, 706
- during pregnancy 662
- of external genitals 662
Variola 57, 60, 92, 506, 592, 706
Varioloid 54, 706
Veins 284, 286, 288, 291, 309, 310, 369, 374, 530, 535, 706
- fullness of, swollen 490, 552
- varicose 178, 208, 289, 310, 369, 374, 529, 522, 580,
Venereal 5, 433, 677, 684, 703
Vertebrae(See also Spine).......200, 216, 511, 701, 706
- tumours of 631
Vertex 45, 71, 128, 135, 184, 191, 216, 301, 306, 373, 375, 377, 467, 468, 590, 606, 614, 565, 653, 655
Vertigo *(See dizziness)* 10, 13, 62, 66, 67, 71, 88, 97, 98, 111, 113, 115, 120, 121, 123, 132, 134, 139, 152, 198, 208, 212, 215, 223-227, 245, 246, 248, 284, 285, 294, 296, 324, 354, 362, 363, 374, 378, 383, 397, 435, 450, 467, 480, 482, 485, 494, 499, 500, 502, 508, 510, 513, 533,

557, 583, 587, 588, 589, 590, 615, 629, 630, 639, 640, 641, 652, 690, 706
Vesication 158, 706
Viscera 119, 283, 607, 637, 707,
Vision 45, 68, 87-89, 134, 136, 139, 167, 179, 191, 246, 264, 294-296, 322, 367, 371, 455, 468, 516, 525, 551, 552, 553, 618, 632, 634, 657, 673, 675, 678, 680, 685, 693, 698,
- disordered 88, 167, 246, 264, 322,
Voice 47, 64, 70, 73, 83, 117, 138, 165, 170, 172, 177, 178, 179, 180, 182, 194, 270, 294, 324, 508, 509, 510, 577, 618, 674, 684, 688
- hoarse 83, 194, 604
- lost 170, 178, 294, 328, 506
- low 47
- nasal 604
Vomiting 13, 15, 21, 25, 34, 44, 49, 50, 51, 53, 54, 55, 68, 72, 76, 80, 109, 110, 132, 133, 134, 136, 137, 148, 182, 198, 199, 213, 216, 224, 225, 237, 241, 242, 258, 261, 262, 265, 269, 280, 284, 285, 286, 289, 295, 336, 340, 342- 346, 363, 365-368, 391, 392, 395, 398, 412, 413, 424, 456, 457, 459, 476, 485, 486, 489, 490, 493-495, 506, 510, 516, 523, 564, 565, 580, 584, 620, 626, 629, 637, 651, 652, 654, 656, 658, 678, 685, 687, 690, 691, 692,
- bilious 258
- of milk, of water 109, 568
- of mucous 55, 68, 237
- of pregnancy 15, 44, 199, 216, 286, 391, 367
Vulva 99, 100, 251, 567, 584, 585, 621, 644, 677, 698, 706, 707
Walking- weeping on 212
Walking late 132
- delay in 588
Warts 5, 44, 47, 48, 49, 66, 95, 132, 178, 181, 184, 185, 198, 274, 275, 369, 374, 394, 411, 447, 450, 461, 466, 494, 500, 514, 542, 552, 570, 580, 604, 605, 615, 625, 641-644, 679, 707
Water-brash 120, 394, 405, 480, 652, 707
Weakness 11, 12, 14, 21, 22, 30, 44, 45, 64, 66, 68, 75, 77, 80, 81, 95, 96, 98, 118, 137, 139, 143, 168, 176, 177, 178, 179, 181, 184, 208, 209, 223, 224, 225, 226, 228, 238, 248, 249, 264, 265, 277, 284, 286, 295, 297, 305, 318, 323, 327, 332, 335, 336, 338, 349, 350, 354, 355, 360, 363, 367,373-375, 377, 379, 384, 393, 406, 423, 429, 439, 440, 448, 454, 456, 465, 467, 471, 473, 475, 487, 500, 501, 503, 510-512, 519, 524, 526, 527, 543, 546, 547, 548, 554, 557, 578, 579, 584, 586, 587, 592, 599, 600, 601, 606, 618, 626, 654, 655, 662, 663, 673, 693, 695
Wens 95, 105, 246, 304, 305, 314, 354, 359, 391, 466, 500, 514, 542, 707
Wheezing 77, 337, 340, 341, 344, 356, 597
White swelling 354, 615
White-leg 258
Whitlow 27, 35, 85, 132, 205, 268, 291, 314, 345, 374, 381, 383, 506, 530, 564, 588, 592, 707
Whooping-cough 10, 27, 44, 47, 54, 70, 76, 98, 117, 120, 162, 178, 182, 188, 198,217, 253, 258, 261, 262, 269, 274, 286, 289, 314, 339,

341, 344, 350, 354, 362, 366, 391, 394, 405, 407, 439, 450, 466, 490, 561, 564, 565, 580, 597, 642, 652, 662, 696, 707
Windpipe 125, 356
Worms 76, 92, 132, 211, 212, 217, 218, 223, 286, 304, 321, 336, 394, 413, 450, 456, 459, 474, 480, 500, 557, 565, 588, 595, 597, 599, 600, 615, 624, 634, 636, 662, 706
- fever 707
Worry 604, 615, 687
Wounds 59, 60, 70, 76, 255, 279, 310, 311, 318, 341, 373, 374, 375, 381, 382, 383, 385, 435, 506, 592, 605, 610
Wrist 57, 522, 523, 546, 554, 560, 704
- boils on 568
- pain in 540
Writer's cramp 407, 588, 645, 707
Yawning 10, 41, 70, 143, 165, 185, 198, 220, 315, 317, 328, 366, 394, 450, 457, 480, 535, 542, 544, 555, 609, 615, 655
- spasmodic 517
Yellow fever 10, 27, 76, 120, 160, 162, 170, 173, 257, 258, 261, 339, 506, 652
Zona 66, 304, 432, 433, 707
Zygoma 378
Zygomata 519

BOOKS OF RELATED INTEREST FROM NAB

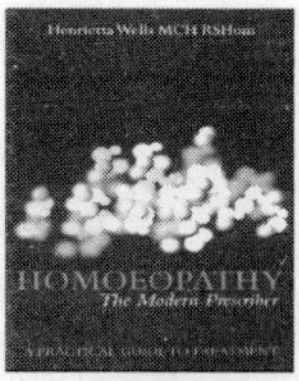

HOMOEOPATHY: THE MODERN PRESCRIBER: A Practical Guide to Treatment — *Henrietta Wells*
Homoeopathy gently stimulates the body's natural healing mechanism, providing a safe alternative to the side-effects and toxicity of conventional medicine. This book covers only those acute ailments which can be dealt with quickly, easily and confidently by the layperson. It does not cover chronic and more complicated conditions.

ISBN: 81-7822-131-4

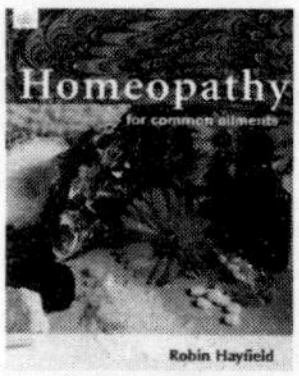

HOMEOPATHY FOR COMMON AILMENTS — *Robin Hayfield*
Gentle, sympathetic and safe, homeopathy is a system of healing that acts deeply to restore the whole person, making lasting cures at all levels—physical, emotional and mental. *Homeopathy for Common Ailments* is a practical, beautifully illustrated guide that explains and demystifies this safe and simple form of treatment.

ISBN: 81-7822-044-x

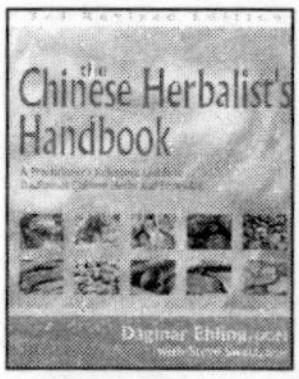

THE CHINESE HERBALIST'S HANDBOOK: Guide to Traditional Chinese Herbs — *Dagmar Ehling*
Within the context of Oriental medicine, Chinese herbal medicine is one of the oldest treatment modalities. Though it is not as well known in the West, it is rapidly gaining popularity. China has achieved full integration of traditional Chinese and Western medicine and practitioners are usually trained in both practices.

ISBN: 81-7822-196-9

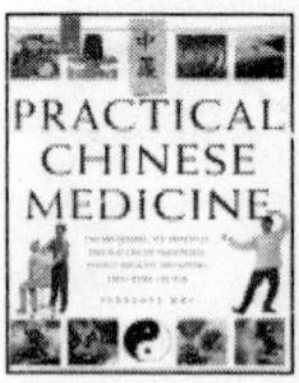

PRACTICAL CHINESE MEDICINE — *Penelope Ody*
Take a holistic approach to your health and discover the ancient art of Chinese medicine which is effective even today. Chinese medicine aims to cure diseases by focusing on the person and the cause, and identifying a range of highly detailed syndromes with specific treatment programmes. It will help you to discover the key to total health and heal yourself and your family of a wide range of common ailments.

ISBN: 81-7822-123-3

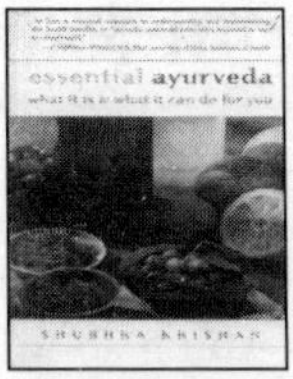

ESSENTIAL AYURVEDA — *Shubhra Krishan*

Simple routines based on the age-old secrets of India's revered sages will bring you home to your body. Ayurveda can help you re-awaken your body's powers to create balance, energy, vitality, and beauty from the inside out. Peppered with healthful recipes and tips, this book includes clear explanation of doshas with exercise, diet, and relaxation recommendations for each type.

ISBN: 81-7822-216-7

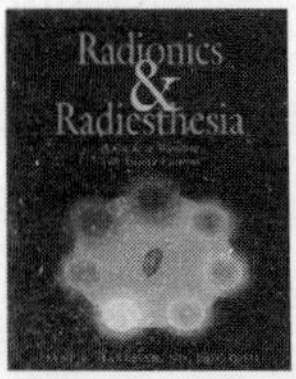

RADIONICS & RADIESTHESIA: A Guide to Working with Energy Patterns— *Jane E. Hartman*

Radionics & Radiesthesia explains this unique therapy, providing insights into the energetic analysis and treatment of ailments affecting humans, animals, plants, and soil. Ultimately, it presents a model that helps us reconnect with our own healing gifts.

Included are step-by-step instructions for working at a distance with color therapy, gem remedies, aromatherapy, flower essences, homeopathy, and other means of restoring patters of well-being.

ISBN: 81-7822-166-7

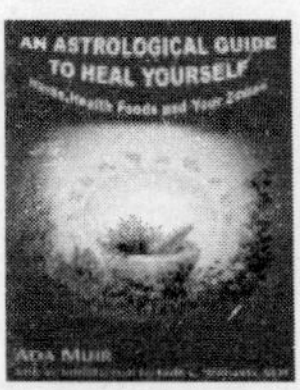

AN ASTROLOGICAL GUIDE TO HEAL YOURSELF: Herbs, Health Foods and Your Zodiac — *Ada Muir*

There used to be a time when every doctor was also an astrologer for knowledge of the zodiac was essential for diagnosing and curing illness. This book of the Zodiac covers the illnesses most often found in each zodiacal sign, along with the herbs attributed to healing them. More than 70 herbs are discussed in all, with illustrations to aid in identification.

ISBN: 81-7822-230-2

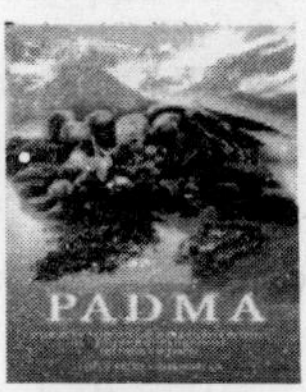

PADMA: The Jewel of Tibetan Remedies—*G. Feyerer*

The book reveals the principles of Tibetan medicine, as well as how its natural herbal remedies work. Plant remedies with many substances represent an aspect of the Tibetan medicine that distinguishes its practical applicability in a special way in the modern world. The formulas have been and continue to be subjected to internationally controlled medical studies for the purpose of distinctly documenting their effectiveness.

ISBN: 81-7822-220-5

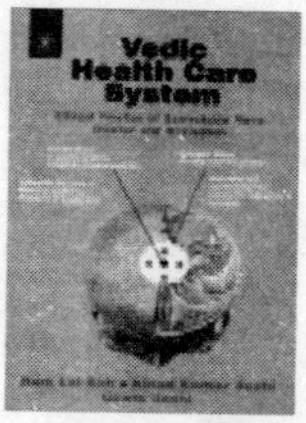

VEDIC HEALTH CARE SYSTEM: Clinical Practice of Sushrutokta Marm Chikitsa and Siravedhan—*Ram Lal Sah, Binod Kumar Joshi & Geeta Joshi*

The book is an attempt to present the Sushrut Samhita in its right perspective. It presents the correct meaning of Sira, Dhamani and Marmas which so far have been misunderstood as vein, artery and tissues to be saved during surgery. Sira and Dhamani are not vein or artery instead they are the channels for the circulation of Rasa. It revives Sushrut Shalya Chikitsa which is lost, to give the right direction to students, clinicians and researchers of Ayurveda.

ISBN: 81-7822-041-5

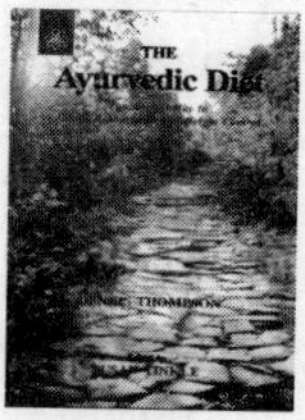

THE AYURVEDIC DIET: The Ancient Way to Health Rejuvenation and Weight Control—*Dennis Thompson*

This book offers practical solutions for everything from chronic health problems and weight control to the proper exercise and life style management. It is essential reading for all who want to lose weight, stay young and be healthy.

ISBN: 81-7822-014-8

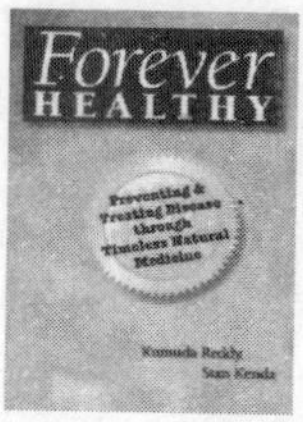

FOREVER HEALTHY: Preventing and Treating Disease through Timeless Natural Medicine— *Kumuda Reddy & Stan Kendz*

If you've ever looked for a more fundamental way to improve your health, look no further. Here age-old principles of health and healing from the Ayurveda tradition are described in clear, simple prose. As the authors explain, there is an inner intelligence within each of us that governs and coordinates all the life processes of the body. The secret of staying forever healthy is to enliven this natural inner intelligence.

ISBN: 81-7822-171-3

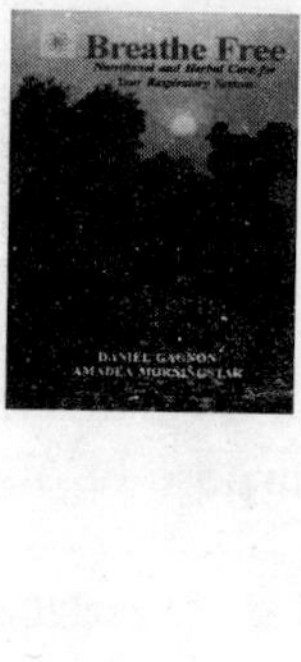

BREATHE FREE: Nutritional and Herbal Care for Your Respiratory System—*Daniel Gagnon & Amadea Morningstar*

It provides therapeutic guidelines for holistic approach, an exposé on respiratory diseases and their natural treatment. It helps you heal and manage: Common Cold, Allergies, Bronchitis and related respiratory infections.

ISBN: 81-7822-018-0